Clinical Trials in Cancer

Clinical Trials in Cancer: Principles and Practice

David J. Girling
Mahesh K. B. Parmar
Sally P. Stenning
Richard J. Stephens
Lesley A. Stewart

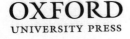
OXFORD
UNIVERSITY PRESS

OXFORD

UNIVERSITY PRESS

Great Clarendon Street, Oxford OX2 6DP

Oxford University Press is a department of the University of Oxford.
It furthers the University's objective of excellence in research, scholarship,
and education by publishing worldwide in

Oxford New York

Auckland Bangkok Buenos Aires Cape Town Chennai
Dar es Salaam Delhi Hong Kong Istanbul Karachi Kolkata
Kuala Lumpur Madrid Melbourne Mexico City Mumbai Nairobi
São Paulo Shanghai Taipei Tokyo Toronto

Oxford is a registered trade mark of Oxford University Press
in the UK and in certain other countries

Published in the United States
by Oxford University Press Inc., New York

A catalogue record for this title is available from the British Library

Library of Congress Cataloging in Publication Data
(Data available)

ISBN 0 19 262959 X

10 9 8 7 6 5 4 3 2 1

Typeset by Newgen Imaging Systems (P) Ltd., Chennai, India
Printed in Great Britain
on acid-free paper by
Biddles Ltd., Guildford & King's Lynn

Preface

This book is a 'how to do it' book on the practicalities of conducting clinical trials, systematic reviews and meta-analyses in cancer, showing how recent developments and current thinking can be implemented. Our aim is to provide a practical and common-sense guide on how to conduct cancer trials from start to finish – from bright ideas to published reports – giving plenty of examples to illustrate key points. Our intention has been to bring together current thinking on the design, conduct and analysis of trials into a single text and also to cover essential related matters such as patients' perspectives, systematic reviews and meta-analyses. We have tried to give emphasis to areas incompletely or inadequately covered elsewhere, including the need to decide and measure realistic target differences in trials, the conduct and interpretation of interim analyses, patient advocacy, good clinical practice, the study of quality of life, the role of meta-analyses, and informed consent and other ethical issues.

The book covers the principles and practice of planning, designing, conducting, analysing, reporting, and interpreting phase III trials, predominantly, but also single-arm and randomized phase II trials. Although many of the basic principles were established many years ago, there have been important developments in all these areas in recent years. Phase I studies, a separate and highly specialized area of clinical research, are only briefly mentioned.

We provide a working and reference text for a wide readership, including medical, statistical, and biological cancer researchers, health care professionals, and researchers in the pharmaceutical industry. We also hope that aspects of the book will prove helpful to a more general readership. Thus, trial sponsors, principal investigators, members of data monitoring and trial supervisory committees, specialists invited to provide independent assessments, and many others involved in research related to clinical trials should, we hope, find this book helpful in understanding and fulfilling their roles.

It might be questioned why a book concerned specifically with clinical trials in cancer is needed. Obviously, many of the issues we discuss here are also relevant to trials in other diseases. Nevertheless, cancer has important features that are distinctive, if not unique. Malignant diseases are serious and often fatal, and have profound effects on patients and their families. The treatments used are often toxic, with small therapeutic indices and with hazards that may outweigh possible advantages. Improvements are often small and temporary. The primary outcome measure is usually the duration of survival, although its quality is also important. The management of patients frequently requires a high level of clinical expertise and supportive care within specialist treatment centres. There is therefore much to be said for a book in which the relevance of all these issues in the planning and conduct of clinical trials is given full weight.

The book is self-contained and we assume no prior specialized knowledge on the part of the reader. In writing it, it has been our intention to provide a coherent text rather than a series of disparate chapters, and so all authors contributed to all aspects of the book. Primary responsibilities for drafting each of the chapters lay as follows: Chapters 1, 7, 8 and 12 DJG, Chapters 3–5 and Chapter 10 SPS, Chapters 2 and 11 LAS, Chapter 6 RJS and Chapter 9 MKBP.

D.J.G., M.K.B.P., S.P.S., R.J.S. and, L.A.S.
Medical Research Council Clinical
Trials Unit, London
June 2002

Acknowledgements

We much appreciated the help and encouragement we received from Ian Chalmers of the UK Cochrane Centre, Mike Clarke of the UK Cochrane Centre, Bec Hanley (formerly) of the consumers in NHS research support unit, Joe Pater of the National Cancer Institute of Canada, and Catherine Barnes of Oxford University Press. We are also very grateful to many people in the MRC Clinical Trials Unit, especially the following, for their help, advice and comments on draft, which were greatly appreciated: Sam Bottomley, Sarah Burdett, Pat Cook, Janet Darbyshire, Gareth Griffiths, Linda Jenkin, Andrew Lewin, Laryssa Rydewska, Jayne Tierney, Barbara Uscinska, and Claire Vale.

Contents

Chapter 1

Introduction

With the best of intentions, medical interventions have the capacity to do harm as well as good, and before any new treatment is accepted into clinical practice it should pass through a series of pre-clinical and clinical evaluations to ensure that it is both safe and has some efficacy. Safety is usually first evaluated in laboratory studies followed by observations of either healthy volunteers or patients. Clinical effectiveness must be evaluated through some kinds of comparisons against no treatment or other competing therapies – on either a formal or an informal basis. Only rarely will an intervention be so obviously effective that formal comparison is not required: for example, defibrillation following cardiac arrest. The effects of most interventions are much more subtle and require careful evaluation to ensure that we are indeed measuring the effect of treatment rather than differences in the prognosis and potential responsiveness to treatment between the individuals being compared [1].

Random allocation in a clinical trial ensures that assignment to therapeutic groups is unbiased. There is no other way of creating comparison groups that has this property, because it can never be assumed that all factors relevant to prognosis and responsiveness to treatment have been distributed between the groups in an unbiased way. Although other methods of assigning treatment can attempt to match for factors that are known, there are always likely to be many unknown, and therefore unmatchable, factors that may influence outcome. There is good empirical evidence that the results of non-randomized studies give results different to those of randomized controlled trials addressing the same question [2–4].

The randomized controlled trial is therefore widely accepted as the gold standard of treatment evaluation, and has been an essential tool of medical research since the 1940s [5]. The first clinical trial in which the treatments were assigned by a genuinely random process was probably a British Medical Research Council trial comparing bed-rest with or without streptomycin in the treatment of tuberculosis [6]. The first randomized trial in cancer was initiated in 1954 and compared two regimens of chemotherapy in the treatment of acute leukaemia [7]. Current emphasis on evidence-based medicine has increased the international awareness and acknowledgement of the importance of randomized trials in reliably comparing the advantages and disadvantages of different treatment policies and for accurately assessing their relative impact on the outcome measures of interest.

While the central role of randomization was established many years ago, the environment in which trials are now conducted has changed enormously since those times, and those responsible for running trials have had to and must continue to adapt. The next chapter after this considers one of the areas of the greatest change, namely the public perspective. When designing trials, we need to be certain that we are addressing questions that are clinically relevant, measuring outcomes that are important to patients and their families, and presenting information concerning participation in trials in an accessible and readily understandable format. It is incumbent upon those who conduct trials to help promote the public understanding of the principles involved and to educate and encourage not only patients but also the healthy public to agree to take part in trials as occasions present. In improving communication with patients and increasing their involvement in trials, we need, perhaps, to question the terms we use. 'Randomized controlled trial', for example, means little to most patients. Much thought needs to be given to explaining randomization in ways that are both accurate and reassuring. There is scope for much wider involvement of the medical and scientific communities, patients and patient advocacy groups in promoting together a high standard of collaborative research to which all groups contribute constructively. Our experience suggests that there is an enormous resource of goodwill among patients that can be harnessed.

The first step in initiating a clinical trial is formulating an idea which typically arises from an individual or small group. Much work is then needed to filter out research questions that have already been answered and to translate ideas into realistic and feasible protocols. In Chapter 3 we discuss the importance of deciding, on the basis of information already available and the type of cancer under study, whether a trial is needed and, if so, what type of trial will best address the question posed. We describe the standard stages in developing a new treatment, from establishing its safety and acceptability, through assessing its potential benefits and hazards compared with other treatments already in use, to monitoring its use in routine practice. Understanding these stages, the need for randomization – including its role in phase II trials, and the advantages and disadvantages of all types of comparative study is essential.

Most new treatments will be evaluated in a randomized trial before they can be accepted into clinical practice. In Chapter 4 we describe how to design a randomized trial, drawing particular attention to the nature and number of treatment groups, the timing and unit of randomization and the practical methodology of randomization.

The results of many randomized trials are inconclusive, often because inadequate numbers of patients were included. In Chapter 5 we describe the need to estimate sample sizes realistically, emphasizing the importance of deciding what difference in primary outcome measure should be targeted and the information that needs to be considered in determining this. Reasons why unequal allocation is sometimes desirable, and why and how sample size may need to be adjusted during an intake in the light of event rates, are also discussed.

The assessment of health-related quality of life is becoming increasingly important in cancer clinical trials; indeed, many of the principles and much of the methodology were developed and continue to be developed in the context of such trials. We review the current status in Chapter 6, and emphasize the importance of formulating hypotheses, deciding what outcome measures to study, and how they should be measured.

In Chapters 7 and 8, we describe how plans are put into practice. Once a trial has been designed, much has to be done before it can be launched. We describe what needs to be done, who does it, and what resources are required. To attract funding from a sponsor and support from the clinical community and patient advocacy groups, the proposal must make a persuasive case for conducting the trial and show that it stands a good chance of answering its questions reliably. For a trial to be run successfully and ethically it generally requires independent data monitoring and supervision, and must conform to the general principles of good clinical practice. It should usually be conducted by a multi-disciplinary group, competent to organize the trial, to elicit and maintain the trust and enthusiastic collaboration of clinicians, to analyse the data, and to present and publish the results.

This book is not the place for presenting analytical and statistical methodology in great detail, or for reviewing statistical packages, for which specialist texts should be consulted. Nevertheless, all those involved in conducting and collaborating in clinical trials need to be aware of the important principles of analysis, which we cover in Chapter 9. This is essential if they are to appreciate the reliability of the findings of trials in which they are involved and to appraise the literature critically. It is of fundamental importance to have a feel for the nature and variety of the data and hence the methods appropriate for analysing them, to appreciate what is required for making informative and reliable comparisons, and to be able to present, communicate and interpret results.

We discuss reporting and interpreting the results of trials in Chapter 10: what information to present, how and where to report it, and when; and how to interpret it. All trials should be reported, with due attention to CONSORT guidelines, including trials that have to be terminated prematurely; and reports must assure readers that the trial was conducted correctly, that the data were fully and relevantly analysed, and that the findings and their interpretation are reliable and unbiased. We also suggest sensible approaches to communicating with the media and preparing press releases.

A single trial, even a large randomized trial impeccably conducted, will rarely change clinical practice internationally. Systematic reviews and meta-analyses, which we discuss in Chapter 11, are therefore essential tools in objectively evaluating all the available evidence on which treatment decisions are based. The requirements for conducting meta-analyses reliably are substantial. We discuss the practical issues involved, from formulating the question, through writing a protocol, collecting or abstracting data, analysing the data, to reporting the results, drawing particular attention to the value of individual patient data analyses compared with those based on published or summary data. We also highlight the need for international registration of all randomized trials.

Finally, in Chapter 12, we describe the characteristics of, and benefits that accrue from, an established trials centre and research group. The potential benefits are great and stem largely from the ability to build up an experienced staff and a group of experienced collaborators, to plan and conduct coherent programmes of trials in collaboration with other groups over many years, and to conduct trials-associated research based on large accumulations of data.

In summary, we hope that this book will not only prove helpful to other researchers but also play its part in encouraging a positive and collaborative attitude to trials, and particularly randomized trials, in the treatment of cancer, in all sections of the community.

References

[1] Kleijen, J., Gotzche, P., Kunz, R.A., Oxman, A.D., and Chalmers, I. (1997) So what's so special about randomisation? In *Non-random Reflections on Health Services Research* (eds. A. Maynard and I. Chalmers), pp. 93–106. British Medical Journal Publishing Group, London.

[2] Chalmers, T.C., Matta, R.J., Smith, H., and Kunzler, A.M. (1997) Evidence favoring the use of anticoagulants in the hospital phase of acute myocardial infarction. *New England Journal of Medicine*, **297**, 1091–6.

[3] Sacks, H., Chalmers, T.C., and Smith, H.J. (1982) Randomized versus historical controls for clinical trials. *American Journal of Medicine*, **72**, 233–40.

[4] Diehl, L.F., and Perry, D.J. (1986) A comparison of randomized concurrent control groups with matched historical control groups: Are historical controls valid? *Journal of Clinical Oncology*, **4**, 1114–20.

[5] D'Arcy Hart, P. (1996) Early controlled clinical trials. *British Medical Journal*, **312**, 378–9.

[6] Medical Research Council Streptomycin in Tuberculosis Trials Committee (1948) Streptomycin treatment of pulmonary tuberculosis. *British Medical Journal*, **ii**, 769–82.

[7] Frei, E., Holland, J.F., and Schneiderman, M.A. (1958) A comparative study of two regimens of combination chemotherapy in acute leukemia. *Blood*, **13**, 1126–48.

Chapter 2

The public perspective

2.1 Introduction

Clinical trials are a special type of research involving human participants, sometimes with healthy volunteers, but often with patients who agree to participate in trials as part of their treatment and medical care. Trials therefore carry particular responsibilities both to ensure the welfare of their participants and to be publicly accountable. In the quest to design, conduct and report the results of the 'perfect' trial, we must not lose sight of the fact that the whole purpose of trials is ultimately to benefit patients and the community at large. Clinical trials cannot be done without patients, and success depends upon establishing effective partnerships between researchers, clinicians and patients.

In the past, patients seldom played an active role in decisions about their treatments, but this is changing rapidly. Although many patients do still wish decisions to be taken entirely by their doctor, in general, people are better informed and want to be more involved in determining their individual health care. This has been facilitated by the availability and accessibility of information over the internet which has made it easier for individuals to learn in detail about their disease and treatment possibilities. It is not unusual for patients to arrive at consultations with downloaded information on the 'latest advances' in the treatment of their particular condition. However, they may need help in evaluating the information that they have found. In particular, because the internet provides health-care advice from a variety of contributors, including academic institutions, self-help organisations, commercial interests and downright cranks, they may need help in sorting the potentially worthwhile from the worthless.

New trials must therefore be planned in the context of an increasingly informed patient population. Historically, many doctors and researchers favoured a paternalistic approach and the public perspective was often neglected. However, this is changing and lay involvement is becoming established at all levels of clinical research. This includes helping to set research agendas, to design trials that are relevant and to ensure that the results of research are reported appropriately. These days trialists must be ready to accept wider responsibilities and to forge new kinds of relationships with the patients included in their trials, with community groups and with the general public.

The public consists of many different stakeholders, all of whom have differing needs for information about clinical trials. Central are those patients, doctors and nurses taking part in the trials. The wider audience includes the pool of all potential participants, others involved in healthcare provision and policy making, and the general public – including politicians and the media. Ultimately, we are all potential trial participants at some point in our lives, and we all need information concerning trials at some level.

If trials are to be successful and achieve their aim of improving public health, then they should be relevant and practical. The accrual rate must not be so slow that the results are overtaken by changing conditions or practice, and results should be disseminated and acted upon appropriately. All of these aspects require public support. This chapter can address only briefly some of the many issues involved. It deals mostly with communication relating to entry to trials. Where possible this is based on the results of empirical research. It differs from other parts of this book in that first-hand experience of lay involvement in the design and conduct of MRC cancer trials is less well developed than for other aspects of trial design, management and analysis. So far, trials in breast and prostate cancer have benefited from lay representation at all stages of trial development and it is an area that we believe to be essential to future progress. Important first steps have been taken and we plan to build on these over the coming years.

2.2   Barriers to taking part in trials

Although many patients are eligible to enter trials of cancer therapy, accrual rates are low and it is estimated that on average around 5 per cent of UK patients [1] and 3 per cent of US patients [2] take part. Trials generally rely on a minority of clinicians who have a particular interest in research and who recruit the majority of patients. However, even among highly committed doctors, accrual rates can be low. For example, a survey of members of the research-oriented US Eastern Cooperative Oncology Group (ECOG) found that doctors overestimated the number of patients they intended to enter in trials by a factor of six. Members entered less than 10 per cent of eligible patients to ECOG trials and 62 per cent did not enter a single patient during the 12-month period of the survey [3]. Although a survey of British oncologists [4] found that almost all of the 65 per cent who responded stated that they were participating in clinical trials, three-quarters of respondents acknowledged that they were entering less than half of all eligible patients. A study of enrolment to trials at a US Cancer Centre, conducted over three separate six-month periods, found that even with a certain level of promotion during which clinicians were reminded of the availability of trial protocols, a relatively low proportion of patients entered trials [2]. Of 276 eligible patients, only 171 were considered for trial entry by the clinician and a suitable protocol was available for ninety-one of them. Out of these, seventy-six met the eligibility criteria of the particular trial for which they were considered, thirty-nine agreed to participate and thirty-six did not. It is worth noting that the greatest numbers were lost at the earliest stage before the clinician had reviewed protocol availability and eligibility criteria.

Similarly, in the ECOG survey [3], doctors appeared to select patients with whom to discuss possible participation in trials according to their own additional eligibility criteria. Those with poor disease status or those thought to have a lack of trust in medicine were not considered for trials, even though the clinicians involved believed that trial patients were given a higher quality of care. Most felt that randomization was a very difficult concept to explain and therefore a powerful obstacle, which limited their own ability to participate in clinical trials. In the UK survey [4] many commented that lack of time or resources were barriers to trial recruitment and others cited difficulties in obtaining informed consent as being a particular problem. Perceived intelligence was cited as the most important factor influencing the ease of communicating about trials with patients. Most doctors indicated that it was easier to approach more intelligent patients, although a minority found that patients with poorer understanding were easier [3]. Likewise, senior oncologists attending communication skills courses have indicated that providing complex information about trials and obtaining informed consent are the most difficult aspects of communicating with patients [5].

Overall, it seems that doctors are relatively pessimistic about the likely reactions of at least a proportion of their patients to invitations to take part in trials. However, studies of public opinion have indicated that the general public is supportive of clinical research. Far larger proportions of people say that, in theory, they would be willing to take part in trials than is suggested by current accrual rates. For example, in a professional survey of over a thousand adults carried out in the UK during the 1980s, two thirds of those interviewed said they would be prepared to participate in clinical trials. This was even in the most demanding of circumstances, trials of lumpectomy versus mastectomy for women and amputation versus bone grafting for men [6]. There was however a strong tendency for younger and more highly educated people to want to have a say in choosing their own treatment, which might preclude them from trials. A criticism of this type of opinion seeking is that people may react differently to hypothetical and actual situations. Faced with a theoretical scenario, many may feel that they would wish to take part in a trial whereas they may well act differently in reality. However, it seems that the views of those who are ill are in broad agreement with the healthy, and are generally supportive of clinical research. For example, in a survey of seventy-five cancer patients carried out in seven oncology centres in the UK, 42 per cent said they would agree to take part in research trials, 10 per cent that they would not, and 48 per cent were uncertain [7]. Those who indicated that they did not want to take part, or were uncertain, said that this was mostly because they would prefer the doctor to make the decision, or that they would worry about receiving a new treatment. The particular aspects of trials that were cited as particularly appealing or unappealing are summarised in Table 2.1. Another study of 325 patients attending two major cancer centres in the UK found that more than 90 per cent of those interviewed believed that patients should be asked to take part in medical

Table 2.1 Characteristics of trials cited as particularly appealing or unappealing by cancer patients (Kemp *et al.* 1984)

Characteristics	Scored greatly (un)appealing %
Appealing	
Greater chance of treatment by doctor with special interest in particular cancer	83
Progress monitored closely	80
Taking part contributes to research knowledge and benefits humanity	75
Likely to obtain more information about condition	75
Greater chance of obtaining new treatments	72
Not appealing	
Don't choose treatment oneself	25
Treatment decided by trial not doctor	24
Greater chance of obtaining experimental treatments	15

research. However, only three-quarters said that they would be prepared to take part themselves, and less than half if the trial was randomized. Encouragingly, when given more details and further explanation of randomization more than half of those who had initially refused, or were unsure about randomization, changed their mind [8].

It seems that a limiting factor to including a greater proportion of eligible patients in trials may be in motivating more doctors to take part in research and to discuss possible participation in trials with more of their patients. Undoubtedly, time and resource issues are involved in clinicians' reluctance, but it also seems that many are uncomfortable about discussing trials and in particular, randomization with their patients. Better training in communication, both generally and specifically relating to trials and randomization, could be a way of tackling this difficulty. The clinical trials community should be ready to initiate and become involved in such educational activities. Ensuring that good written explanations along with other material, such as explanatory videos, are available for all trials may also provide useful support for those at the front-line of discussing trials with potential participants.

The issue of patients' willingness to participate in trials is a key determinant of success. Little is known about what precisely motivates individuals to take part in trials although most studies have indicated that participation is driven more by self-interest than altruism [9]. It is often thought that individuals take part in trials for the public good and improvement of treatment for future patients. Whilst this may be entirely true for some and in part for many, studies of patients' attitudes have revealed that the main motivation is the hope or expectation of gaining a benefit from the new treatment. Published research seems to show that the majority of those who take part in trials are generally satisfied with the experience [10,11]. Furthermore, systematic reviews of research studies, that have compared patients enrolled in clinical trials with those treated outside of trials, have concluded that overall there is evidence (albeit weak and in need of further study) that trial participants have received better care and have had better outcomes [12,13].

Encouragingly, when given appropriate explanation, the majority of the public appear enthusiastic or uncertain about entering trials. Only a small minority are unwilling to participate and we may be relatively optimistic that given the appropriate information, and support, the public will remain strong supporters of clinical research. Ultimately this may have the effect of encouraging consumer pressure on doctors to be more active in clinical trials.

2.3 Informed consent

It is widely, although not universally, accepted that informed consent should be obtained from all conscious patients entered into clinical trials, and the principle of freely given informed consent is emphasized in the Declaration of Helsinki (http://www.cirp.org/library/ethics/helsinki/). The ethical arguments concerning consent have been discussed at length elsewhere and are not repeated in detail here. Commentaries by Doyal [14] and Tobias [15] and the subsequent debate in the *British Medical Journal* (vol. 316, pp. 1000–1011) provide a good overview of the subject as does the subsequent book [16].

The laws concerning consent vary internationally, but informed consent is considered essential under most circumstances by all the major organisations that manage and fund cancer trials. Obtaining such consent is therefore an important aspect of planning and conducting trials and for those run to the International Conference on Harmonisation (ICH) or other good clinical practice, there are specific and detailed guidelines for obtaining and documenting consent (see Section 7.3). Some trialists have pointed out that although rigorous informed consent is required when treating patients with a new treatment within the context of a trial, were they to give this same new treatment to all of their patients outside of a trial, then no such consent would be required [17]. However, this should not be viewed as a reason to make consent for trials any less meticulous. Rather, in an ideal world, consent to all treatment should be as informative and rigorous as the consent required for randomized trials [18].

In practice, consent has not always been as informed as it ought to be [19] and lay people and health professionals alike find it difficult to give the phrase 'informed consent' tangible meaning [20]. A review of publications relating to the ethics of randomized trials [9] found that a considerable number of doctors thought that patients included in their trials may not have fully understood that they were being included in a trial, or the information given to them. The authors suggested that for some doctors informed consent seemed little more than a ritual. Although consent is usually obtained by the medical staff caring for a patient, this does not mean that those designing and co-ordinating trials can abdicate responsibility for this important component of trial procedure. Responsible researchers should make sure that clinical staff are given as much support as possible to help ensure that consent is obtained appropriately and does not become ritualized. The importance of obtaining properly informed consent should therefore be stressed in the trial protocol and also addressed in patient information sheets and consent forms.

2.3.1 Public opinion concerning consent

Whatever the underlying academic arguments, public opinion seems to support properly informed consent. Reported cases of individuals included in trials without their knowledge or full consent have met with considerable outrage. Cases such as that described in Box 2.1 do nothing to promote the cause of trials or engender public confidence.

> 'When scientists have academic arguments about clinical research they should remember that they are dealing with people's lives. We have feelings and opinions. We don't want to be just another statistic; we're real, we exist, and it's our bodies that you are experimenting with'. [21]

Frank explanation about trials and the interventions involved can be difficult and potentially distressing for patients. Undoubtedly, there are those who do not wish to be told such details. However, the costs of avoiding such disclosure, both in terms of the harm to those involved and the damage to trials generally, are great. If full disclosure means that some patients cannot be entered in trials, then it is a price we have to pay. It is to be hoped that in the long term, open discussion between doctors and patients, together with public debate and education about trials, will create an environment within which a greater proportion of patients are willing to become involved in clinical research, on a more fully informed basis. From a purely pragmatic point of view, if trials are to be acceptable to the public who take part in them (and in one way or another fund them), then researchers need to address the issues surrounding informed consent. There is certainly much scope for empirical research into the best ways of going about this.

Box 2.1 View of a woman included in a clinical trial without her knowledge

As a result of radiotherapy treatment given in the late 1980s for cervical cancer, a young woman sustained serious long-term damage. This resulted in over 100 admissions to hospital and twenty-four operations which included: those for adhesion attacks; a hernia operation; a permanent colostomy and urostomy; an operation to remove compacted faeces; formation of and then removal of a rebuilt rectum and those for a mucus fistula and thrombosis. She currently suffers from a vaginal fistula, which intermittently allows faeces to escape through her vagina. She has survived her cancer, but at what price.

When she later learned, through the work of an investigative journalist, that she and others had been included in a clinical trial without knowledge or consent, she described her reaction thus: 'we discovered that we had been guinea-pigs in a clinical trial of a new radiotherapy protocol we felt totally betrayed. We trusted our doctors, yet none had given our written consent, even to treatment (only to the anaesthetic), and we were not given details about possible complications . . . We could hardly believe him: this was Britain in the 1980s not Hitler's Germany.'

She notes that of the many women included in this and similar trials and suffering similar long-term medical problems, many cannot have sexual intercourse, some are housebound through pain and incontinence and some have tried to commit suicide. As a result, marriages have broken up and children have been fostered. All are understandably angry about what has happened to them [21].

2.3.2 How much information should be disclosed?

The amount of information given to patients as part of the randomization and consent process varies greatly. The level of verbal information is often decided by doctors on an individual and sometimes *ad hoc* basis. Whilst some clinicians believe that only total disclosure of all information is ethical, others suggest that information overload can distress the patient unduly. An Australian randomized study, which compared two methods of seeking consent (an individual approach at the discretion of the doctor versus total disclosure) for entry to trials of different standard cancer treatments, found that patients who experienced total disclosure were less willing to enter the trial and were significantly more anxious [22]. A more recent randomized study comparing standard consent methods with the same plus a follow up telephone call from an oncology nurse found that the latter resulted in the patients being better informed about the trial and their treatment. It did not significantly affect anxiety or participation rates [23]. Studies of patients' attitudes have indicated that most (but not all) would like comprehensive information about trials and treatments [6,24] and would prefer to have a combination of written and verbal explanation [24].

2.3.3 Explaining randomization and rationale for trials

A major obstacle to trial participation appears to be explaining the randomization process. Some doctors may find it difficult or awkward to discuss, and participants may find the concept difficult to deal with. One study reported that 63 per cent of patients approached refused entry to a trial because of an aversion to randomization [25], and it is thought that many trial participants do not fully understand the nature of the trials in which they are involved [9]. Other studies, which have paid particular attention to explaining the process of randomization, have suggested that comprehension levels can be good.

The UK population survey described previously, in which interviewers were specifically instructed to ensure that randomization was explained thoroughly, found that most respondents understood the concept of randomization [6]. Likewise, a study, using in-depth semi-structured interviews, of men participating in a randomized trial (CLasP) evaluating the effectiveness and cost-effectiveness of three different types of intervention for the management of urinary symptoms related to benign prostatic disease, found that almost all participants were aware of some aspects of randomization. Most acknowledged the involvement of chance in their treatment, often transformed to lay terms such as a lucky dip or lottery [26].

However, a revealing study that involved interviewing parents who had consented for their critcally ill infants to enter a randomized trial, found that although superficially many appeared to know that the trial was randomized, when questioned further it became clear that few understood either the design of the trial or how or why randomization was done [27]. Agreement to participate was made in one of the most distressing and difficult of situations. Their newly born babies, already perceived by the majority of parents to be dying, were to be randomized to continue with unchanged ventilation or to be transferred to another hospital to receive oxygenation of the blood through an external circuit (ECMO) inserted through a cannula in the neck. The majority of parents found it difficult to accept the idea of clinical uncertainty and thought that the new treatment was obviously better and that they were being offered the chance of taking part because standard care was failing. The trial was viewed as an opportunity to gain access to a new, and implicitly better, treatment, which had only limited availability. Rather than a situation where the two treatments were the focus of randomization, they saw their baby as being at the centre of a decision about access to ECMO (which they were competing with other babies for). Only four parents out of thirty-seven suggested that randomization had been done to obtain a fair comparison between the treatments and only one suggested that the trial was needed to assess associated hazards of ECMO treatment. Interestingly, many of the parents thought that the babies allocated to standard care were not part of the trial and the authors comment that this may have been reinforced by the trial being known as the ECMO trial. Randomization was not fully understood and often focussed on the use of the computer. Some believed that the computer was used to make complex therapeutic decisions, or to check on the availability of an ECMO bed. Some, acknowledging the play of chance, believed that randomization was used as a route to fair rationing rather than treatment allocation – the computer was selecting babies for ECMO rather than the treatment for their particular child. Perceived competition for places on ECMO was described by many parents, and randomization was described as 'unfair' 'tough' and 'heartless.'

Undoubtedly, when discussing trials with potential participants, particular attention needs to be paid to describing the process of treatment allocation, and describing why randomization is necessary. This should perhaps start with a clear statement that new treatments are not necessarily better than existing ones, and that sometimes they may in fact be worse. Information concerning the various treatment options should be accompanied by a clear explanation that treatments are allocated in a way that makes sure that there is a fair test between the treatments and that nobody knows which treatment the patient will be allocated until they are actually entered into the trial or 'randomized.' This may be more important than describing the practicalities of the procedure. A survey that investigated how members of the public rated different explanations of randomization found that the statement that scored best was as follows:

> 'Once you have agreed to enter the trial, you will be allocated to one of two treatments with equal chances of each treatment being the one you will receive.'

This description was favoured over six other statements that included references to tossing a coin, drawing names from a hat, and a computer making a choice at random. The least liked statement was as follows:

> 'Once you have agreed to enter the trial, one of two methods of treatment will be chosen by chance and not by a decision made by the patient or doctor.'

It appeared that preferred wordings were less explicit, perhaps not allowing the mind to dwell too long on the random nature of treatment assignment or on the perceived loss of medical control [24]. Thus, although on the face of it phrases such as 'tossing a coin' may appear to be good ways of describing the process of randomization, they may also appear flippant or uncaring. We perhaps need to question whether such descriptions are actually useful. Thus, explaining *how* the allocation will be done may not be so important, provided that it is made clear that there is no foreknowledge of which treatment will be allocated, and that options are equally likely (or as appropriate for the ratio of allocation).

2.3.4 Patient information sheets

Most trials provide patients with written information sheets as part of the consent process. This ensures that all patients receive the same minimum details [28], which can be supplemented by discussion. The patient can take written material home and the benefits and risks of the trial can be considered in a less stressful environment, perhaps with help from family or friends [29]. Initially such information sheets and consent forms were designed primarily to protect patients from unfairness or exploitation. However, as patient autonomy has become increasingly important, the focus of such documentation has become to help patients make their own decisions about treatment and taking part in trials, based on clear and accurate information. To accommodate this, the information provided has changed from the straightforward disclosure of information to an approach aimed at improving the quality of a patients' understanding of the proposed trial and treatments involved [30]. In order to fulfil this role, information leaflets must be written in clear language that is easily understandable by the majority of patients and should be changed if important new evidence comes to light.

However, a study of consent forms used at a leading oncology centre in the US revealed that most of the forms were too complex to be read by most patients and their families [30]. Another study comparing the reading ability of a sample of patients attending three US clinics found that only 27 per cent had reading skills that would enable them to understand pamphlets produced by the American Cancer Society and by the National Cancer Institute [31]. Other research found that although 80 per cent of participants claimed to have read the consent form only 60 per cent reported that they had understood it. Only half could name all their drugs and just 4 per cent could list all the main side-effects [32].

It is therefore vital that information sheets and leaflets are presented and targeted appropriately. These should be written in plain language and avoid the use of jargon or complicated terminology. Words with specialist meanings in the context of trials should be explained. For example, the men interviewed as part of the ClasP trial found the use of words with common meanings outside of clinical trials to be confusing. The word 'trial' itself, which is usually associated with something that is being tried out or a difficulty, and 'random' which normally means haphazard were cited as being particularly difficult [26]. In the ECMO trial a number of the parents understood 'trial' to mean 'on a trial basis' suggesting assessment of acceptability to the healthcare system rather than measuring potential benefits and hazards.

'Why the hell have we got it on trial when it's been in the States . . . why is the National Health playing around with this' [27]

Similarly, interpretation of 'fulfil the entry criteria for the ECMO trial' was interpreted by some parents as meaning that their baby was likely to be accepted for ECMO. This work raises many questions, not only for neonatal trials, but for trials in general as to whether it is time to rethink some of the terminology that researchers use to discuss and describe clinical research. Perhaps it is time to redefine the language of trials, or failing that to ensure that it is explained thoroughly and understood by those participating in trials. Further research is needed to investigate how we might best communicate the rationale of trials and into ways of adequately explaining randomization using non-pejorative terms.

Providing the right level of information and achieving a balance between avoiding complex scientific language and being patronizing can be difficult. It is important to remember that average reading skills of the public are low, and that participants are not uniform in their skills, experiences or need for information. In the UK, given that the average reading age of the adult population is around nine years, the Plain English Campaign advocates that public information should be written in language that can be understood by a nine year old child. Very few patient information sheets are pitched at this level and indeed such a level would not be appropriate for all individuals. One approach might be to produce a range of participant information material targeted at different types of individual. For example, an MRC/EORTC trial of chemotherapy in osteosarcoma has three separate information sheets one for adults and adolescents, one for children and one for parents. Clearly each requires different types and levels of information. Similarly, those with recurrent disease may be more likely to understand technical language (as they have had time to learn the terminology) than those who have been newly diagnosed. Offering patients a choice of detailed or more straightforward information leaflets, or indeed both, may help doctors consider inviting more patients to take part in trials. Trialists must also be able to harness other methods of imparting information, for example using pictures in information sheets or providing patient information audio or video tapes.

Undoubtedly, providing more written material will mean more work for trialists and trial support staff. However, individual researchers need not attempt to reinvent the wheel with each new trial, as much of the general information required will be similar across trials. As discussed in Chapter 7, there are many sources of guidance, examples and templates available. Such sources are a valuable resource for those writing patient information material. Ideally, drafting of this material should be done in active collaboration with a patient support or advocate group, to ensure that it is appropriately written.

2.4 Informing participants about the results of trials

There is widespread agreement that those asked to participate in clinical research should be given adequate information concerning the aims and design of a trial. However, in cancer it is currently the exception rather than the rule that participants are actively informed of a trial's results by its organizers. Yet, studies have shown that patients have a strong desire to receive feedback about the trials in which they have taken part [33–35].

The way that results of trials are communicated to patients and their families needs careful thought, as results can be complicated, alarming and distressing. It has been suggested that this is particularly true of randomized trials [35] where patients who did not receive the favoured treatment may, in retrospect, feel that they have been deprived of the best treatment or placed at risk. Nonetheless, the indication is that those who take part in trials do wish to be informed of the results, even if the information that they receive can be potentially upsetting. For example, a survey of the parents of surviving babies enrolled in the ECMO trial, described previously, found that even though feedback was emotionally exacting (significant differences in mortality were observed), the parents still wanted this information [36]. Parents seemed to find that, although upsetting, the provision of information about the trial results removed uncertainty, provided a clear end to difficult events, promoted further discussion within the family and acknowledged their contribution to answering an important clinical question.

Providing trial participants with feedback about results may well be particularly difficult in cancer, not least because in advanced disease a large proportion of patients will have died before the close of the trial. The situation is likely to vary according to cancer site and from trial to trial. However, at least in cases where long-term survival is anticipated, there is a strong case for providing details about the results of a trial, written in lay terms, for those who have taken part. So far, this approach has not been used widely in cancer, but it is an issue that should be taken into consideration by those designing new trials. It would be a much more reliable way of reporting the results and implications and more reassuring to those involved than for them to obtain this information through the media. There have been calls for patients to be furnished with trial results in advance of scientific publication or presentation [37]. This stems in part from situations where results of high profile studies have been reported by the media at the same time as, or even before, scientific publication. Those who had taken part learned of striking or controversial results from television news or newspapers. This type of situation can clearly be very distressing for those involved (see Box 2.2), and information received in this way may be a selective or edited version of the results and conclusions of a trial. Although it may be difficult to inform all participants of the results of trials before publication, with careful planning it should be possible for trialists to link the circulation of lay summaries of the results of trials with the date of publication. It is now fairly common practice for the results of trials to be presented, in confidence, to the clinicians involved prior to publication. As well as the scientific advantages of involving participating clinicians

Box 2.2 Example of controversial trial results reported by the press in advance of scientific publication

Results of a trial of complementary treatment offered to women with breast cancer who attended the Bristol Cancer Help Centre [38] published in 1990 were reported in the press three days before the Lancet publication date. The women involved in the trial, who still believed it to be ongoing (they had completed only four of the planned five annual questionnaires that they had been asked to complete), first learned the results from the television news. The news report stated that those of them who had been to the Centre were twice as likely to die and three times as likely to relapse as women who had not been to the centre. This was certainly not the most sensitive way of breaking such news. In fact it later emerged that the study was fundamentally flawed in that those who had chosen to pay to attend the centre in addition to NHS treatments were as a group more ill than the controls. The women involved in the trial challenged the results and complained to the Charities Commission about the conduct of two charities, which had funded the research. Their complaint was upheld.

in early discussions of results, this approach has the benefit of preparing doctors for ensuing discussions with their patients. It seems worth exploring whether this approach could be extended to include lay representatives or advocates. They would be bound by the same confidentiality agreements, could actively participate in discussions, could help in the preparation of lay summaries and where appropriate could prepare their groups for counselling patients. Indeed this type of approach has been very successful with HIV trials [39] where there is an established history of advocate groups being actively involved in disseminating trial results to their membership. A similar approach could be successful in cancer.

Researchers have a responsibility to trial participants that extends beyond their enrolment and treatment in a trial. In the UK, the Royal College of Physicians recommends that patients should receive written thanks for co-operating in a study [40]. However, deciding on the best way to inform patients of the outcome needs to be thought through early in the design stages of a trial. Ideally a policy statement on dissemination of results should be part of the protocol, and perhaps also included in patient information sheets. Further research is needed, to investigate the most appropriate methods of implementing such a policy, and to evaluate its effectiveness, with due consideration of the special difficulties that cancer trials may raise.

2.5 Involving the public in designing trials and setting research agendas

Setting and implementing health research priorities is a complex and sometimes obscure process. Although the aim should be that the views of all stakeholders are considered, with few exceptions (notably the Childbirth and AIDS advocacy movements), patients and consumers have little input to how research is prioritized, funded and monitored [41].

Despite the progressive attitude of organizations such as the Cochrane Collaboration (see Section 11.10), where lay participation is fostered at all levels [42], involving consumers in designing trials and reviews is still seen by some as a hindrance to progress. It has been suggested that lay input to the design of trials is an intrusion that compromises scientific integrity. Yet, there are examples where lay involvement has helped researchers to address important clinical questions. For example, it was the mother of a woman with vaginal adenocarcinoma who first suggested that this could have been caused by the diethylstilbestrol that the mother had been prescribed during pregnancy [43]. It has also been suggested that patients might be more willing to take part in trials if they knew that there had been lay or advocate involvement in the design, as they would be reassured that the questions posed would address their needs and that their interests had been represented [34].

To help encourage researchers to involve lay input at all stages of clinical research, a concerted effort to systematically collect and collate evidence of situations where lay input has improved research proposals or defined new proposals would be extremely useful. Encouragingly, a national survey of UK Clinical Trial Coordinating Centres, carried out in 1999/2000, found that most centres had involved or were planning to involve consumers in their work, and less than a quarter had no plans to do so [44]. Almost a third of trials covered by the survey (19/60) had consumer representation on the Trial Steering Committees (though none were involved in data monitoring). Consumer input was mostly at the level of single trials and largely related to preparing information for patients. This type of representation is typical of UK cancer trials, conducted during the 1980s and 1990s. Individual consumer representatives or groups were usually involved in the development of individual protocols, or as members of advisory committees [45]. Although valuable, with this approach there is the risk that lay representatives become isolated or intimidated, perhaps because they do not have adequate training to allow them to participate fully in technical discussions. Providing specialized training is an area where researchers and advocate/support groups can work together towards enabling informed consumer input to clinical research. A pioneering example of this type of approach is project LEAD (Leadership Education and Advocacy Development). This is a 5-day basic science and leadership training programme for breast cancer advocates, that is organized by the US National Breast Cancer Coalition (http://www.natlbcc.org), and aims to give individuals the training that they need to participate more fully in breast cancer research [42].

Until fairly recently, few cancer research organizations have sought public input at the policy level. However, in the mid-1990s, the US National Cancer Institute (NCI) recognized the need to take a more global view. It took the lead in implementing a policy to include the views of consumers at the highest levels, through the creation of the Directors Consumer Liaison Group – a model that is being used and adapted internationally.

2.5.1 NCI directors consumer liaison group

Although representatives of advocacy groups had participated in a variety of NCI committees for many years, the pool of representatives was relatively small. In 1996 the NCI recognized a need to incorporate the views of the cancer community in a more structured way and embarked upon creating a new entity comprised entirely of consumers. This goal was achieved in August 1998 when the first Directors Consumer Liaison Group (DCLG) was selected, with a remit to provide input to the planning of programmes and future directions of research of the NCI. Setting up the initial DCLG involved careful planning by a group of NCI staff undertaken in collaboration with key cancer advocacy groups. Following response to an NCI call for nominations, fifteen members were selected by the NCI director. Nominees had to meet a series of eligibility requirements (summarised in Box 2.3) and were subject to an objective and pre-defined screening and evaluation process. The planning group recommended that the DCLG should reflect the breadth and depth of the cancer advocacy community and should therefore be multi-culturally diverse and include representation from a range of organizations and a broad mix of cancer sites. The initial membership, which was selected from 136 nominations, comprised mostly cancer survivors, but family members and health professionals involved in cancer advocacy were also included. Collective cancer experience included cancers of the bladder, brain, breast, cervix, kidney, lung, ovary, and prostate and in Hodgkin's disease, leukaemia, multiple myeloma, and sarcoma.

Members of the DCLG serve overlapping terms of three years, and meet at least twice per year. Subgroups charged with specific tasks meet more frequently. Members are responsible for liaising with their constituencies and for seeking and reflecting input from them. The work of the group is supported by the NCI Office of Liaison Activities with the director of this office serving as the DCLG Executive Secretary. Recommendations of the DCLG go directly to the Advisory Committee to the Director of the NCI. Other national and international organizations have established or are establishing similar advisory groups. Following many years of having lay representation on its governing body, in 2000, the British Medical Research Council set up a Consumer Liaison Group to advise Council on ways of promoting effective and appropriate consumer involvement in its activities. The UK National Cancer Research Institute, which was established in 2001 set up its Consumer Liaison Group in parallel with its Clinical Studies Groups as one of its initial priorities.

Box 2.3   Eligibility to serve on the NCI Director's Consumer Liaison Group

Applicants must:

- be involved in the cancer experience: a cancer survivor, a person affected by the suffering and consequences of cancer (i.e. a parent or family member) or a professional/volunteer who works with survivors or those affected,
- represent a constituency with which s/he communicates regularly on cancer issues and be able to serve as a conduit for information both to and from his/her constituency,

If applicants satisfy the above, then assessed for

- cancer advocacy experience, the ability to communicate effectively, ability to represent broad issues and think globally, ability to contribute to an effective group process, leadership ability.

2.6 Education and raising public awareness of trials

Clinical trials involve testing medical interventions on members of the public, function at a societal level and aim to help determine health care policy for the entire community. Yet, the level of public understanding and awareness of trials is poor. The need for clinical trials to establish the value of new and existing therapies is not widely appreciated. Many people believe that trials are offered only as a last resort when other options have failed [46] and a substantial proportion think that doctors know privately which of the treatments on offer in a trial is best [47]. There is therefore an urgent need to raise public awareness about trials – what they are, how they work and why they are important. There is a need to educate the public that 'new' does not necessarily mean better and that there is the very real possibility that new treatments may be less effective or more toxic than standard care. Similarly, we need to reassure those patients who fear that trials always compare an active treatment with a placebo or no treatment [48] that in cancer trials this is seldom the case. It is important to convey the fact that most randomized trials in cancer compare new treatments with the best standard therapy.

Entry to trials would be less stressful and upsetting if patients had a good understanding of trials and awareness of the issues involved before they were invited to participate in a specific trial. This is especially difficult for cancer and other life threatening illnesses because trials are discussed at a particularly difficult time, when there are many other important decisions to be made. Perhaps it would be easier if we each had an idea of whether in principle we would be willing to take part in a trial, should the opportunity arise. It has been suggested that members of the public should carry a 'trials participation card' in the same way that they would an organ donor card [49].

Although open and informed public debate concerning medical research may often accelerate implementation of research findings, the process of rigorous evaluation must not be hijacked by those with vested financial, professional or political interests. An example of such difficulties is illustrated by a controversy regarding breast cancer screening policy for women under fifty in the US. This story which is described in more detail elsewhere [50] and summarized in Box 2.4 highlights some of the difficulties that we are increasingly likely to face as the world of clinical research becomes more open.

Box 2.4 Mammography screening in the US [50]

The rationale

Mammography has been in use since the 1960s. It was used initially for diagnosis and later for screening purposes with the rationale that early detection and treatment would ultimately save lives. However, the small number of deaths prevented by screening needs to be balanced against the disadvantages of the anxiety caused and the potential importance of losing cancer-free years, as well as the impact of false positive and false negative results.

The evidence

Although randomized controlled trials of the effectiveness of mammography screening have found that it reduces mortality in women over fifty, the benefit appears to be smaller and associated with greater harm in women less than 50 years of age. Most of the trials were not

Box 2.4 *(continued)*

designed specifically to address the issue of screening in younger women and included few such participants. Subsequent subgroup analyses did not therefore have sufficient statistical power to detect differences in outcome with reliability and may therefore be criticized (see Section 9.4.7). This lack of benefit in younger women was a source of debate and concern. In consequence a number of meta-analyses, published between 1993 and 1996, were undertaken to try to resolve this issue. However, the meta-analyses varied with respect to the trials that were included and methodology used, and consequently gave varying results. Although all but one suggested a benefit of screening in terms of the relative risk of mortality, the size and significance of the effect depended on the trials that were included and the statistical analyses that were done.

The history

In the US, there had been little debate over the recommendation made in 1977 by the National Cancer Institute (NCI) that women aged over fifty should have regular mammograms. However, over the years, younger women had received conflicting advice from various institutions, associations and organizations. Following an international workshop in 1993 to consider the most recent evidence, the NCI replaced its recommendation for regular screening with the advice that women aged between forty and forty-nine should talk to their doctor before deciding about screening. Most other organizations who had previously issued guidelines on screening disagreed with this and were in favour of women in the younger age group having regular screening as a matter of course. In January 1997, following the publication of results of the most recent trial, the NCI convened a consensus meeting to review the evidence. The unanimous conclusion of the independent panel that they set up was that there was insufficient evidence to recommend routine mammography, and that younger women should decide for themselves, in consultation with a health professional, whether or not they should be screened.

The furore

These recommendations, which were met with surprise and considerable hostility, caused a good deal of controversy in both the scientific and lay press and inevitably the debate entered the political arena. In February 1997 the US Senate passed a resolution urging the NCI to recommend regular mammograms for women aged 40–49, and the Director was urged to reject the consensus panel's conclusions. In turn the Director asked for a recommendation from the National Cancer Advisory Board. Yet even whilst the subcommittee assigned to tackle the issue was considering the facts, the political pressure mounted to the point where it was made clear that decisions on the budget for the National Institutes for Health and the NCI would be postponed until (and by implication depended on) the NCI's final recommendation was issued. In March, a statement was issued by the NCI that had been agreed seventeen to one by the Board that women aged 40–49 at normal risk should be screened every one to two years. [Interestingly, the lone voice of opposition was from a leading scientist in the field of clinical trials, herself a breast cancer survivor.] A joint statement was then released by the NCI and the American Cancer Society stating that 'mammography screening of women in their 40s is beneficial and supportable by the current scientific evidence' thereby completely at odds with the original panel recommendation. Statements of approval by many politicians including the President followed quickly.

Of course clinical research cannot operate in a vacuum and everyone (even politicians) is entitled to their opinion and input. Society should be able to reject the recommendations of the experts. However, the mammography example may highlight the problem that a little knowledge can be a bad thing. The public may have been less aware of the issues than they thought they were and much of what was involved was in fact not well understood. The controversy needs to be seen in the context that the public health message of early detection of cancer is one that has gained widespread acceptance. The prevailing attitude is therefore that screening must be a good thing. When the issues were discussed it was probably not clear to most members of the public that, although there might be a significant reduction in the relative risk of mortality, in absolute terms the potential number of premature deaths avoided is very small – a high proportion of very little is still very little. It emphasises the need for a much better level of public education, and for clear explanation of results to non-researchers to enable a fuller understanding of the facts. Whether or not such an approach would ever circumvent the political coercion that was exerted in this case is of course another question.

There is a need for public education at all levels including specific training for patients advocates and representatives, such as project LEAD, general education in schools and colleges and more general publicity campaigns. There is also a need to work with the press on specific issues to try to ensure that reportage is fair and unbiased. Such public education is a specialist area and detailed discussion is outside the scope of this chapter. However, many of those involved with trials must be ready and willing to take part in open public debate. We must be ready to face the pressures of the press interview, to explain our science to the public and become involved in a public education process.

2.7 Conclusions

Randomized controlled trials are the gold standard in evaluating new cancer therapies. To evaluate new treatments in a timely fashion, and to make progress in treating cancer, trials will almost always need to recruit a large number of patients over relatively short periods of time. Yet, only a small proportion of eligible patients are currently included in trials. A major challenge is therefore to find innovative ways of increasing the number of people who take part in trials. Much of this effort needs to be directed at the clinical community, to persuade more doctors to become involved with research and to invite greater numbers of potential participants to take part in trials. Greater training in communication may be of value to such doctors in order that they are more able to discuss trials and related issues with their patients. Researchers also need to review the ways in which clinical trials are presented to potential participants and we need to undertake further research into alternative methods of inviting patients to volunteer for trials.

Greater and more appropriate communication with those who take part in trials is also needed. Participants need clear information about the reason for the trial, how it will operate and how it may affect them, through good communication with their medical practitioners and by clear and informative literature produced by trialists. Written trial materials need to be produced in patient- friendly formats that can be easily understood by the majority of cancer patients. This is probably best done in collaboration with patient groups or representatives. Investigation of and implementation of appropriate ways of providing feedback on trials to participants is also urgently required.

There is also a clear need for much wider debate to educate the public about the meaning of randomization and clinical trials, ideally before they are in the situation of coping with the news that they have cancer. But, we need to go beyond this, and involve the public more fully in understanding the role of trials and in setting research agendas. This consultation process should not merely be seen as lip service or window dressing, it is a two way process, and one from which researchers and trials can benefit. If trials are ultimately to succeed in changing clinical practice and improving patient care, then they should be relevant to the patient group they serve. Trials must address relevant questions and endpoints and explore treatments that patients would be willing and able to tolerate. Although involving patients in designing trials may add to the burdens of the trial development process, which is already regarded as lengthy and cumbersome by many, we must bear in mind that the conduct of clinical trials is not an academic pursuit in itself, and that this involvement may ultimately lead to more successful trials. The challenge is to find a practical way to forge positive relationships with members of the public. It is to be hoped that, armed with the appropriate information, very many more people will decide to participate in clinical research. Indeed, if the public becomes sufficiently well informed about the need for trials and their role in medical progress, they may well become powerful allies in lobbying for an increased research effort in trials.

References

[1] Stephens, R., and Gibson, D. (1993) The impact of clinical trials on the treatment of lung cancer. *Clinical Oncology*, 5, 211–19.

[2] Lara, P., Higdon, R., Lim, N., Kwan, K., Tanaka, M., Lau, D. *et al.* (2001) Prospective evaluation of cancer clinical trial accrual patterns: Identifying potential barriers to enrollment. *Journal of Clinical Oncology*, 19, 1728–33.

[3] Taylor, K.M., Feldstein, M.L., Skeel, R.T., Pandya, K.J., Ng, P., and Carbone, P. (1994) Fundamental dilemmas of the randomised clinical trial process: results of a survey of the 1737 Eastern Cooperative Oncology Group Investigators. *Journal of Clinical Oncology*, 12, 1796–1805.

[4] Fallowfield, L., Ratcliffe, D., and Souhami, R. (1997) Clinicians' attitudes to Clinical Trials of Cancer Therapy. *European Journal of Cancer*, 33, 2221–29.

[5] Fallowfield, L.J. (1995) Communication skills for oncologists. *Trends in Experimental Medicine*, 5, 99–103.

[6] Kemp, N., Skinner, E., and Toms, J. (1984) Randomized Clinical Trials of Cancer – a public opinion survey. *Clinical Oncology*, 10, 155–61.

[7] Slevin, M., Mossman, J., Bowling, A., Leonard, R., Steward, W., Harper, P., McIllmurray, M., and Thatcher, N. (1995) Volunteers or victims: patients views of randomised clinical trials. *British Journal of Cancer*, 71, 1270–4.

[8] Fallowfield, L.J., Jenkins, V., Sawtell, M., Brennan, C., Moynihan, C., and Souhami, R.L. (1998) Attitudes of patients to randomised clinical trials of cancer therapy. *European Journal of Cancer*, 34, 1554–9.

[9] Edwards, S.J.L., Lilford, R.J., and Hewison, J. (1998) The ethics of randomised controlled trials from the perspectives of patients, the public and healthcare professionals. *British Medical Journal*, **317**, 1209–12.

[10] Henzlova, M.J., Blackburn, G.H., Bradley, E.J., and Rodgers, W.J. (1994) Patient perception on a long-term clinical trial: Experience using a close-out questionnaire in the studies of left-ventricular dysfunction (SOLVD) trial. *Controlled Clinical Trials*, **15**, 284–93.

[11] Suchanek Hudmon, K., Stolzfus, C., Chamberlain, R.M., Lorimor, R.J., Steinbach, G., and Winn, R.J. (1996) Participants perceptions of a phase I colon cancer chemoprevention trial. *Controlled Clinical Trials*, **17**, 494–508.

[12] Braunholtz, D.A., Edwards, S.J., and Lilford, R.J. (2001) Are randomized clinical trials good for us (in the short term)? Evidence for a 'trial effect.' *Journal of Clinical Epidemiology*, **54**, 217–24.

[13] Sackett, D. (2001) How do the outcomes of patients treated within randomised controlled trials compare with those of similar patients treated outside these trials? *Controlled Clinical Trials*, **22**(2S), P64.

[14] Doyal, L. (1997) Journals should not publish research to which patients have not given fully informed consent. *British Medical Journal*, **314**, 1107–11.

[15] Tobias, J.S. (1997) British Medical Journal's present policy (sometimes approving research in which patients have not given fully informed consent) is wholly correct. *British Medical Journal*, **314**, 3111–14.

[16] Doyal, L., and Tobias, J.S. (eds.) (2000) *Informed Consent in Medical Research*. British Medical Journal Publications, London.

[17] Smithells, R.W. (1975) Iatrogenic hazards and their effects. *Postgraduate Medical Journal*, **15**, 39–52.

[18] Chalmers, I., and Lindley, R. (2000) Double standards on informed consent to treatment. In *Informed Consent in Medical Research* (eds. L. Doyal and J.S. Tobias). British Medical Journal Publications, London.

[19] Montgomery, C., Lydon, A., and Lloyd, K. (1997) Patients may not understand enough to give their informed consent. *British Medical Journal*, **314**, 1482.

[20] Baum, M. (1993) New approach for recruitment into randomised controlled trials. *Lancet*, **341**, 812–13.

[21] RAGE. (1997) All treatment and trials must have informed consent. *British Medical Journal*, **314**, 1134–35.

[22] Simes, R.J., Tattersall, M.H.N., Coates, A.S., Raghavan, D., Solomon, H.J., and Smart, H. (1986) Randomised comparison of procedures for obtaining informed consent in clinical trials of treatment for cancer. *British Medical Journal*, **293**, 1065–68.

[23] Aaronson, N.K., Visser-Pol, E., Leenhouts, G.H.M.W., Muller, M.J., van der Schot, A.C.M., van Dam FSAM *et al.* (1996) Telephone-based nursing intervention improves the effectiveness of the informed consent process in cancer clinical trials. *Journal of Clinical Oncology*, **14**, 984–96.

[24] Corbett, F., Oldham, J., and Lilford, R. (1996) Offering patients entry in clinical trials: preliminary study of the views of prospective participants. *Journal of Medical Ethics*, **22**, 227–31.

[25] Llewellyn-Thomas, H.A., McGreal, M.J., Theil, E.C., Fine, S., and Erlichman, C. (1991) Patients willingness to enter clinical trials: measuring the association with perceived benefit and preference for decision participation. *Social Science Medicine*, **32**, 35–42.

[26] Featherstone, K., and Donovan, J.L. (1998) Random allocation or allocation at random? Patients perspectives of participation in a randomised controlled trial. *British Medical Journal*, **317**, 1177–80.

[27] Snowdon, C., Garcia, J., and Elbourne, D. (1997) Making sense of randomization; responses of parents of critically ill babies to random allocation of a treatment in a clinical trial. *Social Science and Medicine*, 45, 1337–55.

[28] Marsh, B.T. (1990) Informed consent – help or hindrance. *Journal of the Royal Society of Medicine*, 83, 603–06.

[29] Dal-Re, R. (1990) Informed consent in clinical research with drugs in Spain: perspective of clinical trials committee members. *European Journal of Clinical Pharmacology*, 38, 319–24.

[30] Grossman, S.A., Piantadosi, S., and Covahey, C. (1994) Are informed consent forms that describe clinical oncology research protocols readable by most patients and their families? *Journal of Clinical Oncology*, 12, 2211–15.

[31] Olver, I.N., Buchanen, L., Laidlaw, C., and Poulton, G. (1995) The adequacy of consent forms for informing patients entering oncological clinical trials. *Annals of Oncology*, 6, 867–70.

[32] Cooley, M.E., Moriarty, H., Berger, M.S., Selm-Orr, D., Coyle, B., and Short, T. (1995) Patient literacy and the readability of written cancer educational materials. *Oncology Nursing Forum*, 22, 1345–51.

[33] Schulte, P. (1991) Ethical issues in the communication of results. *Journal of Clinical Epidemiology*, 44, 57–61.

[34] Marshall, S. (1996) How to get patients' consent to enter clinical trials. Participants should be given feedback about the trial. *British Medical Journal*, 312, 186.

[35] Cockburn, J., Redman, S., and Kricker, A. (1998) Should women take part in clinical trials in breast cancer? Issues and solutions. *Journal of Clinical Oncology*, 16, 354–62.

[36] Snowdon, C., Garcia, J., and Elbourne, D. (1998) Reactions of participants to the results of a randomised controlled trial: Exploratory study. *British Medical Journal*, 317, 21–62.

[37] Goodare, H., and Smith, R. (1995) The rights of patients in research. *British Medical Journal*, 310, 1277–8.

[38] Bagenal, F.S., Easton, D.F., Harris, E., Chilvers, C.E.D., and McElwain, T.J. (1990) Survival of patients with cancer attending Bristol Cancer Help Centre. *Lancet*, 301, 606–10.

[39] Hanley, B. (1999) Involvement works. The second report of the Standing Group on Consumers in NHS Research. NHS Executive.

[40] Royal College of Physicians. (1990) Research involving patients. London:RCP.

[41] Liberati, A. (1997) Consumer participation in research and health care: making it a reality. *British Medical Journal*, 315, 499.

[42] Bastian, H. (1998) Speaking up for ourselves: the evolution of consumer advocacy in health care. *International Journal of Technology and Assessment in Health Care*, 14, 3–23.

[43] Chalmers, I. (1995) What do I want from health research and researchers when I am the patient? *British Medical Journal*, 310, 1315–18.

[44] Hanley, B., Truesdale, A., King, A., Elbourne, D., and Chalmers, I. (2001) Involving consumers in designing, conducting, and interpreting randomised controlled trials: questionnaire survey. *British Medical Journal*, 322, 519–23.

[45] Thornton, H. (1998) Alliance between medical profession and consumers already exists in breast cancer. *British Medical Journal*, 316, 148.

[46] Ellis, P.M., Dowsett, S.M., Butow, P.N., and Tattersall, M.H.N. (1999) Attitudes to randomized clinical trials amongst out-patients attending a medical oncology clinic. *Health Expectations*, 2, 33–43.

[47] Cassileth, B.R., Lusk, E.J., Miller, D.S., and Hurwitz, S. (1982) Attitudes towards clinical trials among patients and the public. *Journal of the American Medical Association*, 248, 968–70.

[48] Ellis, P.M., and Butow, P.N. (1998) Focus group interviews examining attitudes to randomised trials among breast cancer patients and the community. *Australian and New Zealand Journal of Public Health*, 22, 528–31.

[49] Lindley, R.I. (1998) Thrombolytic treatment for acute ischaemic stroke: consent can be ethical. *British Medical Journal*, 316, 1005–07.

[50] Wells, J. (1998) Mammography and the politics of randomised controlled trials. *British Medical Journal*, 317, 1224–30.

Chapter 3

What type of trial is needed?

3.1 Introduction

In this chapter, we provide an overview of the general process by which a new treatment is evaluated; from initial clinical investigation through to widescale clinical practice. We review the factors which may determine, at each stage, whether or not a new clinical trial is warranted. Crucial to this is knowing what you want to have achieved by the time each stage is completed.

Ideas for new therapies and for new trials may emerge from many sources, but all will have in common the hope that they will – in some way – lead to a better therapy for a given condition. They may be anticipated to improve survival, to provide a better toxicity profile, to be more convenient or more widely applicable than standard therapy or perhaps to offer a combination of these factors. To establish whether or not the new therapy really does bring these benefits will ultimately require a direct comparison with the current best standard treatment in a large group of patients, not least because there may be a fine balance between gains and losses with a new therapy. However, a large multi-centre trial is a major undertaking which should only be embarked upon if the case for doing so is strong. The questions addressed must be clinically important, scientifically informative and ethically sound, and must be accorded high priority by the clinical and patient communities involved. A 'screening process' is therefore necessary to ensure a high chance that therapies which are ineffective, impractical or inappropriate for whatever reason are rejected at an early stage. Typically therefore, new therapies go through many stages of testing, both pre-clinical and clinical. We begin by describing a widely used categorization of clinical trials which mirrors the typical process of development of therapies from the first clinical developments to widescale use in clinical practice.

3.1.1 Phases of clinical trials

The categorization of clinical trials into phases I–IV (see Box 3.1) has its origins in drug development, but serves as a useful framework to describe the typical stages of development of any form of treatment. It is, however, increasingly rare that a new therapy would be evaluated in just one trial of each phase, and the distinctions between the phases have perhaps become less clear in practice than the conventional description would suggest. The main focus of this book is the randomized phase III trial. However, in this chapter we discuss some of the issues in the design of phase II studies and non-randomized phase III trials which do not appear elsewhere and which set the discussions

Box 3.1 Conventional framework for drug development trials

Phase I – Clinical pharmacology and toxicity
Phase II – Initial investigation of treatment activity
Phase III – Full-scale comparative treatment evaluation
Phase IV – Post-marketing surveillance

concerning randomized phase III trials in context of the entire treatment development process.

3.2 Phase I – Clinical pharmacology and toxicity

Following on from laboratory studies and pre-clinical investigations, phase I trials represent the first use of a new agent or combination in humans. In the case of most new cancer therapies, the subjects will be cancer patients, usually with advanced disease (not necessarily with a single common primary) which is not suitable for treatment with any established therapy. In other (non-cancer) settings, initial phase I investigations will often include healthy volunteers. On the assumption that – for most treatments – activity increases with dose, the primary aim of a phase I trial is to determine the maximum tolerated dose (MTD). Thus, small groups of patients are treated at different dose levels and the degree, timing and duration of toxicity observed. The starting dose will be based on pre-clinical observations. A number of schemes to determine dose escalation are in use, but the essential elements are that the initial escalations are large while no toxicity is observed, becoming smaller once toxicity-inducing levels are reached. Each of the early dose levels will typically include 4–6 patients, increasing slightly when toxicity is reached and with the first patient at each level observed carefully for several weeks. The definition of maximum tolerated dose is somewhat subjective and is likely to be affected by the previous treatments a patient has received. The dose taken forward to phase II testing may not be the MTD, but often the preceding dose, described by Carter [1] as the dose which causes moderate, reversible toxicity in most patients. A detailed discussion of phase I trials in cancer is beyond the scope of this book, but a special article from the American Society for Clinical Oncology [2] provides a useful reference for further information.

3.3 Phase II – Initial investigation of treatment activity

3.3.1 General aim

Once phase I trials have determined an appropriate 'therapeutic' dose, the first real evaluation of the treatment's anti-tumour effect comes with the phase II trials (see Box 3.2). The aim here is to assess the activity, feasibility and toxicity of a given dose and schedule and thus to screen out insufficiently active treatments. Individual phase II studies will usually focus on a specific cancer type. This will influence the stage of disease for which a patient is considered suitable for such a study, the outcome measure used to

Box 3.2   Key roles of a phase II trial

- ◆ Assess activity
- ◆ Assess feasibility
- ◆ Assess toxicity
- ◆ Screen out inactive treatments

assess activity, and the level of activity that the agent needs to demonstrate if it is to be considered potentially useful.

For cytotoxic agents, phase II studies are often carried out in patients with metastatic disease, with tumour response as the activity measure. Wherever possible, standard outcome measures should be used to facilitate comparison across studies; response is often assessed by the 'RECIST' criteria [3], the key features of which are described in Box 3.3.

3.3.2   The importance of prospective conduct

There are several widely used designs for phase II studies and we review them briefly here. Whatever the design though, a key, but sometimes neglected, feature of a phase II trial is the importance of *prospective* conduct. Any phase II study should aim to register its target number of patients prospectively, as this is the only means by which one can be sure that the results of the study apply to a defined cohort of patients who all began the treatment with the intention of being evaluated. It is often the case that a number of patients will have received the treatment under investigation outside of a formal trial setting, before the trial starts, and there may be understandable enthusiasm for such patients to contribute data in some way, particularly when the disease is rare. However, allowing patients to be registered retrospectively has serious drawbacks. Without systematic records and careful monitoring, it is difficult to determine whether those patients who are registered retrospectively comprise all relevant patients from that centre, or perhaps a highly selected group who did particularly well, or particularly badly, on the trial therapy. The former is perhaps the most common problem, since an obvious selection criterion is to register only surviving patients who could give their consent for their data to be used. Selecting patients for inclusion in a phase II trial *on the basis of their characteristics* is inevitable and does not represent a bias in assessing treatment activity. Selecting patients for inclusion *on the basis of their response* does introduce bias, but can be avoided by registering prospectively and accounting for all registered patients in the analysis.

3.3.3   Common phase II designs

Here we give a brief introduction to the most widely used phase II trial designs; sample size formulae and examples are given in Chapter 5.

The simplest phase II design involves treating and assessing a predefined number of patients, and determining overall 'success or failure' on the basis of a hypothesis test

Box 3.3 Essential features of the RECIST response criteria

For full details see: http://www3.nci.nih.gov/bip/RECIST.htm

1. Definitions

Measurable disease – the presence of at least one measurable lesion. If the measurable disease is restricted to a solitary lesion, its neoplastic nature should be confirmed by cytology/histology.

Measurable lesions – lesions that can be accurately measured in at least one dimension with longest diameter ≥ 20 mm using conventional techniques or ≥ 10 mm with spiral CT scan.

Non-measurable lesions – all other lesions, including small lesions (longest diameter <20 mm with conventional techniques or <10 mm with spiral CT scan), i.e., bone lesions, leptomeningeal disease, ascites, pleural/pericardial effusion, inflammatory breast disease, lymphangitis cutis/pulmonis, cystic lesions, and also abdominal masses that are not confirmed and followed by imaging techniques.

2. Baseline documentation of 'Target' and 'Non-Target' lesions

- All measurable lesions up to a maximum of five lesions per organ and ten lesions in total, representative of all involved organs should be identified as *target lesions* and recorded and measured at baseline.

- Target lesions should be selected on the basis of their size (lesions with the longest diameter) and their suitability for accurate repeated measurements (either by imaging techniques or clinically).

- A sum of the longest diameter (LD) for *all target lesions* will be calculated and reported as the baseline sum LD. The baseline sum LD will be used as reference by which to characterize the objective tumour response.

- All other lesions (or sites of disease) should be identified as *non-target lesions* and should also be recorded at baseline. Measurements of these lesions are not required, but the presence or absence of each should be noted throughout follow-up.

3. Response evaluation

Response Criteria	Evaluation of target lesions
* Complete Response (CR)	Disappearance of all target lesions
* Partial Response (PR)	At least a 30 per cent decrease in the sum of the longest diameter (LD) of target lesions, taking as reference the baseline sum LD
* Progressive Disease (PD)	At least a 20 per cent increase in the sum of the LD of target lesions, taking as reference the smallest sum LD recorded since the treatment started or the appearance of one or more new lesions

Box 3.3 *(continued)*

Response Criteria	**Evaluation of target lesions**
* Stable Disease (SD)	Neither sufficient shrinkage to qualify for PR nor sufficient increase to qualify for PD, taking as reference the smallest sum LD since the treatment started.
	Evaluation of non-target lesions
* Complete Response (CR)	Disappearance of all non-target lesions and normalization of tumour marker level
* Incomplete Response/ Stable Disease (SD)	Persistence of one or more non-target lesion(s) or/and maintenance of tumour marker level above the normal limits
* Progressive Disease (PD)	Appearance of one or more new lesions and/or unequivocal progression of existing non-target lesions

of the form, 'what is the probability that the true response rate exceeds x per cent?' One such design, introduced by Fleming [4] takes as a starting point the assumption that for any new treatment, there will be a level of response, p_1, below which – in the light of response rates for standard therapy – the treament would not be considered for further study, and a higher level, p_2, above which the treatment would certainly warrant further investigation. The sample size is determined by the need to minimize the probability of concluding that the response rate is greater than p_1 when that is false and to minimize the probability of concluding that the response rate is less than p_2 when that too is false.

However, as in many clinical situations, summarizing the results of a study simply in terms of a p value from a hypothesis test is of limited value. Given the twin desires of treating as few patients as possible with an insufficiently active treatment, while treating enough patients to gain a reasonably precise estimate of efficacy, the first phase II trials of a new treatment may often be conducted in two stages. Gehan [5] proposed such a design where, in the first stage, the aim is to screen out insufficiently active treatments. A set number of patients are treated (the number is determined by the minimum acceptable response rate and the maximum acceptable probability of rejecting an effective treatment); if no responses are seen, the trial proceeds no further. If any responses are seen, the trial continues to the second stage in which sufficient patients are treated to estimate the response rate with a given level of precision.

An alternative two-stage design is given by Simon [6]. This takes as its premise the point of view that the aim of a phase II trial is simply to screen out inadequate treatments at as early a stage as possible, that large numbers are needed to provide reasonably precise estimates of response rates, and therefore that estimation should not be the main aim of a phase II trial. Therefore the design allows either the number of patients in the first stage, or the total number of patients to be minimized if the treatment has an inadequate response rate, subject to specification of the error rates. As for the Fleming single-stage design, this requires specification of an unacceptable level of activity (p_1) and an activity level above which there would be interest in taking the treatment forward for further testing (p_2).

3.3.4 Choice of design

How would you choose between designs in a given situation? There is no clear-cut answer. Deciding factors include the importance of stopping early if a treatment is clearly insufficiently active – this might be high if there is an alternative treatment, in which case one may wish to avoid a single-stage design such as Fleming's. On the other hand, if you have good reason to expect a response rate above 50 per cent, the Gehan design is perhaps unappealing; the first stage would require only between two and four patients at conventional error rates. Both the Gehan and Simon designs allow early stopping if a treatment is inactive; the Simon design provides a numerical rule for deciding, at the end of the second stage, whether the treatment is worth pursuing. Although this may be useful, the final decision will also need to incorporate the information gained on toxicity and general feasibility and the structure of the Gehan design may sit more comfortably with the less prescriptive aims of many phase II trials. Finally, the benefit of early stopping is lost if the outcome measure is not a short-term outcome such as response. In cancers for which radiological response is particularly difficult to assess, it may be appropriate to use a later endpoint such as progression-free survival. In such situations, the Fleming design may be most appropriate; an example of such a trial in stage I testicular teratoma is given in Box 5.1.

3.3.5 Limitations of conventional phase II trials

The decision is not, however, limited to these three options. The fact that so many of the treatments which reach phase III testing fail to demonstrate clinically important differences suggests some problems with the conventional wisdom of phase II studies. The value of tumour response as a predictor of long-term efficacy might be questioned in some cancer sites, particularly when the phase II study involves patients with advanced disease – possibly heavily pre-treated – but the treatment is intended ultimately for use in the adjuvant setting. Perhaps, though, the key problem is that patients in phase II studies are typically highly selected, and the impact of such selection is perhaps not always well understood. How would standard therapy have fared in exactly the same set of patients? The typical phase II design makes an implicit assumption that this is known and invariable, but this may well be questionable.

Alternative designs have been developed to attempt to tackle this latter point, for example, designs which formally incorporate historical data to quantify the size and variability of the minimum acceptable response rate have been proposed – these are described by Thall [7].

Randomized phase II trials

While there probably remains a place for the conventional, non-randomized, phase II trial early in the development of a treatment, there has been a welcome extension of this phase of testing to include some early, small, randomized studies. The description 'randomized phase II trial' is widely misused, often applied to what is simply a small randomized phase III trial, or a larger randomized phase III trial in which response or an alternative 'early' endpoint is the primary outcome measure but where, in both cases, the aim is to compare the outcome in the treatment groups, and this has been used to determine the study size. As shown in Box 3.1 and discussed below, the characteristic feature of the *phase III* trial is that it is comparative. A true randomized phase II trial is NOT primarily intended to be comparative, and it is certainly not powered, statistically, to be comparative. Rather, it should be seen as a combination of two or more parallel phase II trials in which conventional phase II sample size selection and stopping rules, such as those described above, are applied to one or more of the individual arms [8]. Typically, one would design a standard single arm phase II trial of a new therapy, but would then add an additional arm by randomizing patients equally between the standard therapy and the new therapy until the required sample size for the new therapy is achieved. The response rate on the standard therapy is not used to determine whether or not to stop the phase II trial early, but provides a check on the extent to which patient selection alone accounts for the results in the experimental group. This is then used, rather informally, to aid decisions about whether a new treatment is sufficiently promising to be taken forward into a phase III trial. An example of a trial in which such an approach was taken is given in Box 5.3. This example illustrates another of the benefits of a randomized phase II design in that, if the experimental treatment shows sufficient activity to be taken into a phase III trial, patients from the randomized phase II can contribute to the overall sample size.

Randomized phase II trials can be particularly useful when good data on response to standard therapy are lacking, perhaps because the disease is rare; where there is limited knowledge of prognostic factors and their potential impact on outcome, or where several potential new therapies require testing. In the latter case, the aim is to eliminate inactive treatments, not compare arms, and the Simon design seems to lend itself well to this situation as the determinant of sample size.

With randomized phase II trials, as indeed for any small randomized trials, it is important to use a method of treatment allocation which ensures balance for the most important prognostic factors; these are described in Chapter 4.

3.4 Phase III – Full-scale comparative treatment evaluation

Phase III trials are the first, direct comparison between the new treatment and the current standard (which may sometimes be no active treatment). In most cases, patients will be allocated to the alternative treatments using a chance mechanism, leading to *randomized controlled clinical trials* (often referred to simply as RCTs). '*Randomized*' means that patients are allocated treatments within the trial prospectively, by an unpredictable (usually random) means. '*Controlled*' implies comparative in some sense, but does not always imply 'randomized' or prospective. Indeed as we discuss later, something referred to as a randomized trial may not in fact mean truly randomized. The randomized controlled phase III trial is the established gold standard for determining the relative value of a new therapy, and it will be a rare treatment indeed which becomes established therapy without having successfully passed through at least one randomized phase III trial. Chapter 4 is devoted to this most important phase; here we discuss the importance of randomization and the problems associated with non-randomized comparisons.

3.4.1 The importance of randomization

The goal of good trial design is to enable a clinical question to be answered reliably, in particular to estimate the effect of treatment without bias, and with adequate precision. If a trial is designed appropriately it should always be possible to extract useful information. If the design fails to ensure this, even the most sophisticated analysis cannot guarantee to extract an unbiased estimate.

To identify the ways in which bias can enter a trial design, it is useful to consider why the treatment effect observed within a trial may differ from the true, underlying effect which it aims to estimate.

In fact, observed effect = true effect + 'error', where the 'error' term can be broken down into two components:

◆ Systematic error or bias – this can be controlled if not eliminated by good trial design, the most fundamental aspect of which is the allocation of patients to treatment groups by a means which does not systematically select patients with different characteristics to go in different groups and which is unpredictable to the person deciding whether to invite a patient to enter a trial – randomization.

◆ Random error – this is simply the play of chance which is always present to some degree when the number of patients being studied is finite. In a randomized trial it can be minimized by randomizing large numbers of patients, and to some degree controlled by the method of randomization chosen.

Good design will address systematic error by ensuring that the patient groups being compared differ overall only in the treatment they received – this generally means ensuring that they are randomized appropriately – and that the trial outcome measures are assessed without bias. It will address random error by ensuring, through appropriate sample size calculation, that the impact of random error will be small in relation to the size of effect the trial aims to detect. Sample size issues are addressed in Chapter 5; here though we discuss the potential for systematic bias to be introduced through non-randomized comparisons.

3.4.2 Non-randomized comparisons – an introduction

While randomized trials are regarded as the gold standard, they are not always easy to perform and in some cases may be infeasible. The typical trial will take many years from the initial idea to the final publication of results. During this time one must agree the trial design, negotiate and secure support from participating clinicians and funding bodies, submit the trial for scientific and ethical review, recruit, treat, assess and follow-up patients, analyse the results and pass peer review before publication. Each of these steps present (necessary) obstacles of varying difficulty, and consequently the structure and commitment required to see a trial through from beginning to end should never be underestimated.

Where problems concerned with conducting randomized trials are considered insurmountable, some form of comparison is often still necessary. Here, and perhaps in the early stages of drug development when phase II data alone do not justify a randomized trial and more data are needed, there are essentially two options. A comparative control group is necessary, and this can be non-concurrent (historical) or concurrent.

3.4.3 Historical controls

Here, a new treatment is tried on a group of patients and results are compared with a 'similar' group of patients previously treated on a standard therapy. Previously treated patients might include

- literature controls – a comparison with published results of similar trials
- consecutive groups of patients treated within the same hospital over different time periods

There are problems with both approaches, first and foremost that of patient selection. Early trials may well assess the impact of treatment in patients with very advanced disease, but will eventually consider those patients (possibly with much less advanced disease) for whom the treatment is actually intended. It is understandable that such early studies will focus on those patients who, through disease characteristics and general fitness, would be expected to respond most positively. Identifying a control group in whom the same selection criteria have been applied is more difficult. A well established treatment is likely to have been applied to a much wider variety of patients in more recent years.

Even if patients are unselected, other factors may have changed over time (for example, supportive care or antibiotic use). The criteria for assessing 'response,' including staging procedures, may have changed over time – or data on the historical group of patients may not have been recorded in sufficient detail for comparison with current patients to be made. The type of patient being seen may have changed. This might occur through specific changes in referral practice, for example specialist centres may be referred more 'difficult' cases. Perhaps even more difficult to account for are changes in the overall pattern of disease stage, for example the shift towards presentation at an earlier stage resulting from screening for breast, prostate or bowel cancer.

Two examples follow, the first illustrating a fairly typical example of the impact of patient selection, the second a more subtle issue.

Example 1: Treatment of malignant brain tumours. In the late 1980s, the MRC was considering a new trial in high-grade glioma, which would address whether or not some form of chemotherapy could improve survival when given in addition to the standard treatment of surgery followed by radiotherapy. One of the options was a new drug which had undergone phase II testing in one UK hospital. There was a considerable amount of data, both from previous MRC trials and other sources, establishing the 2-year survival rate on standard therapy at no more than 10–15 per cent. The new drug study showed a 2-year survival rate of approximately 35 per cent. Clearly this was very encouraging. However, the previous trials had not only provided data on the expected survival on standard therapy (Fig. 3.1a), they had also provided data on prognostic factors. In particular, data from two previous MRC trials had been used to derive a prognostic index [9] which was able to classify patients into six groups with varying probabilities of survival (Fig. 3.1b).

When the patients on the new drug were assessed and categorized into the prognostic groups defined by this index it was clear that they fell into the best prognostic groups, and that their survival did not differ substantially from that expected in patients with similar characteristics but undergoing conventional treatment. While this alone did not

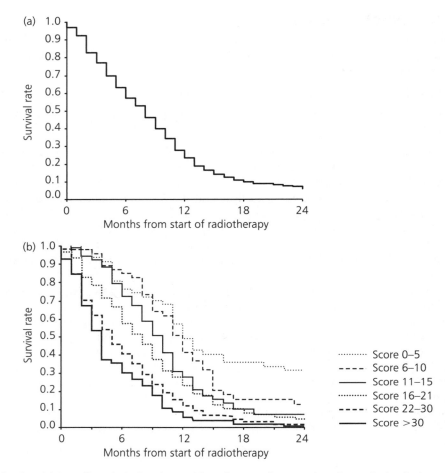

Fig. 3.1 (a) Overall survival of patients with malignant glioma undergoing radical radiotherapy. (b) Survival according to prognostic group.

eliminate the new drug as a potential component of the new trial, it did identify the need for cautious interpretation of the pilot study data.

Such situations are common, although good data on baseline survival and on prognostic factors against which new data can be assessed are unfortunately not always available. While this situation is one in which the potential biases involved in historically controlled studies are fairly easy to anticipate, the issues are not always so clear.

Example 2: Testicular cancer. The outcome of treatment for metastatic testicular germ cell tumours improved substantially during the 1970s through the introduction of the drug cisplatin. During the 1980s combination chemotherapy regimens were developed and these too, possibly combined with increased experience in treating the disease, led to improvements in outcome. More recently, with standard treatment established as the BEP (bleomycin, etoposide, cisplatin) regimen, there have been no clear improvements in outcome. Meanwhile, post-operative surveillance had become a widely accepted form of management for early stage disease. In such a situation, one might consider the following proposal:

- Between 1990 and 1993, every patient with stage I disease (disease confined to the testis) at a particular hospital was treated by surgery alone.
- The same hospital treats the next 100 stage I patients with surgery followed by BEP chemotherapy.

This is a rare disease in which randomized trials might be thought difficult. Some of the usual concerns with the use of historical controls appear to be absent – for example, overall survival has not changed recently, the type of primary treatment (surgery) has remained the same, and the endpoint – survival – is clear and objective. It might therefore seem reasonable to assume that, if survival improves, it must be due to the treatment, because the patients are unselected, and no other aspect of treatment has changed.

However, there is possibly a more subtle bias here. Patients undergo radiological procedures to establish their disease stage. In recent years, this would include chest CT to look for lung metastases, whereas in the past this would more often have been done using chest X-rays. If chest CTs are able to identify patients with lung metastases too small to be identified using chest X-rays, then a group of patients who would previously have been classified as stage I, but who would have developed obvious lung metastases in due course, would in the present day be reclassified as having advanced disease immediately. The prognosis of the present-day group of stage I patients is better than that of 'historical' stage I patients because a high-risk group is now excluded. However, the prognosis of the present day advanced disease group may also have improved, because the additional patients now falling into this group have minimal disease. It is possible in this situation for survival in both subgroups (stage I and advanced disease) to improve, while overall survival stays the same. Although this seems counter-intuitive at first, we are simply shifting patients from one group to another. A hypothetical numerical example will illustrate this.

Box 3.4 shows survival rates by disease stage for 1000 patients treated in the 1980s and another 1000 patients treated in the 1990s.

We see that in the 1990s, fewer patients are classified as stage I, but those that are have a slightly higher survival rate (99 per cent) than those diagnosed as stage I in the 1980s (95 per cent).

Box 3.4 Number of patients by year and stage at diagnosis (3-year survival rate in brackets)

Period	Stage I	Stage II–IV	All patients
1980s	800 (95%)	200 (70%)	1000 (90%)
1990s	600 (99%)	400 (76%)	1000 (90%)

The overall survival rate can be calculated, approximately, as a weighted average of the survival rates for stage I and stage > I patients as follows:

$$\frac{800 \times 0.95 + 200 \times 0.7}{1000} = 0.90,$$

$$\frac{600 \times 0.99 + 400 \times 0.76}{1000} = 0.90.$$

In both cases, overall survival remains at 90 per cent. However, it is clear that a comparison of stage I patients treated in the 1980s with stage I patients treated perhaps differently in the 1990s would identify a difference in survival which could be attributed erroneously to changing treatments.

This illustrates a phenomenon known as stage migration, often referred to as the 'Will Rogers phenomenon' [10]. Will Rogers was an American humourist famously reported as saying of the 1930s Gold Rush, 'when the Okies moved from Oklahoma to California, they raised the IQ in both states,' implying that even the least intelligent people in Oklahoma were more intelligent than the typical Californian.

This example serves to illustrate a real difficulty in interpreting the results of treatment comparisons involving historical controls, and one in which adjustment for prognostic factors can do nothing to help.

3.4.4 Concurrent controls

In an attempt to avoid some of the problems associated with time-related changes, some non-randomized comparisons may make use of concurrent controls. Here, all patients are treated and assessed prospectively, but receive different treatments by a non-random mechanism. Typical examples include comparing the results of a treatment given in one hospital with those of a different treatment given in a different hospital. Clearly though, there may well be other systematic differences between hospitals; for example, in the type of supportive or ancillary care they provide or in the type of patient being referred. As another example, it has been suggested that treatments can be compared more fairly if patients are allowed to choose which treatment they wish to receive. The assumption is that patients will not harbour the biases or pre-conceptions of their doctors. However, even if these biases have not been expressed to the patient, the 'volunteer' effect is well known – patients feeling fitter or more confident opting perhaps for the new treatment whilst those feeling less robust prefer to receive the established standard therapy for their condition. The groups of patients selecting specific treatments may also differ in more subtle ways and again these may be very important with respect to treatment outcome, but not necessarily quantifiable.

In recent years there has been a great deal of interest in recording common datasets on all newly diagnosed cancer patients. The suggestion that these might be used to make treatment comparisons crops up with a degree of regularity with proponents arguing that because registration is complete, treatment effects can be estimated using statistical models to adjust for the imbalances in important patient characteristics. Unfortunately, such comparisons may still suffer from problems associated with both historical and concurrent controls:

- The treatments patients have received are the result of clinical judgement as to what was appropriate. The factors determining that choice may not be quantifiable, and even if quantifiable, may not be recorded.
- As with historical controls, patients will not necessarily have been identified or evaluated in a consistent manner.
- Adjusted (or matched) analyses can be used (see Section 9.4.3) but the important prognostic factors may not be known or agreed, or even if agreed, recorded in an appropriate manner. There are many possible adjusted analyses which could be carried out, each potentially resulting in a different treatment effect. Finally, the assumptions underlying such multivariate models may not always be met, adding to the difficulty of determining which is the 'best' estimate of treatment effect.

Thus the difficulties in interpreting treatment comparisons from non-randomized studies are considerable. They may generate hypotheses, or provide useful supplementary data to non-randomized studies in order to determine if a randomized trial might be worthwhile (e.g. [11]), but they cannot provide an accurate estimate of treatment effect. If they are truly the only feasible form of comparison, patient characteristics must be taken into account in the analysis and careful consideration given to all the possible biases relevant to the particular comparison, including the direction in which they are most likely to act.

3.5 Phase IV – Post-marketing surveillance

A new treatment may become established with relatively little knowledge of its long-term effects. 'Phase IV' evaluation usually refers to the study of adverse events and late morbidity and mortality in cohorts of patients who have undergone such treatment. These studies perhaps assume most importance when treating non-fatal conditions, where adverse effects may be relatively rare and/or may not become obvious until some time after the efficacy of the treatment has been determined. Many phase III cancer trials are evaluating the impact of treatment on survival and necessarily follow patients for most of their life; in this situation, evaluation of late effects is actually an integral part of the phase III trial.

3.6 'Positioning' your trial

In deciding whether a clinical trial of a therapy is warranted, it is important to know what has been done before, in particular what phase of development the treatment has reached. Systematic searching for relevant systematic reviews and trials is therefore an essential pre-study requirement. The first step should be to find out whether a systematic review or meta-analysis has already been done. The Cochrane library (see Chapter 11) is a good starting point as it includes Cochrane Collaboration systematic reviews in the Cochrane Database of Systematic Reviews (CDSR) and also abstracts of systematic reviews done outside of the collaboration in the DARE database. Literature searches may reveal additional systematic reviews. If no systematic review has been done, a systematic search for relevant trials should be carried out (see Section 11.5.4) to identify both

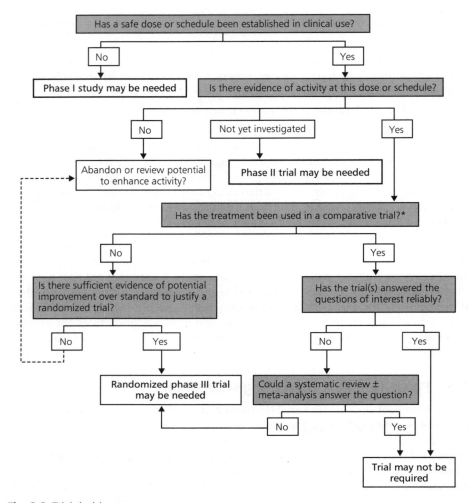

Fig. 3.2 Trial decision tree.
* Search for or/and conduct systematic review to identify trial.

published and unpublished trials. This information is essential in justifying a new trial as it would be unethical to embark on a new trial if there is already sufficient information from completed trials to answer the question posed, and possibly impractical if similar trials are already ongoing.

Fig. 3.2 gives an outline of the questions to ask in determining whether a trial is needed, and if so, the type. Points to consider in answering the questions are described below.

Has a safe dose been established in clinical use?

If a new therapy has yet to be used in humans, then a phase I dose-finding study of some form is almost always needed; such a stage may even be needed if a treatment is in clinical use, but is being evaluated as part of a new combination therapy.

Is there evidence of activity?

If a therapy has been subject to some clinical evaluation to determine an appropriate dose and schedule, then it may be appropriate next to conduct a phase II study, particularly if none have yet been performed. If phase II studies have been performed, but have failed to demonstrate a useful level of activity, then options are to abandon the treatment, or conduct another phase II study. Careful thought is needed before taking either path, and certainly it is worth considering if there is any potential to enhance activity before doing so.

Has the treatment been used in a comparative trial?

Chapter 11 describes search strategies for identifying randomized trials in the published literature, and sources of information which may identify unpublished trials. Searching for non-randomized comparative studies requires a more *ad hoc* approach but is nonetheless important; such studies may help build a case for or against a randomized trial.

Is the case for a phase III trial sufficiently strong?

If systematic searching has failed to identify any comparative studies involving the new therapy, then it should not automatically be concluded that a phase III trial should be performed. Given the limitations of phase II trials with respect to identifying active (as opposed to inactive) treatments, it will generally be the case that even after one or even more have been completed, uncertainty will remain about the potential benefits of a treatment. Simply repeating a phase II trial in a similarly small group of patients may bring limited data to help this process, but may well be necessary if existing trials have been flawed in some way – perhaps toxicity recording was inadequate, or the group were not registered prospectively. Other reasons for repeating a phase II study might include the need to look at different patient populations or the performance or practicalities of a therapy under different health care systems. If the treatment you wish to study has been modified in some way compared with the previous studies, then it will often be a clinical judgement as to whether the degree of modification is sufficient to warrant a further phase II trial, or whether the existing data are sufficient.

Has the trial(s) answered the questions of interest?

If other phase III trials have been done or are ongoing, the question is, is another phase III trial required? Repetition and replication are important principles of most scientific disciplines. Essentially, clinical research is no different, but the particular ethical requirements surrounding clinical rather than laboratory or theoretical research demand that the case for repetition should be carefully made. There is often a good case for repetition; as was mentioned in the context of repeating phase II trials, there may be a need to repeat what is essentially the same trial in a different – perhaps broader – group of patients, or in a different health care system where other aspects of patient care may differ. More often, a decision is taken to conduct a further randomized trial because it is felt that existing trial data are in some way inadequate. There are several reasons why this conclusion may be reached, each of which is discussed in more detail in the following sections.

- *Previous phase III trials were not randomized.* As we have explained earlier, a 'phase III' trial is comparative, but not necessarily randomized. Non-randomized comparisons can suffer from serious bias and problems in interpretation; their limitations are discussed in Section 3.4.

- *Previous phase III trials did not compare the new treatment with the existing 'gold standard'.* The appropriate choice of control arm is a major issue in trial design and, while the choice may sometimes appear obvious, it may not always be so and in fact it may be in some people's interest to compare a new treatment with a sub-standard control. This issue is discussed further in Chapter 4.

- *Previous phase III trials were underpowered for clinically important differences.* As discussed earlier, it is rare that a new treatment will pass through just one trial of each phase before becoming accepted. This is particularly true of phase III. In some situations, small or moderate treatment effects can be very important clinically, but may require trials of several thousand patients if such effects are to be detected reliably. It will often be the case that a smaller trial is performed first. This might be as a planned feasibility study for a subsequent larger trial, but perhaps more commonly smaller trials are done either because those conducting them had limited resources, or because they believed the impact of the new treatment would be substantial. Thus, although otherwise designed to assess the impact of a new treatment in clinical practice, existing trials may simply not have been large enough to produce reliable results. Chapter 5 discusses ways of determining how large a trial should be. In this situation, however, it might be appropriate to ask whether a formal systematic review and meta-analysis could answer the question without needing another trial.

- *Data on potentially important outcome measures are lacking.* A more difficult situation is perhaps where previous randomized trials have shown evidence of potentially useful efficacy over other treatments with respect to one outcome measure, but data on other relevant outcomes were not collected. Randomizing further patients in this situation may be difficult ethically, but equally may be important; first one needs to consider how extreme the differences between treatments must be with respect to other outcome measures – perhaps toxicity or quality of life – before they would overwhelm the benefit shown with respect to the primary outcome measure. If the differences would have to be substantial, it is possible that a carefully designed non-randomized study may provide sufficient data. If small or modest differences in the secondary outcome measures could be important, then a further randomized trial collecting such data may be appropriate.

- *The trial population was highly selective.* Perhaps a treatment has shown efficacy in a particular type of patient, or perhaps in a particular setting, and the question arises as to whether the results can be extrapolated to other patients or settings. Sometimes, treatments pass through two broad stages of phase III trials in a planned manner; an early one on a modest scale designed with the aim of giving a new therapy the best possible chance of showing improved efficacy levels and a later, often larger scale trial, aimed at assessing impact in routine clinical practice. These two broad types of trials have been termed 'explanatory' and 'pragmatic' [12], and their different aims can have a major impact on many aspects of trial design, conduct and analysis. These issues are discussed further in Chapter 4, but one characteristic concerns patient selection.

For the explanatory trial, the patients who are considered most likely to demonstrate a difference in response to the alternative treatments are chosen; for the pragmatic trial one would include any patient who might be considered for the experimental treatment outside of the trial. For example, one might choose higher risk patients (who have most potential to benefit) for the early trial but be interested more generally in the impact on lower risk patients should the treatment prove effective. There are no hard and fast rules for determining when a trial result can be extrapolated and when it cannot. More often than not, the differences will be of degree and not direction, and thus it will be a question of asking by how much would the treatment effect have to differ in a broader population before it was no longer considered worthwhile.

Could a systematic review or meta-analysis answer the question?

A systematic search of the literature alone may reveal a considerable quantity of relevant data pertaining to the treatment of interest, but the usual situation is that the results are to some degree at least, apparently conflicting. After all, if there were unanimity, you probably wouldn't even be considering the trial (unless you were very out of touch with the field). In this situation, it may often be that a systematic review and formal combination of the data from all relevant trials is appropriate. Chapter 11 describes the motivation and methods for systematic reviews and meta-analyses, and the pros and cons of using only published data to do this. If the systematic review indicates that the new therapy is already of proven benefit, or the evidence against a clinically worthwhile benefit is sufficiently strong, then a further trial is unlikely to be needed. If it demonstrates that a potentially useful effect may be obtainable, but perhaps the number of patients and events in previous trials is insufficient to be conclusive, then a new trial may be warranted and the findings of the systematic review may be helpful in designing the trial. We describe in Box 3.5 two such situations in which a meta-analysis was used to guide decisions about future trials.

Box 3.5   Examples of the role of meta-analyses in determining the need for a trial

1. Pre-operative radiotherapy for oesophageal cancer

When the MRC set up a new Oesophageal Cancer Working Party in 1990, this working party considered conducting a randomized trial of surgical resection with or without pre-operative radiotherapy. A small planning group was given the task of pursuing this idea, but, having consulted widely and conducted a literature search, were aware that a number of randomized trials had already investigated this question. The results of these trials appeared conflicting, however, and none of the trials was large enough to provide a reliable answer. The planning group therefore suggested that a meta-analysis would be more appropriate, and this was carried out by the MRC CTU meta-analysis group. The results [13] did not show a clear role for pre-operative radiotherapy, nor did they show sufficient promise to generate enthusiasm for a further trial.

> **Box 3.5** *(continued)*
>
> ## 2. Intraportal fluorouracil for colorectal cancer
>
> In 1989, the UK Coordinating Committee on Cancer Research identified improving survival of colorectal cancer patients as a national priority, and set up a working group to develop trial proposals. This group conducted a systematic review [14] of published adjuvant chemotherapy trials, and also contacted other trials organisations to find out about ongoing trials and to obtain, where possible, unpublished data. This review identified portal vein infusion of fluorouracil given immediately post-operatively for one week as a highly promising treatment; six trials had evaluated this treatment and together they suggested a striking, and highly statistically significant, reduction in the annual odds of death. However, the total number of patients included in the trials was only 1500 (only 300 of whom had died) and a high proportion of randomized patients were excluded from the published analyses which may have biased results in favour of chemotherapy (see Section 9.4.1). The data were therefore considered promising, but inconclusive, and led to the design of AXIS (Adjuvant X-ray and 5FU Infusion Study), a 4000-patient trial powered to look for modest but clinically worthwhile improvements in survival through the use of intraportal fluorouracil [15].

3.7 Conclusion

This chapter has covered the issues involved in 'positioning' a new trial; establishing the need or otherwise for a new trial in the context or previous and current work and clarifying the broad goals of a trial. The real work on the trial now begins. The design must be finalised and the appropriate sample size determined; Chapters 4 and 5 cover the key issues with respect to these aspects. Equally important are the practical issues. Even at this stage, a number of people may have been closely involved in formulating the idea for the trial. Many of them will form the embryo 'Trial management group,' who will ultimately be responsible for running the trial. The role and functions of this group are described in Chapters 7 and 8.

References

[1] Carter, S.K. (1977) Clinical trials in cancer chemotherapy. *Cancer*, **40**, 544–57.

[2] American Society of Clinical Oncology (1997) Critical role of phase I clinical trials in cancer treatment. *Journal of Clinical Oncology*, **15**, 853–9.

[3] Therasse, P., Arbuck, S.G., Eisenhauer, E.A., Wanders, J., Kaplan, R.S., Rubinstein, L., Verweij, J., Van Glabbeke, M., van Oosterom, A.T., Christian, M.C., and Gwyther, S.G. (2000) New guidelines to evaluate the response to treatment in solid tumors. *Journal of the National Cancer Institute*, **92**, 205–16.

[4] Fleming, T.R. (1982) One sample multiple testing procedure for Phase II clinical trials. *Biometrics*, **38**, 143–51.

[5] Gehan, E.A. (1961) The determination of the number of patients required in a preliminary and follow-up trial of a new chemotherapeutic agent. *Journal of Chronic Diseases*, **13**, 346–53.

[6] Simon R. (1989) Optimal two-stage designs for phase II clinical trials. *Controlled Clinical Trials*, **10**, 1–10.

[7] Thall, P.F., and Simon, R. (1995) Recent developments in the design of phase II clinical trials. In *Recent Advances in the Design and Analysis of Clinical Trials* (ed. P. Thall) pp. 49–71. Kluwer, Norwell, Massachusetts.

[8] Simon, R., Wittes, R.E., and Ellenberg, S.S. (1985) Randomized phase-II clinical trials. *Cancer Treatment Reports*, 69(12), 1375–81.

[9] Stenning, S.P., Freedman, L.S., and Bleehen, N.M. (1990) On behalf of the MRC Brain Tumour Working Party. Prognostic factors in malignant glioma – development of a prognostic index. *Journal of Neuro-Oncology*, 9, 47–55.

[10] Feinstein, A.R., Sosin, D.M., and Wells, C.K. (1985) The Will Rogers phenomenon, stage migration and new diagnostic techniques as a source of misleading statistics for survival in cancer. *New England Journal of Medicine*, 312(25), 1604–08.

[11] Beyer, J., Stenning, S.P., Fossa, S.D., and Siegert, W. (2002) High dose vs conventional-dose chemotherapy as first salvage treatment in patients with non-seminomatous germ cell tumours: a matched pair analysis. *Annals of Oncology*, 13(4), 599–605.

[12] Schwarz, F., and Lelouche, A. (1967) Explanatory and pragmatic attitudes in therapeutic trials. *Journal of Chronic Diseases*, 20, 637–48.

[13] Arnott, S.J., Duncan, W., Gignoux, M., Girling, D.J., Hansen, H.S., Launois, B., Nygaard, K., Parmar, M.K.B., Roussel, A., Spiliopoulos, G., Stewart, L.A., Tierney, J.F., Wang, M., and Zhang, R.G. (1998) Preoperative radiotherapy in esophageal carcinoma: A meta-analysis using individual patient data (oesophageal cancer collaborative group). *International Journal of Radiation Oncology Biology Physics*, 41, 579–83.

[14] Gray, R., James, R., Mossman, J., and Stenning, S.P. (1991) Guest editorial: AXIS – A suitable case for treatment. *British Journal of Cancer*, 63, 841–45.

[15] Stenning, S.P. for the AXIS Collaborators (1994) The AXIS colorectal cancer trial: randomization of over 2000 patients. *British Journal of Surgery*, 81, 1672.

Chapter 4

Design issues for randomized trials

4.1   Introduction

In this chapter we describe the main design issues specific to randomized trials; these
include issues of trial philosophy as well as the choices to be made concerning the number
of arms, the number and timing of randomizations and the choice of control arm. The
chapter ends with a section on the practical methodology of randomization.

4.2   Key design decisions

4.2.1   Choice of arms

Most randomized trials can be categorized into one of two types; those that compare
A with B (for example surgery versus radiotherapy for oesophageal cancer, carboplatin
versus cisplatin for advanced ovarian cancer), and those which compare A with A + B
(for example surgery alone versus radiotherapy followed by surgery for rectal cancer;
radiotherapy with or without prophylactic anti-emetics in patients undergoing abdominal radiotherapy). The former types compare entire treatment policies, the latter, one
aspect of treatment. In both cases, A is the control treatment and B the experimental
treatment. Pure scientific method might suggest that only one aspect of management
should ever vary between the treatment groups, as only then can differences in outcome
be attributed solely to this one change in treatment. In practice absolute purity is hard
to achieve and rarely necessary. There is often a good argument for making the most
extreme comparison – which might involve several changes over standard therapy – first
rather than attempting to justify each change through carefully controlled trials in which
only one aspect of treatment changes each time. Making the most extreme comparison
first means that if no worthwhile benefit is shown, there is rarely a need to go back and
examine the individual components for potential efficacy. If on the other hand the most
extreme comparison finds a worthwhile benefit, then one can choose whether or not
to go back and examine the individual components from the happy position of having
improved outcome. In general, in designing a trial one should take time to consider for
each possible design what conclusions could be drawn from each of the possible trial
outcomes, and where they will lead; this kind of 'options appraisal' can help determine
which comparisons should be made first.

The process of treatment development means that the choice of experimental treatment will generally be clearly defined before a randomized trial is considered. However,
the choice of control arm perhaps gets less consideration than it might.

Box 4.1 Declaration of Helsinki 2000 on choice of control arms

'The benefits, risks, burdens and effectiveness of a new method should be tested against those of the best current prophylactic, diagnostic and therapeutic methods. This does not exclude the use of placebo, or no treatment, where no proven prophylactic, diagnostic or therapeutic method exists.'

In general, a new therapy should be compared against best standard practice, as described in the 2000 revision of the Declaration of Helsinki (see Box 4.1 and http://www.wma.net/e/policy/17-c_e.html). To identify whether your control arm represents 'best standard therapy', consider whether or not there is evidence from randomized trials to support or refute it (this may require a systematic review – see Chapter 11). Consider also whether it represents an international, or national standard. It goes without saying that to choose an inferior control arm with the intention of enhancing the apparent benefit to a new treatment is unethical. However, knowingly choosing as your control arm a therapy that has been shown to be inferior to another treatment may sometimes be justified if, for example, financial or practical reasons make the 'better' treatment of limited use.

There are occasions when the choice of control arm is not entirely straightforward and it is sometimes the case that no internationally agreed standard therapy exists. In this situation, trials addressing similar questions, but using different control arms, may produce conflicting results (see for example Box 4.2).

It may also be the case that two (or more) 'standard' therapies may be considered approximately equivalent with respect to efficacy, but with different centres preferring one over the other for reasons perhaps of cost, toxicity or local practicalities. Minor

Box 4.2 Control arms in advanced ovarian cancer trials

In the late 1990s, several chemotherapy regimens were in use in the treatment of advanced ovarian cancer. In the US, both cisplatin (P) alone and cyclophosphamide + cisplatin (CP) combinations were standard, although evidence from a meta-analysis of trials comparing CP with CAP (cyclophosphamide, doxorubicin, cisplatin) showed a survival benefit to the 3-drug combination [1]. The US Gynaecological Oncology Group (GOG) used CP as the control arm in one trial evaluating a paclitaxel-based combination [2] and P as the control in another [3]. The former trial showed striking benefits to the paclitaxel arm, which were at odds with the results of the European ICON3 trial [4]. ICON3 compared a similar paclitaxel combination with a control group comprising either CAP or single agent carboplatin. This choice followed from the results of the ICON2 trial [5], which demonstrated the clinical equivalence of adequately dosed carboplatin and CAP. ICON3 did not find a benefit to the paclitaxel combination, and detailed analysis of the data from all the relevant trials identifies the most likely explanation for the conflicting results to be the inadequacy of the CP control arm.

variations which cannot conceivably have a large impact on outcome can and should be accommodated if a trial is to achieve widespread accrual. But can more substantial differences, completely different chemotherapy regimens for example, be accommodated in the design? Perhaps the first thing to consider is the weight of evidence in favour of 'equivalent efficacy.' Is there an opportunity to test this by including a randomization between the competing control arms? If equivalence has already been established through randomized trials, then is it necessary to distinguish between them at all? Given that the choice between the experimental arm and standard therapy may well be influenced by the very things influencing the choice of standard therapy (toxicity for example), then the answer is yes. If there is no good reason to believe the potential control therapies differ in efficacy, and randomizing between them is (for whatever reason) not appropriate, then it can be helpful to allow a choice of control arms, provided the choice is made before randomization, and randomization is stratified for that choice. One example of such a trial is the ICON3 trial in advanced ovarian cancer, described in Box 4.2. Effectively, this means that the trial can if necessary be considered as two separate trials. Indeed, it is appropriate, if not essential, to estimate the treatment effect separately in the two subgroups, and formally test for heterogeneity (Section 9.4.8) before calculating an overall estimate of the treatment effect.

4.2.2 Efficacy, equivalence or non-inferiority?

The conventional clinical trial compares a standard treatment with a new treatment which, it is hoped, may improve outcome; this we refer to as an 'efficacy' trial. In some situations, a new treatment may be expected to have a similar, rather than better, effect on outcome to the standard treatment, but perhaps to have other advantages; for example, a better toxicity profile, a more convenient means of administration or a lower cost. A trial comparing these treatments would aim to show that the difference in impact on the primary outcome measure lies within a pre-specified acceptable range, and would present data on the other outcome measures that would, it is hoped, demonstrate the advantages that the new treatment brings. This is an 'equivalence trial,' so called because one is attempting to demonstrate the clinical equivalence of two treatments. This is different from absolute equivalence – that is, an identical outcome in the two groups – which can never be demonstrated in a clinical trial with a finite number of patients. The term 'clinical equivalence' implies that, on balance, the costs and benefits associated with the treatment options are such that both treatments provide acceptable alternatives.

A 'non-inferiority trial' is a specific type of equivalence trial in which one compares a standard treatment to a new treatment, which is not necessarily expected to be better than standard with respect to the most important outcome measure, but perhaps as good or slightly worse, within a carefully specified range. Again, the new treatment is expected to bring other benefits, and the new treatment would be defined as equivalent (or non-inferior) if any disadvantage with respect to the major outcome measure is sufficiently outweighed by the benefits it brings. In cancer therapy trials, this often brings about a situation in which a trade-off is made between possible gains for *all* patients allocated a particular treatment (e.g. reduced toxicity) and possible losses for *some* patients, for example a higher recurrence rate. This is clearly a very difficult balance to strike, and one which patients, doctors, and those designing trials may see very differently. In Chapter 5, we discuss some ways in which the information necessary to design such trials might be elicited. It is important to note that a non-inferiority trial should only be considered if there is sufficiently strong evidence that standard therapy is better than no treatment. Where this is not the case, demonstrating non-inferiority of a new therapy over standard therapy will not necessarily have proved that it is better than no treatment.

Both equivalence and non-inferiority trials have perhaps their greatest role where cure rates are high, but there is a wish to reduce as far as possible the morbidity of treatment without compromizing efficacy (for example, stage I testicular seminoma) or where survival rates are very low, and the aim is to provide the best palliation while again avoiding adverse effects on already low survival rates (for example, poor prognosis small cell lung cancer patients).

It is important to make the distinction between efficacy, equivalence and non-inferiority when developing a trial since it should affect the design, not least the trial size. If the aim is really to show that two treatments are equivalent, then the size of difference the trial must be powered to detect (or exclude) logically must be less than the size of difference that would be considered sufficient to prove the efficacy of one of the treatments (it is predominantly this fact, more than technical differences in the way sample sizes are calculated, that makes 'equivalence' trials generally much larger than efficacy trials).

4.2.3   Explanatory or pragmatic?

Chapter 3 began by reviewing the traditional classification of trials from phase I to IV. The fact that a promising treatment will rarely pass through just one trial in each phase was pointed out. This is particularly true of the phase III setting, where it may well be appropriate to consider a division of the phase III randomized trials into 'early'/'developmental' trials and 'late'/'public health' trials. The former are designed in a manner which gives the treatment under investigation the best possible chance of showing its potential. This may mean testing new treatments in situations which do not reflect the nature or breadth of routine clinical practice. Only if they succeed in this setting are they likely to pass through to the latter stage, in which their effect in routine clinical practice is assessed. As stated in Chapter 3, this distinction almost entirely mirrors a classification of clinical trials introduced by Schwartz and Lellouch [6] – they referred to trials being either explanatory or pragmatic, the former having the aim of determining the precise action of a treatment in a defined setting, the latter answering the question – is the treatment of any practical use?

This is a somewhat idealized division, and it is not essential that all new therapies are evaluated in this way, but it can provide a useful framework for considering many design aspects of a randomized trial. In fact, the somewhat different aims of explanatory and pragmatic trials may affect the clinicians involved, the patients involved, the type of ancilliary care that patients receive, the type and amount of data that are collected, even the way the trial is analysed. These issues are summarized in Box 4.3, and described in more detail below. The basic principle is that the different types of trials value variability differently. In the early trial, which will generally be of modest size, it is a source of random error, which can limit the ability of a trial of modest size to detect a true underlying difference between treatments. All aspects of the design therefore aim to limit the sources of variability. When the issues turn to those of practical benefit of a treatment in clinical practice, heterogeneity can be a good thing – it can be explored in

Box 4.3   Two approaches to trial design

	Explanatory	Pragmatic
Aim	Determine precise action of a treatment in a defined setting	Is the treatment of any practical use?
Patients	Homogeneous – those most likely to respond as we would 'like'	Heterogeneous – representative of those to whom the results would be extrapolated
Clinicians	Those with most experience, most likely to get the 'best' out of a new treatment	Representative of those who would use the treatment outside of the trial
Treatments	All aspects of patient care clearly defined	All other aspects of patient care as for normal practice
Randomize	As close as possible to the time at which treatments diverge	At the time when treatment policy would be decided
Monitoring	May require specific specialized tests – intensive surveillance	Only investigations used in routine clinical practice
Data	Large amounts to identify protocol deviations and monitor compliance	Minimum required to answer question posed by trial
Analysis	May concentrate on those eligible on blind review	Analyse all patients

order to identify any clear evidence of qualitative or quantitative treatment differences and in the absence of this, confirm that the overall treatment effect is the best estimate of the effect in any individual patient.

Patient eligibility

Eligibility criteria can in general be divided into two types – safety and efficacy criteria. Safety criteria are used to select patients who are fit to receive any of the treatments under consideration. Requirements for specific haematological and biochemical values address safety issues as, for example, do the exclusion of patients with immune-deficient diseases from chemotherapy trials, and the tumour size limit on patients being considered for stereotactic cranial irradiation. The efficacy criteria aim to identify patients with the potential to benefit from the new treatment. These include, for example, the common criteria of no previous or concurrent serious disease – if a patient is more likely to die from a disease other than the one the trial is aiming to treat, they are less likely to contribute to the trial than a patient with no obvious, immediate risk of a competing event. There are many other factors which nominally come under this category – things such as age, stage of disease and histology. Trials will often have eligibility criteria based on such things. But it is rare that one of these factors will actually distinguish a patient who will respond from one who will not, it is more a question of degree, or of anticipated quantitative differences, rather than qualitative differences in response. Older patients may be more likely to suffer toxicity limiting the completion of some treatments with consequent effects on their efficacy. But receiving three courses rather than six is not likely to cause harm rather than benefit, rather minimal versus maximal benefit. Hence it is these efficacy criteria which should be considered most carefully in explanatory and pragmatic trials. Explanatory trials might impose stringent limits in an effort to obtain a group of patients thought most likely to respond the way we hope they will. The pragmatic trial will aim to include in the eligibility criteria all those patients who might be considered for treatment outside of a trial setting.

The 'uncertainty principle' gained recognition with the first 'mega trials' in cardiovascular diseases and then cancer [7]. This states that if you feel there is a definite indication or contraindication to one of the treatments under study, then the patient should not be entered into the trial. Only if the doctor and patient are uncertain as to the benefit should a patient be randomized. It is naïve to assume that all trials only involve clinicians with complete uncertainty, and more generally it can be sufficient to have a balance of uncertainty (clinical equipoise) in the clinical community as a whole [8].

Interpreted in its broadest sense, the uncertainty principle is a necessary, if often unwritten, eligibility criterion for any randomized trial. In some situations – for example a widely used treatment – it may be the only eligibility criterion which is required, since it covers both the safety and efficacy criteria. However, it must be remembered that clinical trial protocols will often be testing new treatments with which many collaborating clinicians will have limited experience. Additional guidance on eligibility may often therefore be necessary. For example, a randomized trial evaluating the role of portal vein infusion of fluorouracil (AXIS) used the uncertainty principle as its only eligibility criterion; however, to steer less experienced clinicians the protocol specified additional guidelines as to contraindications (see Box 4.4).

Eligibility criteria have rightly come under more intense scrutiny in all stages of trials, and the assumptions about homogeneity of anticipated response questioned. For example, it is now uncommon for trials to include an upper age limit. In the past this was often used as a surrogate for fitness to receive treatment and risk of intercurrent

Box 4.4 Supplementary notes on eligibility in the AXIS colorectal cancer trial

Contraindications are specified not by the protocol but by the responsible clinician and might include:

- Intra-abdominal sepsis
- High blood urea
- Insulin-dependent diabetes
- Pregnancy
- Marked hepatic impairment
- Major life-threatening disease other than colorectal cancer

death. However, continuous variables such as age can never be dichotomized in a way which precisely defines fit and unfit, and other measures of 'fitness' are probably more appropriate.

Non-randomized treatments

The specific treatments being randomized will rarely be the only treatments which the patient receives, but these 'other' treatments constitute another source of variability which might be controlled or encouraged. They range from ancillary or supportive care such as antibiotics or antiemetics to more fundamental aspects of treatment. For example, in high grade glioma trials comparing the addition of adjuvant chemotherapy to standard treatment, there are possible sources of variability in standard treatment, for example the extent of surgery a patient had, and the radiotherapy schedule they received. Should any of the 'other treatments' be controlled? It is useful to consider the extremes. The early, exploratory, trial aiming to limit variability wherever possible, might choose to do so – specifying a prophylactic anti-emetic schedule or a specific radiotherapy dose and fractionation, or even imposing a strategy for supportive care which is identical in both arms of the trial, even if this would not be done out of the trial setting. The pragmatic trial would need to consider what would happen outside the trial – is there really any evidence that these variations in non-randomized treatments have an impact on outcome? The MRC BA06 trial in locally advanced bladder cancer [9] addressed the question – does CMV (cisplatin, methotrexate, vinblastine) chemotherapy, in addition to local therapy, improve survival? Internationally, opinion was and is divided on the best local treatment, some centres performing cystectomy, others radical radiotherapy and still others combining both treatments. These differences in routine practice have evolved, as such things do in the absence of trials. However, because there was no clear evidence of superiority of one over the other and, as importantly, no clear evidence that the impact of chemotherapy would differ in a patient undergoing cystectomy as local treatment and one undergoing radiotherapy, the trial permitted any of these forms of local treatment. This added a source of variability, but also doubled the number of centres which could take part and was one of the reasons why the trial recruited so successfully. It also helped us to provide evidence on the value of adding chemotherapy to both local treatments. These issues crop up regularly in relation to meta-analysis, in which a common concern is the combination of trials addressing the same basic question, but perhaps in different groups of patients and against a background of different non-randomized treatments. In meta-analysis this is addressed by ensuring that comparisons are only made within trials, and the within–trial differences are effectively combined. In an individual trial, this is accomplished by stratifying randomization appropriately and, if necessary, stratifying the analysis too.

Clinicians

A further source of variability is the clinicians taking part, a source which may not be entirely explained by the variations in ancillary and standard treatments which they employ. An early trial of a new treatment may wish to involve only those clinicians experienced in the use of the new treatment, who might be expected to 'get the best out of it.' The public health trial, however, would need to recognize that the best treatment identified in a trial will be used in general practice by a wide range of clinicians with a wide range of experience, and that any difficulties resulting from this need to be recognized at an early stage, by having an inclusive policy as regards participating clinicians.

Randomization

A good principle in any randomized trial is to carry out randomization as near as possible to the time at which the treatments diverge – the shorter the time between treatment being allocated and being administered, the less room for factors interfering with the goal of giving treatment as allocated. For example, in rapidly progressing cancers such as malignant glioma, a delay of a few weeks between randomization and starting treatment might mean a not insubstantial proportion of patients become too ill for radical treatment. The only exception to this rule, and one that would apply more often to the pragmatic trial, is that there may be situations where treatment policy would be decided at an earlier stage. For example, in an MRC/EORTC trial in malignant glioma, patients received conventional radiotherapy alone, or followed by a stereotactic radiotherapy boost. As the boost was to take place after conventional radiotherapy, it would have been preferable to carry out randomization on completion of conventional radiotherapy. However, with stereotactic facilities available at only a limited number of centres, many patients had to be referred to other centres if allocated the stereotactic boost. Without advance warning of a potential patient, the need for review of scans and for securing a place on the waiting list for treatment could have led to a substantial delay between the completion of conventional radiotherapy and the start of the boost course. Therefore, for practical reasons, randomization took place immediately before the conventional radiotherapy course was due to start, and the sample size allowed for possible drop-outs.

In general, there may be aspects of the treatments that are common to all arms which would be modified to some extent if it was known that a specific additional treatment would or would not follow. If this is accepted as appropriate in routine clinical practice, then the public health trial would need to consider accommodating this by randomizing before the common treatments commence.

Data and monitoring

Another practical issue concerns the amount and type of data collected. In an early trial, it may be necessary to collect detailed data on compliance and toxicity. Even if the ultimate aim is to improve survival through the use of a new treatment, it may be important to collect data on intermediate outcome measures such as recurrence or progression. As the public health trial will generally be larger, it should be designed to make participation as easy as possible and onerous data collection is known to be a major deterrent. Investigations which are not part of normal practice should be limited or eliminated if they are not (or no longer) necessary for assessing safety and outcome. The very minimum which might be collected is basic patient identification, allocated treatment, and outcome. If the main outcome is survival, then this can, in some countries, be obtained through central population records with no need, in theory, to collect any further data. While this extreme is rarely realistic, it serves as a good starting point for deciding what data to collect.

Analysis

The intention-to-treat principle (see Chapter 9) is always applicable in a randomized trial, and, as discussed in later chapters, the exclusion of any patients from an analysis may have the potential to bias the results. A possible exception is exclusion based on some form of review – perhaps histological or radiological – which is carried out blind to the patients' allocated treatment and to their outcome. Pathology review is often carried out and there are inevitably a proportion of cases where discrepancies between the local and review diagnosis are apparent. Again it is useful to consider the extremes of approach. The explanatory trial might exclude those patients found ineligible on blind review, on the basis that their inclusion introduces another source of variability, if the outcome or response to treatment of the 'ineligible' patients is anticipated to be substantially different from that of the truly eligible patients. However, the pragmatic trial would have to recognize that in routine clinical practice, the great majority of patients will be treated on the basis of local diagnosis, and thus it is appropriate to quantify the impact of treatment in the type of patients who would be treated outside of the trial on the basis of local diagnosis – in other words not to exclude patients on the basis of conflict with review diagnoses. It therefore follows that central review need not be an essential component of a large-scale pragmatic trial. One exception to this rule might result from consideration of the educational value of the review. If there is an opportunity to identify and resolve problems for the future by systematically comparing local and review diagnoses, then this may be valuable. However this adds an organizational burden to the trial participants, and the impact and value of this therefore needs to be considered.

4.3 Timing of randomization and consent

As discussed above, and as a general rule, patients should be randomized as close as possible to the time at which treatment policies diverge, as this minimizes the chance of drop-out before the allocated intervention can be administered. There is, however, another issue concerning the timing of randomization, or more specifically the timing of consent in relation to the timing of randomization. In a conventional trial, the process of randomization consists of assessing a patient's eligibility for a trial, obtaining their consent to be in the trial while explaining that in doing so neither they nor their doctor will know in advance which treatment they will receive, obtaining the randomized allocation, and then informing the patient. Patients are treated and analysed according to their allocated group, as shown in Fig. 4.1.

4.3.1 Problems with the conventional order of events

Studies have shown that the proportion of patients entering cancer clinical trials is generally low – a few per cent – with the exception of those treated in specialist centres. Different studies reveal different reasons for this, and perhaps the most common is simply that patients are not asked (see Chapter 2). However, a recurring, and understandable reason, is that patients refuse consent. In an effort to limit the impact of patient refusal, an alternative randomization design was introduced by Zelen who had considered whether there might be alternative, ethical designs which could increase the number of patients going into trials.

4.3.2 Alternative randomization procedures

Zelen's central thesis [10] was that patients receiving exactly the same treatment within a trial that they would have received outside of a trial did not necessarily need to be aware that they were in a trial. He therefore proposed what became known as Zelen's single consent design, which is illustrated in Fig. 4.2.

In this design, patients who are eligible for the trial, and fit to receive any of the treatments which may be allocated, are randomized without their consent. Those patients

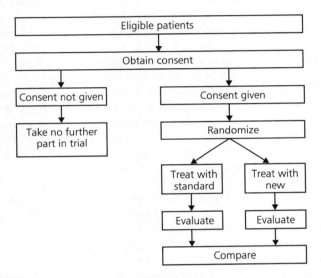

Fig. 4.1 Design and analysis of a conventional randomized clinical trial.

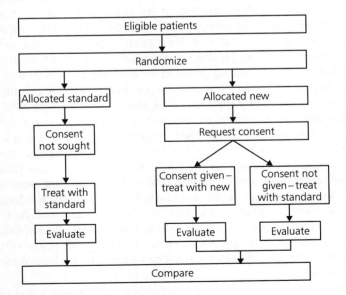

Fig. 4.2 Zelen's single consent design.

who are allocated the standard treatment, which they would have received outside of a trial, are not told that they are in a trial and so do not have an opportunity to refuse. Those who are allocated the new treatment are told that they are in a trial, and that if they choose to remain within it they would receive the new treatment. The doctor is then able to explain about the treatment and its side effects. The patient may refuse the new treatment for any reason and would then generally receive the standard treatment. Because the number of patients who can refuse to be in the trial is reduced, the number being randomized is increased, possibly considerably. This would benefit future patients in that the trial is completed, and the conclusions become available and can be implemented, more rapidly. However, there are both ethical and practical concerns with this design. The first concerns the need to analyse a trial in a way which avoids the introduction of bias, and the core of this is analysis by intention-to-treat, namely the process by which each patient randomized in a trial is analysed according to the treatment they were allocated, whether or not they actually obtained that treatment in full or part. This is discussed further in Section 9.4.1. In Zelen's single consent design, this means that patients allocated the new treatment must be analysed in this group, whether or not they consented to the treatment. Clearly, if a substantial proportion of patients allocated a new treatment refuse it, the comparison of the two groups becomes somewhat muddied. The sample size calculation must take this into account, and if the refusal rate is such that the increase in sample size necessary to enable the size of difference anticipated between the two groups to be estimated reliably outweighs the increase in sample size obtained through limiting the consent process, nothing has been gained. There is therefore a reliance on the tendency for patients to adhere to the treatment they are first told about – and even perhaps pressure on the doctor advising the patient to give information in a way which encourages them to view the new treatment more favourably than they might had the consent process taken place at a time when a patient must be willing to receive either treatment. A further issue is one of data privacy – data on the standard-arm patients must be collected and held centrally for analysis. If the trial is to be analysed in an unbiased manner, then the minimum data required to enable the main outcome measures of the trial to be analysed are required at least. Thus there is a sense in which no patient can withdraw entirely from a trial. However, patients who have actively objected to being part of a trial may well be unwilling to attend for investigations which are necessary to determine a specific outcome measure. If data on an outcome are missing, then that patient is effectively excluded from the analysis. Finally, on a practical note, it is clearly not possible to carry out blind/masked trials with this design.

The single consent design is widely used in screening trials, for example the occult blood screening trial for bowel cancer [11]. Here subjects may be identified from GP lists and randomized to receive an invitation to be screened or not. As patients would not be offered screening outside of the trial, and as the outcome measures and further data required are no more than would be obtained for routine audit, this design has been considered acceptable. In addition, this type of approach means that control patients truly represent patients in normal clinical practice. This can be particularly important in, for example, trials of dietary intervention, in which knowledge of the trial's experimental arm, and the effect that the intervention is hoped to have, may lead the control group to alter their diet anyway.

However, in the context of cancer treatment trials, most sponsors and many ethics committees require all patients entered into a trial to give informed consent and so this design has not been widely used in treatment trials. To get around this problem, a design known as the double randomized consent design was introduced [12]. In this, the procedure up to and including the point of randomization is as above. However, patients in both arms of the trial are told they are in a trial and which treatment they would receive if they remained within it. Again they may not wish to give their consent to stay within the trial. It is not always clear which treatment a patient allocated standard treatment might receive in this situation, since the new arm may not always be open to them. The same ethical issues remain as above, in terms of the ability of a patient to withdraw entirely from a trial once randomized. In addition, the potential problems with analysis and interpretation remain. There are now opportunities for patients in both arms of the trial to refuse their allocated treatment. If half the patients in each allocated group refuse their treatment, and if refusers are given the 'other' treatment, then the two randomized groups become indistinguishable in terms of treatment received, and an analysis by intention to treat is pointless. Even much lower degrees of refusal can have a substantial impact on the sample size required. The calculation takes the following form.

We assume an outcome measure with a yes/no result, for example response rate, and represent the proportion of responders expected with the standard and new treatments by P_s and P_n respectively and the proportion refusing their allocated treatment by R_s and R_n, respectively. We also assume that we plan to randomize $N/2$ patients to each group. If all patients receive their allocated treatment, then the difference in response rates is simply

$$D = P_n - P_s,$$

however, taking account of refusers, the actual difference that would be observed is

$$D^* = [P_n(1 - R_n) + P_s \times R_s)] - [P_s(1 - R_s) + P_n \times R_s]$$
$$= (P_n - P_s)(1 - R_n - R_s),$$

which will always be less than D when either R_n or R_s are non-zero. A trial that is powered to detect a difference, D, will have reduced power to detect a smaller difference D^*. Roughly speaking, sample size is proportional to the square of the difference in outcome between the treatment groups (see Chapter 5); therefore an approximate indication of the sample size required to retain the power of the study with no refusal is given by

$$N^* = N \times D^2/D^{*2}$$
$$= N \times 1/(1 - R_n - R_s)^2.$$

Thus, for example, a refusal rate in both arms of 10 per cent requires the overall sample size to be increased by a factor of 1.56 to maintain the original power to detect the same underlying treatment effect. Altman *et al.* [13] discuss these issues in greater depth. In surveying the use of randomized consent designs in cancer, they found that most often they were introduced part way through trials which were struggling to recruit, but rarely increased accrual to an extent which compensated for the dilution effect. This suggests a limited role for such designs in cancer treatment trials.

4.4 Unit of randomization – individuals or groups?

All the discussions above have assumed that an individual patient will be the unit of randomization, and for most cancer treatment trials this is certainly the most appropriate approach. In other settings, particularly primary care and hence in cancer screening and prevention trials, an alternative design has sometimes been used in which, rather than randomizing individual patients, groups of clearly defined patients are randomized. For example, one might randomize primary care practices, such that every patient within a given practice receives the same treatment. This is known as a cluster- (or group-) randomized trial. While there are situations in which this might be appropriate, it is far from problem-free. The use of this design in many of the trials of screening for breast cancer, and the consequent difficulties in interpretation of the results has contributed to the confusion over the impact of breast screening on breast cancer mortality.

It is worth emphasizing that the 'randomization units', 'experimental units' and 'observation units' may be quite different in a cluster randomized trial compared with a conventional trial. In a conventional individual patient-randomized trial, the randomization unit, experimental unit and observation unit are all the individual patient, that is, the patient is randomized, treated individually and their individual outcome data contribute to the overall assessment of treatment. With cluster randomized trials, the randomization unit is a defined group, but the 'experimental' unit may be an individual – for example the primary care physician responsible for that group of patients might be randomized to receive or not to receive an education package. The observation unit may be the group as a whole, or the individual patients. Even if individual patient outcome data are used, the effect of the original cluster-randomized design cannot be ignored in the analysis.

4.4.1   What are the advantages of cluster randomization?

The two main reasons why such a design might be used, rather than individual randomization, relate to resources and contamination. Ethical issues are sometimes raised as a third motivating factor, but are just as often cited as adverse features of cluster randomized trials.

Resources

It may be practically and/or financially difficult to set up the means required to deliver an intervention in all the centres taking part in a trial – for example, it may be possible to set up only a limited number of centres with access to screening facilities when their value has yet to be evaluated in a formal trial. In such situations, individual GP practices might be randomized to be screening centres or not. The Edinburgh trial of breast cancer screening used such a design [14].

Contamination

In a trial in which an individual or group is allocated to receive or not to receive an intervention, 'contamination' is essentially defined as the influence of an intervention on a subject not intended to receive the intervention. For example, suppose patients within a GP practice are randomized to receive or not to receive dietary advice aimed at reducing their risk of bowel cancer. If individual patients allocated no intervention become aware that others are being treated differently, then they may seek out and act on the advice which the other group is intended to receive. If this is a major problem, then the power of the trial to detect a difference between groups is clearly reduced. A certain amount of contamination is a potential problem with many individually randomized trials, but where the danger is acute, a cluster randomized design may, if it substantially reduces the chance for cross-group contamination, be a useful alternative. Suppose, for example, one wishes to assess the impact of an education package delivered through a GP on patients with a certain condition. If individual patients were randomized to receive or not receive the information, the GP would have to 'unlearn' for some patients, and this may be very difficult. A similar difficulty applies when attempting to assess the impact of organizational changes. Moher *et al.* [15] report a cluster randomized trial comparing three methods of promoting secondary prevention of coronary heart disease (CHD) in primary care. The three interventions were (a) audit and feedback at a practice meeting on the prevalence of CHD in the practice, number of patients with myocardial infarction, angina and revascularization and the proportion of patients with adequate assessment (b) information as for (a) but with discussion on guidelines for secondary prevention, and advice on setting up a register and recall system for GP-led review of patients with CHD and (c) information and advice as for (b) but aimed at nurse-led clinics. Thus the unit of randomization was the GP practice, the experimental units were the practice staff and the observation unit was the individual patient, with the primary outcome measure being evidence of 'adequate assessment' of the relevant patients at 18 months.

Consent issues

It is not always clear how consent issues – relating to the administration of an intervention and the collection and analysis of patient data – are handled in a cluster randomized trial. In this respect they have issues in common with the Zelen designs described in Section 4.3. They may potentially involve no individual patient consent at all; certainly if individuals are asked to consent to receive (or not) an intervention, the very reasons for setting up a cluster-randomized trial may mean it is not possible to offer them the alternative. These issues are discussed further by Hutton [16].

4.4.2 What are the disadvantages of cluster randomization?

It is not possible to analyse a cluster-randomized trial as though individual patients had been randomized. The difficulty arises because the experimental unit is different from the observation unit, and conventional statistical methods are predicated on these being one and the same. In an individually randomized trial, one can consider each patient's outcome to be independent of that for the other patients in the trial. In a cluster-randomized trial, that is not possible, as patients within a cluster are more likely to have similar outcomes than a random sample of patients from all the clusters. The trial analysis must take this into account, as must sample size calculations. The consequence is that a cluster-randomized trial requires more (often many more) patients than an individually randomized trial; in other words a cluster-randomized trial of N patients will have less power than an individually randomized trial of N patients. In fact, the power of the trial is determined by the number and size of the clusters; the smaller and more numerous the clusters, the less the impact on power. This fact makes it important to use these designs only when they are absolutely essential.

4.4.3 Further reading

Further consideration of the design and analysis of cluster-randomized trials are given by Donner [17]. To raise the standard of reporting of cluster-randomized trials, guidelines as for conventional randomized trials (see Chapter 9) have been proposed, and these are described by Elbourne *et al.* [18].

4.5 Designs for randomized trials

4.5.1 Introduction

It is perhaps too often the case that the design of a trial is established from the first discussions about potential treatments and remains unchallenged thereafter. There are few trials which would not benefit from taking a step back and reviewing whether the trial is as good as it can be. Time pressures are often against this, as the process of gaining funding and ethical approval for a trial can be lengthy and replete with deadlines. But given the time, effort and expense which go into the planning, conduct and analysis of a clinical trial, and the continuing struggle to enter more cancer patients into trials, a little more time spent considering whether opportunities are being exploited can be time well spent. The following sections discuss alternative designs, beginning with the simplest, and looking at each stage at questions which should be asked about the number of treatment arms and the number and timing of randomizations.

4.5.2 Parallel groups

The simplest form of randomized trial is known as the parallel group trial. This follows the basic design illustrated in Fig. 4.3. Eligible patients are randomized to two or more groups, treated according to their assigned groups, subsequently assessed for their response to treatment and the groups are compared in a manner appropriate to the data.

There are numerous examples, one being the first MRC trial of radiotherapy in rectal cancer [19]. In this trial, eligible patients (those with potentially operable rectal cancer) were randomized to one of three treatment groups: surgery alone, surgery preceded by low-dose radiotherapy or surgery preceded by higher-dose radiotherapy. Following treatment, patients were followed up until death, and the overall survival rates were compared.

The parallel group design is simple and widely applicable. In theory, the number of treatment arms is unlimited. In practice, however, the number of groups may be limited either because there are only a small number of treatments which people are

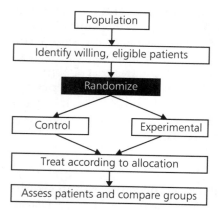

Fig. 4.3 Parallel group trial.

interested in comparing, or because the number of patients available limits the number of treatments which can be compared while achieving a sample size sufficient to give useful results over a reasonable timeframe. In the latter case, attempting to answer several questions at once may lead to none being adequately powered to provide convincing evidence. Where neither of these constraints apply there remain two other issues worth considering; the quantity of information for a patient considering the trial to absorb, and the practical difficulties in the clinic of having many possible treatments in the same group of patients at one time. Although these are reasonable concerns, there is now empirical evidence to suggest that neither need be a bar to embarking on a multi-arm trial [20].

For many trials with more than two arms, questions may arise concerning the necessity for all patients to be randomized with respect to all arms. There may, within the medical community, be sufficient uncertainty about a number of treatments to warrant their study in a trial, but often practical difficulties if not frank disagreement mean that some clinicians would be unwilling to randomize patients with respect to all the arms. Indeed, multi-arm trials sometimes evolve for this very reason. One possibility is to allow participants to opt out of some of the arms. Although this may be a practical solution in some cases, it needs careful thought, making sample size planning difficult. In general, it is often best to begin with a requirement that patients should be randomized with respect to all arms, and only relax this requirement if accrual proves particularly difficult. Given choice from the start, it is perhaps inevitable that patients and clinicians may avoid the 'difficult' arms (for example, 'no treatment' control arms) if they can still contribute to a trial. In the 1980s, the EORTC brain tumour group planned a trial to evaluate the role of post-operative radiotherapy in the treatment of low grade gliomas. There was no compelling evidence of benefit to radiotherapy; nevertheless, sufficient clinicians argued that they could not participate in a trial with a 'no-treatment' control arm that two trials were launched: the 'believers' trial randomized patients between two radio-therapy doses [21]; the 'non-believers' trial randomized patients between immediate post-operative radiotherapy (at the higher of the two doses) and radiotherapy deferred until disease progression [22]. The former recruited at three times the rate of the latter while both were open to accrual; it found no survival benefit to the higher dose. The non-believers trial finally completed its planned accrual after 11 years, the rate of accrual picking up notably on closure of the competing trial; it found no survival benefit to immediate radiotherapy over deferred radiotherapy. One can only speculate at the rate of accrual which might have been achieved in the non-believers trial had this been the only trial available.

If the reasons for comparing several groups are compelling, then there are designs which are more efficient than a simple parallel group trial in that they enable a reliable result to be obtained with fewer patients than would be required in a multi-arm parallel group trial. Sections 4.5.3 and 4.5.4 describe two such designs.

4.5.3 Factorial designs

Motivating example

In the late 1980s a major new trial in colorectal cancer was being planned under the auspices of the UK Coordinating Committee on Cancer Research [23]. For patients with rectal cancer, the standard treatment at the time was surgery alone. Two treatments held promise for improvements in survival – peri-operative radiotherapy (XRT), and loco-regional chemotherapy namely portal vein infusion of fluorouracil (FU). There were a number of possible trial designs. Comparing surgery + XRT and surgery + FU directly in a two-arm trial is a simple approach, but one which fails to provide any comparison with standard treatment. Conducting two separate trials, one comparing surgery alone to surgery plus FU, the second comparing surgery alone to surgery + XRT was an alternative. Although simple in approach, having trials running simultaneously which are competing for patients is not a good idea, and may lead to neither achieving sufficient patients to give useful results. Conducting the same two trials sequentially leads to what is likely to be a long delay before answers to both questions are obtained, given the need for adequate follow-up. A more attractive option was a three-arm trial, surgery alone versus surgery + XRT versus surgery + FU. This is more efficient, in that the control patients are effectively used twice, once in the comparison with XRT and once in the comparison with FU. It enables both questions to be addressed simultaneously and also allows a direct comparison of surgery + XRT and surgery + FU (if adequately powered). However, perhaps surprisingly, the most efficient design of all is a four-arm trial, including the three arms above plus the fourth in which patients receive both XRT and FU in addition to surgery. The four arms can be thought of as arising by subjecting a single patient to two, simultaneous, randomizations (see Fig. 4.4), hence its other name the 2 × 2 design: in the first they are randomized to radiotherapy or no radiotherapy, in the second they are randomized between chemotherapy and no chemotherapy. Thinking of the design this way shows where the increase in efficiency comes from – now all patients, not just those in the control arm, are used twice; they are randomized twice and so contribute to two questions.

We estimate the benefit to FU by comparing all the patients allocated no FU with all the patients allocated FU. Importantly though, the analysis is stratified by the radiotherapy allocation such that we only directly compare arms that differ only by the addition of FU. Thus arm A would be compared with arm C, and arm B would be compared with arm D. This gives two estimates of the treatment effect which we then combine to give

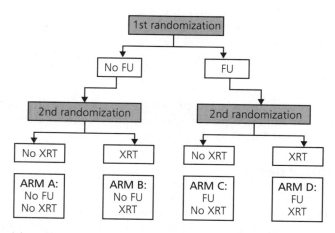

Fig. 4.4 Factorial randomization in the AXIS trial.

an overall estimate. Similarly, comparing arm A with arm B, and comparing arm C with arm D would assess the impact of radiotherapy. The assumption here is that the effect of adding FU will be approximately the same when it is added to surgery alone, and when it is added to radiotherapy. If this is not the case, then combining the two estimates to give one overall estimate is inappropriate. This is known as an additivity assumption, and is one of the key requirements for a factorial trial discussed below.

General requirements Although these designs are appealing, and should perhaps be considered more, there are three practical considerations which must be met:

+ it must be practically possible to combine the treatments,
+ the toxicity of combined treatment must be acceptable,
+ the anticipated treatment effects must be approximately additive.

With respect to the last point, the analysis of a factorial trial in the manner described above is only appropriate when the individual treatment effects are approximately additive. In the AXIS example, we would say the treatment effects were approximately additive if the estimate of the effect of FU on survival was approximately the same amongst those patients who do and do not receive radiotherapy. Where this is not the case, there is said to be an interaction; the effect of the combined treatments compared with the control group will be very different from the effect that would be expected, based on the comparison of the individual treatment effects. It could be much less than the individual effects, suggesting antagonism between the treatments, or much greater, suggesting synergy. Designing a trial as a factorial design provides the opportunity to investigate evidence for interaction. This will often be of interest, but unfortunately where it exists, the trial must be analysed in a way which loses the efficiency for which the design was chosen. Taking the AXIS example, if we found synergy between radiotherapy and FU, such that the effect of FU in patients receiving radiotherapy in addition to surgery was very much greater than the effect in patients receiving surgery alone, it would be best to present the treatment effect in these subgroups separately. However, the subgroups, having half the number of patients anticipated for the main effect, will have much lower power to detect true treatment differences.

Figure 4.5 illustrates possible sets of survival curves from a factorial trial in which patients are randomized between radiotherapy or no radiotherapy and between chemotherapy or no chemotherapy. In Fig. 4.5(a), two possible scenarios are illustrated in which there is no evidence of interaction. On the left-hand side of the figure, both treatments are effective on their own, and the effect when the two are combined is as expected under the additivity assumption. On the right-hand side of the figure, chemotherapy is effective, but radiotherapy is not; therefore the combined effect of radiotherapy plus chemotherapy compared with control is similar to that of chemotherapy alone versus control.

In Fig. 4.5(b) are examples suggesting interaction. On the left-hand side panel, neither treatment is effective on its own, but rather than having no effect as would be expected under additivity, the combination in fact shows substantially improved survival. On the right-hand side panel the opposite applies. Each treatment is, on its own, effective, but the combination does no better than the individual treatments. This might be seen for example if two different treatments are effectively attacking the same target.

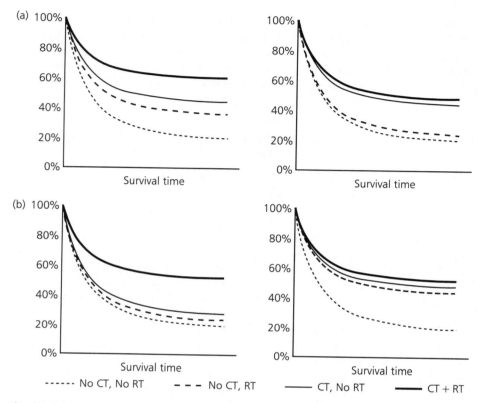

Fig. 4.5 (a) Hypothetical factorial trials with no interaction. (b) Hypothetical factorial trials with interaction.

AXIS was considered an appropriate setting for a factorial trial. FU was given directly into the hepatic vein, and was primarily aimed at preventing liver metastases. Radiotherapy was given either pre-operatively, before any chemotherapy, or 4–6 weeks post-operatively after completion of radiotherapy with the primary aim of preventing local recurrence. Therefore it was practical to combine treatments, there was no expectation of enhanced toxicity, and it was considered clinically unlikely that the treatments would interact.

In general, where there is a reasonable expectation that two treatments may interact, a factorial design may still be appropriate, but the sample size should be calculated to anticipate the possibility, and to provide sufficient power for treatment comparisons in subgroups if necessary.

Because each patient is 'used' twice, the sample size required for a factorial design with two treatments is very similar, or even identical, to that for a simple 2-arm trial. This economy can be extended further when there are three or more (say, n) treatments of interest; again each patient is randomized to receive or not receive each treatment and consequently can be allocated any one of 2^n treatment combinations.

4.5.4 Cross-over trials

A further design which can require fewer patients than the corresponding parallel group design is known as the cross-over trial. Here, every patient receives all the treatments under investigation (which may include a placebo), but the order in which they receive them is randomized. The general, simplified, design of a cross-over trial is shown in Fig. 4.6. In the case of a two-treatment cross-over trial, eligible patients are randomized to receive either A followed by B or B followed by A. An example is given by a trial in patients with chronic cancer-related pain [24], in which patients were randomized to receive contolled-release oxycodone or morphine for seven days, then switched to the alternative treatment for the next seven days. Pain levels were recorded by the patients on a 0–100 mm visual analogue scale, and within-patient differences in pain levels on the two treatments compared.

The benefit of such a design is that each patient acts as their own control, effectively halving the number of patients required when compared to a conventional parallel group design. In addition, because comparisons are made within-patients, intra-patient variability is eliminated which can also lead to a requirement for a smaller sample size. A further benefit is that the patients are in a position to express a treatment preference, having experienced both.

In a trial such as this where each patient is intended to receive two or more treatments in succession, and where the efficiency of the design requires that patients do so, there are naturally constraints. It is only appropriate for chronic conditions, which are stable at least over the time period of the study; there must be a negligible risk of death whilst

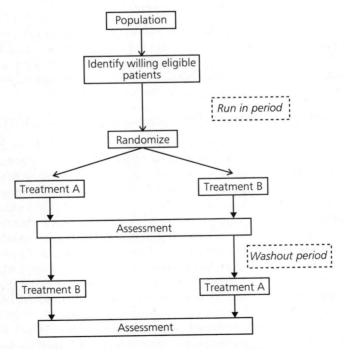

Fig. 4.6 General design of a 2-treatment, 2-period cross-over trial.

on study. It cannot involve treatments which cure the condition, they must only alleviate symptoms, and finally the treatment effects must be short-lasting, such that the effect is ended by the time the next treatment starts. In practice, this is achieved by having a 'wash-out' period between the treatments.

There are a number of potential problems with this design which can mean that only the first period of treatment can be used. These include:

- drop-out after the first treatment, which may be related to treatment,
- carry-over of treatment effect from the first period which is not eliminated by the wash-out period,
- treatment by period interaction – in which the effect of a treatment is substantially different in the two periods – making their combination inappropriate.

Where these problems exist, data from the first period can be used, but the trial effectively becomes a parallel group trial and the sample size is effectively halved – thus, as for the factorial design, the final treatment comparison can be underpowered. Hills and Armitage [25] provided a general rule for determining whether to use a parallel group or cross-over design:

- if an unequivocal result is required from a clinical trial and enough patients are available, then a simple parallel trial should be carried out (this will be approximately twice the size of the cross-over trial to have the same statistical power);
- if the number of patients available is limited and a cross-over design is chosen, results should be presented giving evidence that the basic assumptions are fulfilled and if necessary, basing conclusions on the first period only.

The design requirements make cross-over trials inappropriate for most comparisons of cytotoxic treatments for cancer and there are few examples to be found. However, it can potentially be a useful design when evaluating treatments for symptoms which are either chronic or occur at predictable times such as treatment-related nausea. Detailed discussion of cross-over trials can be found in the book by Senn [26].

4.6 Sequential randomizations within and between trials

In factorial designs, patients are subject to two or more randomizations, but all take place simultaneously. As a consequence, there is no possibility that the outcome of one randomization could influence the decision to take part in another. When designing a trial in which patients may become eligible for further randomizations with respect to some aspect of their treatment, at some time after the initial randomization, some caution is needed, particularly with respect to the impact of *subsequent* randomizations on the outcome assessments of *earlier* randomizations. These issues also arise when considering patients for more than one trial. The fundamental question is, is entry into the second trial (or second randomization) more likely amongst patients allocated one arm rather than another? If the answer is yes, then one needs to consider the impact of this on the endpoints of the first trial. For example – suppose the first trial randomizes between chemotherapy and no chemotherapy and the second trial randomizes between radiotherapy and no radiotherapy. If there is a tendency for more patients allocated no chemotherapy to enter the radiotherapy trial, then there is a potential for the two arms in the first trial to differ not just by whether or not they receive chemotherapy, but also in the proportion of patients receiving radiotherapy, i.e. they would be confounded. If radiotherapy was only available, or would only be considered in the context of the trial, and if radiotherapy proves effective, a false negative could arise in your chemotherapy comparison. It is of course always important to consider what happens in the real world. Suppose in this example radiotherapy was freely available; ethical considerations will always permit the use of any additional treatment which is felt to be in the patient's best interest and so patients could receive radiotherapy in an uncontrolled manner. Is this actually any less problematic than a formal randomized comparison?

To illustrate some of the issues, we review the discussions on the design of an MRC trial in advanced colorectal cancer, CR06 [27], in which the intention was to evaluate two issues. The first was a specific question: which of three chemotherapy regimens is most effective? The second was a more general question: in patients who do not have progressive disease after three months of chemotherapy, should chemotherapy be given continuously until progression is noted, or should chemotherapy stop, recommencing only when progression is noted? Importantly, in both cases, the main outcome measure was survival.

There are three main design options here. The first is to randomize patients between the three chemotherapy options initially, and carry out the second randomization at three months, in the group of patients who do not have progressive disease. The second is to randomize patients with respect to both questions at the same time, as in a factorial design. The third is to conduct two completely separate trials in different groups of patients.

Option 1: Randomize patients between the three chemotherapy options initially, and carry out the second randomization at three months

This option follows the clinical course of events most closely, and ensures that only those patients to whom the question is relevant are randomized. The 'stop or continue' question was relevant to all the chemotherapy regimens, and any difference in survival in the two arms was not expected to differ across the chemotherapy arms (i.e. no interaction between chemotherapy regimen and duration was anticipated). Thus there appear no obstacles to the planned analysis of survival time (measured from the date of the second randomization) according to stop or continue. In fact this is generally true of the last randomization in any trial involving multiple randomizations. The potential problems are generally limited to the interpretation of the earlier randomizations. Here, entry to the second randomization would depend upon response to the initial chemotherapy regimen. As response rates associated with the different regimens might well vary, the proportion of patients in each chemotherapy arm who proceed to the second randomization could also vary. Even if response rates did not vary across the three chemotherapy arms, patients' willingness to be randomized might, particularly if one regimen was found to be more toxic or inconvenient than the others, and the prospect of being randomized to (potentially) continue did not appeal. To assess whether differences across the chemotherapy arms in the proportion of patients being randomized to stop or continue causes any problems in the interpretation of the comparison of survival by chemotherapy arms, we need to consider a number of 'what if's.

The first, and most straightforward, scenario is to assume that there is no difference in survival according to stopping versus continuing. Here, there is no concern about the impact of the second randomization on the first. However, if continuing does indeed improve survival, there is a potential impact; to consider the degree, one needs to consider what happens to patients who do not have progressive disease at three months in practice, out of the trial. If they routinely stop treatment, then randomizing introduces an inequality in the proportion of patients continuing treatment in the trial and this will be highest in the chemotherapy arm with the best response rate, hence the survival of this whole group of patients will be further improved, compared with the other chemotherapy arms. It may not, however, be possible to determine whether the improvement is due to the initial chemotherapy regimen or its duration or both. If on the other hand patients without progressive disease routinely continue treatment out of the trial, then the proportion of patients continuing treatment in the trial will still be highest on the arm with the best response rate, but the absolute difference in the proportions continuing will have been reduced by the randomization. Consequently, the impact of the second randomization will be less.

This may seem a serious limitation to this design. However, it is possible to perform numerical sensitivity analyses, (see Box 4.5) to attempt to determine the impact that a range of differences in the proportion of patients being randomized in the three arms could have on the survival comparison, under the assumption that there is a survival difference according to stop or continue (the size of this difference could also vary, but it would be reasonable to take the size anticipated in the trial design).

Option 2: Randomize patients with respect to both questions at the same time

Here all patients who consent to both randomizations are randomized 'up front' to their chemotherapy regimen and its duration, and so the choice of whether or not to be randomized with respect to duration does not depend on their experience of the initial chemotherapy regimen nor its effectiveness. However, since the question of stopping or continuing is relevant only to those who achieve a response or stable disease (and continuation of the same regimen in the face of progressive disease would not be considered appropriate), it is apparent from the start that a number of patients will not follow their allocated treatment. For example, approximately 50 per cent of patients in all the chemotherapy arms were expected to have progressive disease at three months. Therefore, half of those randomized to continue would in fact have progressive disease, and would not continue. Here then, the major effect could be on the stop versus continue randomization – analysis by intent to treat will mean comparing two groups in which the proportions stopping and continuing may be much more similar than you would like. It would then be necessary to assess the appropriate sample size, which will certainly need to be larger than under option 1 to account for the 'muddying' (the calculation follows the same lines as that described under Zelen randomization in Section 4.3 under assumptions of varying levels of non-compliance). Depending on the proportion of drop-outs, it may be that the sample size required for the stop versus continue question becomes larger than that for the primary question. On the plus side, it might well be argued that patients randomized upfront and knowing their overall treatment plan may have greater levels of compliance with stopping or continuing (where their response makes this question relevant) than patients given the option of a later randomization.

Option 3: Conduct two completely separate trials in different groups of patients

If two independent trials are conducted, cross contamination is eliminated though it may be necessary to provide guidelines concerning duration of chemotherapy in each of the three arms of the first trial. However, the trials will take longer than if the questions were combined in a single trial and, on a practical note, data collection is increased.

The option chosen for CR06 was option 1, having performed sensitivity analyses. These assumed a 10% difference in survival for stop versus continue in those patients whose disease had not progressed at three months, and showed that even for unrealistically extreme differences in the proportion of patients achieving a response (or agreeing to be randomized) at three months across the three chemotherapy arms, the estimated differences in survival between any two of the three chemotherapy arms would be increased or decreased by less than 1%. Some of the calculations are detailed in Box 4.5. Similar orders of effect were found when allowing for a number of other scenarios including different long-term survival rates for patients with responding and stable versus progressive disease at three months, or for different response rates across the regimens. The conclusion was that the impact of the varying assumptions was minimal, and that this design was the most appropriate. However, both of the trial randomizations were kept

---

Box 4.5   Example of the type of calculations performed to aid the design of CR06

If the assumptions underlying the sample size calculations are met, then:

◆ 50% of patients (on any of the three regimens) will have stable or responding disease at twelve months (this was an equivalence trial)

◆ the 18-month survival rate of patients with progressive disease is 10%

◆ the 18-month survival rate of patients with stable or responding disease allocated 'stop' chemotherapy is also 10% (previous trials showed no difference in the long-term survival rate of patients who had stable/responding disease compared to those with progressive disease at three months)

◆ the 18-month survival rate of patients with stable or responding disease allocated 'continue' chemotherapy is 20%

Assuming all eligible patients proceed to the second randomization, of 300 patients on any arm:

◆ 150 will have progressive disease at twelve weeks, and 10% 18-month survival,

◆ seventy-five will be randomized to stop chemotherapy and will have 10% 18-month survival,

◆ seventy-five will be randomized to continue chemotherapy and will have 20% 18-month survival.

This gives an overall 18-month survival of 12.5%

> **Box 4.5** *(continued)*
>
> Suppose on one arm the response rates are similar, but only 80% of eligible patients (i.e. 40% rather than 50% of the total) proceed to the second randomization:
>   Of 300 patients,
>
> - 150 will have progressive disease at twelve weeks, and 10% 18-month survival,
> - sixty will be randomized to stop chemotherapy and will have 10% 18-month survival,
> - sixty will be randomized to continue chemotherapy and will have 20% 18-month survival,
> - thirty will choose not to enter the second randomization
>   (a) if they all choose to continue, 18-month survival would be 20% and the overall survival would be 13%,
>   (b) if they all choose to stop, 18-month survival would be 10% and the overall survival would be 12%.
>
> Thus taking the extremes, the overall survival rates would vary by only ±0.5%

under review by the same data monitoring and ethics committee which was empowered to recommend modifications to the trial design if necessary.

4.7 Allocation methods for randomized trials

4.7.1 Introduction

The most appropriate methods of allocating patients to treatments in trials must fulfil two major requirements; they must avoid systematic bias, and they must be unpredictable. Assigning treatment by a means that employs the play of chance – randomization – aims to ensure that patients assigned to each treatment are balanced for both known and unknown factors which could influence their response to treatment. Making sure that the treatment to be allocated cannot be known in advance, or guessed with a degree of certainty – concealment – ensures that particular types of patients cannot be chosen to receive (or avoid) a particular trial treatment. Both these aspects are equally important; a properly produced randomization schedule loses all its value if it can be found by the person responsible for deciding whether or not to enter a patient into a trial, since knowledge of which treatment that patient would be allocated could affect the decision about whether or not to enter the patient. It is therefore a means by which systematic bias could be introduced. The method used should not only meet these requirements, but it must be *shown* to meet these requirements. Tossing a coin is a perfectly good method of allocating one of two treatments in an unbiased and unpredictable way – but it is very hard to prove to a sceptical referee that the first toss was used, and not the second, or the best of three, or whatever it took to allocate that patient the treatment for which you or they had a preference. With respect to a principle as important as randomization, it is reasonable for a reviewer to take the position that the randomization or concealment method was inadequate unless there is a clear statement to the contrary.

The principle of unpredictability immediately calls into question some methods of 'randomization' used extensively in the past, less so now, namely the use of a patient-related characteristic such as odd or even date of birth, or hospital number, or alternate allocation as patients enter a clinic say, to allocate treatments. For each of these methods, the person responsible for randomizing a patient knows what treatment the patient will be allocated should they agree to enter the trial. They then have a choice as to whether to offer the patient the trial – and thus the treatment – or not, and that decision may be based on patient characteristics which could determine their outcome to therapy in either a blatantly biased, or possibly quite subtle, way. This can make an apparently randomized trial simply a comparison of two groups of patients chosen for different treatments, which have a high chance of differing systematically in some respects. The evaluation of treatment may therefore be confounded with these differences in patient characteristics, and impossible to interpret.

There are a number of simple methods of true randomization which can either be prepared in advance (and held by an appropriate, independent person) or which use patient characteristics dynamically. Computer-based randomization methods add an additional degree of unpredictability and concealment over pre-prepared paper lists and should therefore be used whenever possible. However, it is important to understand the underlying methodology in order that the method of randomization appropriate to a particular trial is used. The next sections illustrate 'manual' methods of randomization which can be set up quickly and simply, requiring only a table of random numbers (one can be found at http://www.rand.org/publications/MR/MR1418). All these methods can, of course, be programmed for computer-based allocations.

4.7.2 Simple (pure) randomization

Simple randomization is a slightly more sophisticated form of coin-tossing, being a method in which each treatment allocation is based purely on chance, with no attempt being made to adjust the scheme to ensure balance across specific patient characteristics.

(a) Two treatments

Random number tables list the digits 0–9 in random order, with each digit equally likely to occur. With two treatments, simply decide in advance which digits will denote treatment 1 and which will denote treatment 2, for example

$$0\text{–}4 \Rightarrow \text{allocate treatment 1}$$
$$5\text{–}9 \Rightarrow \text{allocate treatment 2}$$

(b) More than two treatments

With more than two treatments, the method is simply adapted. Select an equal number of digits from 0 to 9 to represent each treatment. In situations where 10 is not equally divisible by the number of treatments, the remaining numbers can simply be ignored, without introducing any bias, as in the example below

$$1\text{–}3 \Rightarrow \text{allocate treatment 1}$$
$$4\text{–}6 \Rightarrow \text{allocate treatment 2}$$
$$7\text{–}9 \Rightarrow \text{allocate treatment 3}$$
$$0 \quad \Rightarrow \text{ignore, take next number}$$

ID no.	TRT	Patient initials	Hospital
1001	3		
1002	2		
1003	3		
1004	3		
1005	1		
1006	3		
1007	3		
1008	1		
1009	2		
1010	2		
1011	3		
1012	1		
1013	1		
1014	3		
1015	2		
1016	3		
1017	3		
1018	3		

Fig. 4.7 Allocation sheet, simple randomization.

(c) Unequal randomization

Where treatments are to be allocated in a ratio other than 1 : 1, for example 2 : 1, 3 : 1 (meaning that three out of every four patients are allocated one of the treatments), this can be effected by allocating the digits 0–9 in a ratio which mimics the treatment allocation ratio, for example if 2 : 1 randomization is used:

$$0,1,2,3,4,5 \Rightarrow \text{allocate treatment 1}$$
$$6,7,8 \Rightarrow \text{allocate treatment 2}$$
$$9 \Rightarrow \text{ignore, take next number.}$$

(d) Example

A particular random number table, read from the top left-hand corner, generates the digits : 75792 78245 83270 59987 75253.

Suppose we have three treatments, and we aim to have equal numbers on each, and thus use the digit allocation described in section (b) above. This would give the treatment allocation sheet shown in Fig. 4.7.

Note that here, while wishing to have equal treatment allocation, we actually have four patients each on treatments 1 and 2, but 10 on treatment 3. In practice with trials of 10s or 100s of patients, simple randomization may by chance lead to such imbalances, or to fairly long runs of the same treatment. In very small trials, the impact on the overall power of the study can be substantial, but in general you may wish to have slightly more control over the overall treatment allocation than is possible with simple randomization. A number of methods are available to permit this, while maintaining the essential elements of randomization; these are described in Sections 4.7.3—4.7.5.

4.7.3 Block randomization (random permuted blocks)

This is a method to ensure that after the entry of every x patients into the trial, the number of patients on each treatment will be equal; 'x' is referred to as the block size.

For example, in a trial of two treatments with a block size of four, we can ensure that of every four patients, two will receive treatment A and two will receive treatment B. The random element comes from considering all the possible arrangements of, in this example, two As and two Bs within a set of four, and then randomly choosing the order in which the sets are used to form a randomization list. Again using the example above, there are six possible permutations of two treatments (A and B) within a block of four:

1. AABB   2. ABAB   3. ABBA   4. BBAA   5. BABA   6. BAAB

To implement blocked randomization, allocate a digit (0–9) to each block, and use random numbers to choose the order of the blocks to be used in the randomization schedule.

For example, given the random number sequence 1843712 . . .

$\Rightarrow$ AABB (ignore 8) BBAA ABBA (ignore 7) AABB ABAB

More than two treatments, unequal allocation

This method can be adapted to more than two treatments, or to unequal randomization. For multiple treatments, simply choose a block size that is a multiple of the number of treatments (if the allocation ratio is equal). For unequal allocation choose a block size that is a multiple of the sum of the treatment allocation ratio – for example, with 3:2 randomization use a block size of 5, 10, or 15.

Choice of block size

The choice of block size is clearly very important – with any block size the last treatment allocation of the block is always predictable, and a maximum of half the allocations will be predictable (for example with two treatments and a block size of 10, if the first five treatments within a block are treatment A, the next five must be treatment B). To avoid this predictability

+ never reveal the block size to participants,
+ avoid using the smallest possible block size,
+ consider using varying block sizes.

Bear in mind, however, that the aim of block randomization is to keep a slightly tighter control on the overall balance of treatment allocations than is possible with simple randomization – yet the larger the block size, the less the control. For two treatments, equally allocated, a block size of 8–10 is usually adequate. If for any reason a long run of the same treatment allocation needs to be avoided, then remember that the maximum run is equal to the block size, being achieved when a block in which all the allocations for a particular treatment appear at the end is followed by a block in which they all appear at the beginning.

4.7.4 Stratified randomization

In multi-centre trials, it is good practice to ensure that within a hospital, or perhaps an individual clinician, a roughly equal number of patients are allocated each treatment. This might be because variability between centres in some aspect of patient care might be anticipated – for example surgical technique – or perhaps because of the cost or difficulty of one of the treatments. One may also want to ensure that important known prognostic factors are balanced between treatments (randomization does not *guarantee* this – particularly in small trials). In many cancer trials, it may well be the case that differences in outcome according to factors such as stage or age are much larger than the anticipated differences due to treatment. In small trials, therefore, imbalances in prognostic factors may occur across treatment groups which could obscure, or lead to over-estimation of, differences due to treatment itself if a simple unadjusted analysis is performed.

To avoid such imbalances, a widely used method is 'stratified randomization'. With this method, blocked randomization is used, but instead of a single randomization 'list', a number will be prepared such that there is a separate list for each combination of the important stratification factors. For example, if you wish to balance treatment allocation by one factor only, say hospital, simply prepare a block randomization list for each hospital using the methods described previously.

If you wish to balance treatment allocation across a number of factors, for example hospital (A versus B) stage (I/II versus III/IV) and age (<50 versus ≥50), then you must prepare blocked lists for each combination of factors – here there are eight combinations:

> hospital A, stage I/II aged <50;   hospital B, stage I/II aged <50;
> hospital A, stage I/II aged ≥50;   hospital B, stage I/II aged ≥50;
> hospital A, stage III/IV aged <50;   hospital B, stage III/IV aged <50;
> hospital A, stage III/IV aged ≥50;   hospital B, stage III/IV aged ≥50.

Note that using stratified randomization without blocking serves little purpose – without blocking you would simply have random treatment allocations for each of the eight lists, possibly with fairly small numbers of patients on each list, and balance across treatments cannot be guaranteed.

Clearly, if there are many stratification factors, or some factors with many categories, this method may become impractical, even if computerized. In the previous example, if the number of hospitals was twenty rather than two, there would be eighty combinations of factors, meaning eighty 'lists.' For those randomizing without the aid of a computer this is time-consuming, but there are potential problems even with computerized stratified randomization. The larger the number of lists, the smaller the number of patients likely on each. With a moderately large block size and trials which stop when a specified total number of patients is reached, rather than when specified numbers are achieved on each list, each list can be imbalanced at the time of stopping, and potentially large overall imbalances in treatment allocation could occur. They would have to be substantial to affect the power of the study considerably, but even moderate imbalances can give the impression of a poorly conducted study which may even affect its publication.

Also, it has been pointed out [28] that in general we are less interested in whether the number (proportion) of patients aged <50, with stage II disease, from hospital X are balanced between treatments, and more interested in whether the individual factors are balanced – i.e. the number (proportion) aged <50 is balanced and the number with stage II disease is balanced across treatments. *Minimization* is a method of treatment allocation that ensures this in a more direct manner than stratification.

4.7.5 Minimization

In minimization, the treatment allocated to a patient depends on the allocations given to all previous patients with the same characteristics, and the allocation is done in a manner which minimizes the treatment imbalance in each of those characteristics – hence the name.

For example, suppose in a trial comparing treatment A and treatment B, we wanted to ensure balance across three age groups, <50, 50–60, >60. Suppose also that currently fourteen patients aged <50 have been allocated A and twelve have been allocated B. If the next patient is aged <50, then we allocate them to the treatment which minimizes the treatment imbalance for this age group – in this case, we would allocate B. An element of pure randomization must be introduced whenever the current allocations for a given group are exactly balanced, including the first allocations within an age group, but can be introduced at any stage (see later in this section).

More often, just as with stratified randomization, you wish to balance a number of factors. The method here is to sum the imbalances across all the factors, and allocate the treatment which minimizes the sum of the imbalances. This is best shown by an example.

Example 1: Suppose sixteen patients have been randomized into a trial, and their characteristics are distributed as in Table 4.1.

Suppose the next patient is from hospital X, aged 38 and has stage II disease. Currently:

$$
\begin{aligned}
&\text{for hospital X there is no treatment imbalance,} && A - B = 0, \\
&\text{for age} <50 && A - B = -2, \\
&\text{for stage,} && A - B = +1.
\end{aligned}
$$

The overall imbalance, $A - B, = -1$, therefore we allocate treatment A. This is equivalent to simply summing the number of previous patients with the same characteristics on each treatment and allocating the patient to the group with the lowest total:

allocated treatment A: $4 + 3 + 3 = 10$,   allocated treatment B: $4 + 5 + 2 = 11$.

Table 4.1 Example of treatment allocations by stratification factors

		Treatment	
		A	B
Hospital	X	4	4
	Y	3	2
	Z	1	2
Age	<50	3	5
	≥50	5	3
Stage	I/II	3	2
	III/IV	5	6

Manual implementation

A practical method to implement minimization manually is through the use of a series of cards, one for each level of each minimization factor, as shown in Fig. 4.8. Each card is divided vertically into columns, the number equalling the number of treatments. The first patients must be randomized using a list prepared using simple randomization (Section 4.7.2). A patient ID number is written on to the cards which correspond to the patient's characteristics, in the appropriate column. Thereafter, as each new patient is entered, take out the cards corresponding to their characteristics, sum the number of patients in each treatment column across all the cards, allocate the patient to the treatment with the smallest number and write their ID in the appropriate places. If at any stage the treatment allocations are balanced, then allocate the treatment at random (using pre-prepared randomly generated lists for example).

Unequal allocation

As for the other methods of randomization, unequal treatment allocation can be accommodated. For example, suppose we wished to allocate two out of every five patients to treatment A and three out of every five patients to treatment B. Work through the procedure as above until the totals for each treatment allocation are obtained. Then, multiply the treatment A total by three and the treatment B total by two (if the allocations to date are in perfect balance the resulting numbers will be equal). Treatment allocation can then proceed as before, assigning the new patient to the treatment with the lowest (adjusted) total score, or allocating at random if the adjusted totals are balanced.

Is minimization true randomization?

Minimization as applied above is NOT random, and DOES depend on the patient characteristics and so appears to contradict the basic definition of randomization. However, it does meet the requirement to avoid systematic bias in allocating treatments, and where it is impossible for the person considering randomizing a patient to have full knowledge of the characteristics and treatment allocations of all previous patients (and this would usually be the case in multi-centre trials) minimization fulfils the concealment aspect of randomization too in that the next treatment allocation is not predictable.

Bearing in mind the earlier statement that randomization must not only be correct, but must be seen to be correct, this form of minimization may not be an appropriate method to use in a single centre study. However, where predictability is a concern, it is possible to include a random element into minimization. To do this, instead of always allocating the treatment which minimizes the imbalance, that treatment is allocated with a certain probability $p(p < 1)$, for example $p = 0.75$.

To do this in practice, one can prepare a random number list on which 0 to 5 ='allocate the treatment which minimizes imbalance' and 6 and 7 = 'allocate the other treatment' (ignore 8 and 9 and take the next digit ≤ 7). This ensures, on average, that the allocation which minimizes the imbalance is chosen 75 per cent of the time. Having worked through the 'summing' procedure as described above, consult the list to see if the next patient should be allocated the treatment which minimizes the imbalance or not, remembering to strike through each number on the list as it is used.

Minimization is widely used in oncology, perhaps because of the multi-centric nature of many cancer trials – stratifying by centre and other factors does, as described above,

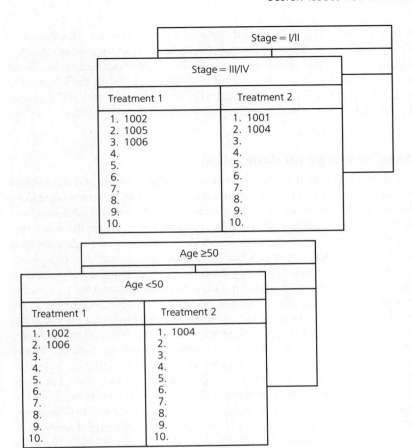

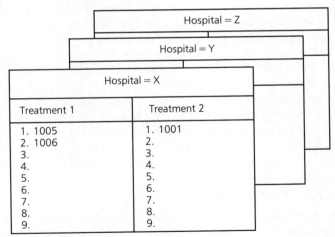

Fig. 4.8 Minimization cards for manual allocation.

become impractical and may not provide the overall balance required. However, it is not accepted universally, and those conducting licensing trials should ensure that the relevant licensing body accepts minimization as a valid method of randomization. Some organizations (of which the Food and Drug Administration (FDA) in the US and the Medicines Control Agency in the UK are perhaps the ones of most note), will certainly require that every allocation method, including minimization, has some form of random element.

4.7.6 Sealed envelope randomization

Since patients to be randomized may present at unpredictable times, and the interval between their agreement to be randomized and the allocation to treatment should be kept to an absolute minimum, access to randomization should be maintained throughout normal clinic hours at least, and this often requires dedicated staff. Where this is impractical, or in emergency situations where treatment decisions must be made extremely rapidly, 'sealed envelope' randomization may be a practical, though not completely infallible, solution. This involves compiling a randomization sequence of treatment allocations and identification numbers, using simple or block randomization, for each centre taking part in the trial. Usually, for simplicity, patient characteristics are not taken into account, although this can be done. The central list is retained. Opaque envelopes are prepared – it is useful to print a copy of the registration form recording the necessary patient information on the envelope. A sheet containing the treatment allocation and identification number is placed in the envelope which is then sealed, the identification number is then written on the outside of the envelope so that they can be placed in order. When a patient is being considered for randomization, the registration sheet should be completed and the next envelope opened *in sequence* to obtain the treatment allocation, which in turn should be written onto the envelope, together with the date of randomization. The original envelope should be returned to the trials office immediately. The office can then check that the patient ID and treatment allocation tally, and that the dates of randomization are consistent with the envelopes being opened in sequential order. With rigorous checks, the potential for bias (opening envelopes until the treatment allocation 'desired' is reached) can be minimized – for example recording the time as well as date of randomization may provide data which can be checked against hospital records of, for example, operation times. This remains, however, theoretically open to abuse – for example as the envelopes must be prepared in advance, they could be opened in advance and operating lists arranged to suit. Random visits to centres to check that there are no opened but as yet unused envelopes can help, but in general, sealed envelope randomization is best used only as a method of last resort. The situation in which rapid telephone access to the randomization centre is truly impossible must be increasingly rare.

4.7.7 Practical issues

To maintain the integrity of randomization, it is always advisable to ensure a degree of separation between those responsible for entering patients into trials, and those responsible for setting up the randomization schedule. This is best achieved when randomization can be performed by contacting a central office, either by telephone or through remote access to a computer-based randomization system. As a minimum, when pre-prepared randomization lists are to be used in a trial, they should be prepared and kept by someone *not* involved in treating trial patients. For local studies, a computer-based system may provide an extra level of security, though issues concerning maintaining the integrity of randomization – such as concealing the block size used – still apply when setting these up. The system should therefore not be set up by the person who will be responsible for inviting patients to take part in the trial.

Whenever a computer-based system is used, a back-up system is useful in case of computer failure. Ideally this should comprise pre-prepared randomization lists, but for very occasional emergency use, it is possible simply to throw a dice or toss a coin. The patient's details and allocated treatment should always be recorded and added to the main system as soon as possible.

4.8 Allocation concealment – blinding/masking

4.8.1 Definitions

Randomization alone is not sufficient to guarantee an unbiased trial. Systematic bias may still be introduced if the method of assessment of outcome is subjective or in some other way open to interpretation. To address this, consideration should be given to whether aspects of the trial can be 'blinded' or 'masked.' With respect to treatment allocation, there are three levels of blinding possible.

- single blind – the patient does not know which treatment they have been allocated,
- double blind – neither patient nor doctor/evaluator knows which treatment the patient has been allocated,
- triple blind – neither the patient, nor the doctor, nor those reviewing the interim results and deciding on continuation of the trial know which treatment the patient has been allocated.

In addition, even if treatments are not blinded, the assessment of eligibility or response can in some situations be carried out without knowledge (or 'blind') of the treatment allocation, for example by using an independent reviewer.

Why blind the patient?

Knowledge of treatment allocation

- may affect motivation to comply with treatment,
- may also affect response.

Why blind doctors/carers/evaluators?

Knowledge of treatment allocation

- may affect the way patients are monitored, for example for side effects or disease progression, possibly leading to earlier diagnosis of failure and initiation of alternative therapy in one treatment group than the other;
- may affect level of reporting of adverse effects, for example over-reporting of effects in patients undergoing a relatively new treatment, while the same events might not be reported in someone undergoing standard care;
- may affect the patient's response, if the doctor has different levels of 'enthusiasm' for the different treatments;

- may affect the evaluators – for example those measuring tumour volumes to assess treatment response may be subtly influenced by knowledge of treatment allocation, perhaps giving the 'benefit of doubt' more readily to one group than the other.

Why blind those conducting interim reviews?
- must be objective,
- knowledge of treatment may affect judgement.

While these are the reasons generally given in favour of blinding, there are strong arguments against. If an independent committee reviewing interim data is blinded to the treatment allocation, then it follows that they are expected to consider the trial in isolation, ignoring any previous trials. It is now widely accepted that before a treatment can be adopted as standard, it is necessary to conduct a systematic review of all the available evidence (see Chapter 11). If a DMEC are to make an informed and clinically relevant decision about the continuation or otherwise of a trial, then they should also be aware of how the present trial fits in with existing data. An example of a trial in which the DMEC's decisions at each stage were always informed by consideration of how the trial would impact on existing data and opinions is given in [29].

4.8.2 Placebos

The use of blinding is traditionally associated with the use of placebos in which one group of patients receive the active treatment, and the other receives an inactive treatment or 'placebo' which must be identical in appearance and packaging and, if given orally, taste. The intention in using placebos is to eliminate the impact of the so-called placebo effect; patients may feel they have improved simply because they are being treated – or believe they are. Therefore, if an open trial compares a group allocated a new treatment with a group who receive no active care, and a benefit is seen in the treatment group, it may not be clear how much of the effect is attributable to a genuine, physical, impact of the treatment on the disease and how much is a psychological effect of simply 'being treated'. If, instead, the 'no active treatment' group receive a placebo, the difference in treatment effect between the two arms cannot be accounted for by the placebo effect, since it is affecting both arms. Of course, exactly the same problem may occur if a trial is comparing two or more active treatments. In this case, it is possible to conduct a double-blind trial without the need for placebos, provided that the treatments can be made indistinguishable. Trials can in principle sometimes be blinded even if the treatments are given in very different ways – for example it is possible to compare an oral drug versus an intravenous drug using the double dummy technique. Here each patient is given two treatments, one group receives the active iv treatment and an oral placebo while the other receives the active oral agent and iv placebo treatment.

While discussion about placebos often focuses on drug therapy, in principle the need to consider blinding applies equally to any form of treatment. Ethical issues may, however, determine the extent to which treatments can be blinded, since one must avoid putting a patient at risk through any procedure which is unlikely to benefit them in any objective sense.

4.8.3 Practicalities of using placebos or blinded treatments

As with the term 'randomization,' a trial which is said to be double-blind may by anything but. Despite best efforts, treatments may not be perfectly matched [30]. Whether this is a problem or not may depend on the curiosity and motivation of the subjects. For example, a group of patients within a trial could compare their capsules and look for differences in internal or external appearance. While not being able to tell which is active and which placebo, pooling and dividing the capsules so that each patient has some of each could satisfy the desire of a desperate patient to have at least some active treatment. If this happened on a large scale, it would make the trial impossible to interpret.

This hypothetical example illustrates the need for great care in matching treatments and gives an indication of the additional level of complication and potentially considerable cost which treatment blinding may bring to a trial. In addition, as discussed below, if the side effects of the treatments being compared are known to be very different, it will soon become clear which patients are on which treatment. For the purposes of blinding the clinician therefore, it would not be sufficient simply to label the treatments A or B, since it takes only one patient with a 'classic' reaction to drug B to unblind the trial to the trial physicians at least. Rather, the randomization list should be prepared such that each patient in the trial is allocated a code, and a separate list (often held by an independent member of the pharmacy staff) identifies which codes correspond to which treatment. There must be a facility to break the code – not just for the final trial analysis, but also in case of emergencies. One example is the unanticipated need to give a patient treatment, perhaps for an unrelated condition, which may interact badly with one of the trial therapies even if they are stopped (naturally any patient for whom such a need is a known possibility should not have entered the trial in the first place since they were not 'fit to receive either treatment,' an eligibility requirement for any trial – see Section 4.2.3). This again emphasizes the need for a complex coding system for which knowledge of one patient's true allocation does not reveal any other patient's allocation.

4.8.4 General guidance

The real need for treatment blinding should therefore be carefully considered, with general guidance given below.

In general, blinding in trials is

- *desirable* for 'soft' endpoints, such as pain, anxiety, depression (subjective),
- often *unnecessary* for 'hard' endpoints, such as survival (objective),
- *useless* if treatments are known to have very different side effects which would make objective assessment impossible,
- *dangerous* if other treatments the patient may receive could react badly with one of the blinded treatments.

Example 2: The US study of tamoxifen for breast cancer prevention [31] was a double-blind placebo-controlled trial which randomized patients at 'high risk' of breast cancer to receive five years of tamoxifen or placebo. The main outcome measure of the trial was breast cancer incidence with secondary outcomes being the incidence of fractures and cardiac events – which tamoxifen would be expected to have a beneficial effect on – and also endometrial cancer and thrombotic events – which tamoxifen would be expected to have an adverse effect on. Was blinding necessary here? In its favour, it avoids the possibility of patients being investigated for breast cancer more closely or frequently in one arm. If, for example, control patients were seen more frequently, any breast cancers which occurred would be detected earlier than they would in the active treatment group, leading to an apparent benefit to tamoxifen even if the total number of breast cancers was the same in the two groups. Does the same argument apply to the secondary outcome measures? Given the known potentially adverse effects of tamoxifen, a patient being treated outside the trial might receive anti-thrombotic treatment, which might prevent thrombosis, or undergo additional screening for endometrial cancer which may identify cases at an early stage. However, within the blinded trial it would be impractical to apply such prophylaxis to all patients and it could be argued that this therefore puts patients at a greater risk than would be the case if they received tamoxifen outside the trial.

Blinding may also for instance affect compliance – a woman who is unaware of whether she is receiving active treatment or placebo may be less or more assiduous than one who knows she is taking an active treatment and again this may introduce a difference between the effect of the treatment on a woman within the trial compared with one who receives the treatment outside of the trial. In general, use of blinding can take the administration and monitoring of treatments away from the 'real life' setting and the importance of this needs to be taken into account in deciding whether blinding is necessary or desirable.

4.9 Conclusion

Randomization is the cornerstone of good trial design and, as has been shown here, can be implemented using a range of practical and more technical methods, such that arguments against its use on the basis of practicalities are unfounded. There will rarely be a situation in which the simple parallel group design for a randomized trial is inappropriate, but as has been illustrated here, there are often opportunities to make better use of a limited pool of patients. Such opportunities should always be investigated.

References

[1] Buyse, M. (1991) Cyclophosphamide plus cisplatin versus cyclophosphomide, doxorubicin, and cisplatin chemotherapy of ovarian-carcinoma – a meta-analysis. *Journal of Clinical Oncology*, 9 (9), 1668–74.

[2] McGuire, W.P., Hoskins, W.J., Brady, M.F., Kucera, P.R., Partridge, E.E., Look, K.Y., Clarke Pearson, D.L., and Davidson, M. (1996) Cyclophosphamide and cisplatin compared with paclitaxel and cisplatin in patients with stage III and stage IV ovarian cancer. *New England Journal of Medicine*, 334(1), 1–6.

[3] Muggia, F.M., Braly, P.S., Brady, M.F., Sutton, G., Niemann, T.H., Lentz, S.L., Alvarez, R.D., Kucera, P.R., and Small, J.M. (2000) Phase III randomized study of cisplatin versus paclitaxel versus cisplatin and paclitaxel in patients with suboptimal stage III or IV ovarian cancer: A Gynecologic Oncology Group study. *Journal of Clinical Oncology*, 18(1), 106–15.

[4] The International Collaborative Ovarian Neoplasm (ICON) Group. (2002) Paclitaxel plus carboplatin versus standard chemotherapy with either single-agent carboplatin or cyclophosphamide, doxorubicin, and cisplatin in women with ovarian cancer: the ICON3 randomised trial. *Lancet*, 360, 505–15.

[5] The ICON2 Collaborators. (1998) Randomized trial of single-agent carboplatin against three-drug combination of CAP (cyclophosphamide, doxorubicin, and cisplatin) in women with ovarian cancer. *Lancet*, **352**(9140), 1571–6.

[6] Schwartz, F., and Lellouch, A. (1967) Explanatory and pragmatic attitudes in therapeutic trials. *Journal of Chronic Diseases*, **20**, 637–48.

[7] Stenning, S.P. (1992) Selection of patients for cancer clinical trials – the uncertainty principle. In *Introducing New Treatments for Cancer* (ed. C.J. Williams). pp. 161–72, Wiley, New York.

[8] Freedman, B. (1987) Equipoise and the ethics of clinical research. *New England Journal of Medicine*, **317**, 141–5.

[9] International Collaboration of Trialists. (1999) Adjuvant cisplatin, methotrexate, and vinblastine chemotherapy for muscle-invasive bladder cancer: a randomized controlled trial. *Lancet*, **354**(9178), 533–40.

[10] Zelen, M. (1979) A new design for randomized clinical trials. *New England Journal of Medicine*, pp. 1242–5.

[11] Krongborg, O., Fenger, C., Olsen, J., Jorgensen, O.D., and Søndergaard, O. (1996) Randomized study of screening for colorectal cancer with faecal-occult-blood test. *Lancet*, **348**, 1467–71.

[12] Olschewski, M., and Scheurlen, H. (1985) Comprehensive cohort study: An alternative to randomized consent design in a breast preservation trial. *Methods of Information in Medicine*, **24**, 131–4.

[13] Altman, D.F., Whitehead, J., Parmar, M.K.B., Stenning, S.P., Fayers, P.M., and Machin, D. (1995) Randomized consent designs in cancer clinical trials. *European Journal of Cancer*, **31**A, 1934–44.

[14] Alexander, F.E., Anderson, T.J., Brown, H.K., Forrest, A.P.M., Hepburn, W., Kirkpatrick, A.E., McDonald, C., Muir, B.B., Prescott, R.J., Shepherd, S.M., Smith, A., and Warner, J. (1994) The Edinburgh randomized trial of breast cancer screening: results after 10 years of follow-up. *British Journal of Cancer*, **70**, 542–8.

[15] Moher, M., Yudkin, P., Wright, L., Turner, R., Fuller, A., Schofield, T., and Mant, D. (2001) Cluster randomized controlled trial to compare three methods of promoting secondary prevention of coronary heart disease in primary care. *British Medical Journal*, **322**(7298), 1338–42.

[16] Hutton, J. (2001) Are distinct ethical principles required for cluster randomized controlled trials? *Statistics in Medicine*, **20**, 473–88.

[17] Donner, A. (1998) Some aspects of the design and analysis of cluster randomized trials. *Applied Statistics*, **47** (1), 95–113.

[18] Elbourne, D.R., and Campbell, M.K. (2001) Extending the CONSORT statement to cluster randomized trials: for discussion. *Statistics in Medicine*, **20**, 489–96.

[19] Medical Research Council. (1984) The evaluation of low-dose pre-operative X-ray therapy in the management of operable rectal cancer; results of a randomly controlled trial. *British Journal of Surgery*, **71**, 21–5.

[20] Seymour, M. on behalf on the MRC Colorectal Cancer Group and all the participants. (2001) An update on the MRC FOCUS/CR08 trial: the first 300 patients. *British Journal of Cancer*, **85** (suppl 1), 44 (abs P.45).

[21] Karim, A.B.M.F., Maat, B., Hatlevoll, R., Menten, J., Rutten, E.H.J.M., Thomas, D.G.T, Mascarenhas, F., Horiot, J.C., Parvinen, L.M., vanReijn, M., Hamers, H.P., Gaspar, L., Noordman, E., Pierart, M., vanGlabbeke, M., vanAlphen, A.M., Jager, J.J., and Fabrini, M.G. (1996) A randomized trial on dose-response in radiation therapy of low-grade cerebral glioma: European Organization for Research and Treatment of Cancer (EORTC) study 22844. *International Journal of Radiation Oncology Biology Physics*, **36** (3), 549–56.

[22] Karim, A.B.M.F., Afra, D., Cornu, P., Bleehen, N., Schraub, S., De Witte, O., Darcel, F., Stenning, S., Pierart, M., and Van Glabbeke, M. (2002) Randomized trial on the efficacy of radiotherapy

for cerebral low-grade glioma in the adult: European Organization for Research and Treatment of Cancer study 22845 with the Medical Research Council study BRO4: An interim analysis. *International Journal of Radiation Oncology Biology Physics,* 52(2), 316–24.

[23] Gray, R., James, R., Mossman, J., and Stenning, S.P. (1991) Guest editorial: AXIS – A suitable case for treatment. *British Journal of Cancer,* 63, 841–5.

[24] Bruera, E., Belzile, M., Pituskin, E., Fainsinger, R., Darke, A., Harsanyi, Z., Babul, N., and Ford, I. (1998) Randomized, double-blind, cross-over trial comparing safety and efficacy of oral controlled-release oxycodone with controlled-release morphine in patients with cancer pain. *Journal of Clinical Oncology,* 16(10), 3222–9.

[25] Hills, M., and Armitage, P. (1979) The two-period cross-over clinical trial. *British Journal of Clinical Pharmacology,* 8, 7–20.

[26] Senn, S. (1993) *Cross-over Trials in Clinical Research.* John Wiley, Chichester.

[27] Maughan, T.S., James, R.D., Kerr, D.J., Ledermann, J.A., McArdle, C., Seymour, M.T., Cohen, D., Hopwood, P., Johnston, C., and Stephens, R.J. For the British MRC Colorectal Cancer Working Party. (2002) Comparison of survival, palliation, and quality of life with three chemotherapy regimens in metastatic colorectal cancer: a multicentre randomized trial. *Lancet,* 359, 1555–63.

[28] Pocock, S.J., and Simon, R. (1975) Sequential treatment assignment with balancing for prognostic factors in the controlled clinical trial. *Biometrics,* 31, 103–15.

[29] Parmar, M.K.B., Griffiths, G.O., Spiegelhalter, D.J., Souhami, R.L., Altman, D.G., and van der Scheuren, E. (2001) Monitoring of large randomised clinical trials: a new approach with Bayesian methods. *Lancet,* 358(9279), 375–81.

[30] Hill, L.E., Nunn, A., and Fox, W. (1976) Matching quality of agents employed in 'double blind' controlled clinical trials, *Lancet,* I, 352–56.

[31] Fisher, B., Costantino, J.P., Wickerham, D.L., Redmond, C.K., Kavanah, M., Cronin, W.M., Vogel, V., Robidoux, A., Dimitrov, N., Atkins, J., Daly, M., Wieand, S., Tan-Chiu, E., Ford, L., and Wolmark, N. (1998) Tamoxifen for prevention of breast cancer: Report of the National Surgical Adjuvant Breast and Bowel Project P-1 Study. *Journal of the National Cancer Institute,* 90, 1371–88.

Chapter 5

Trial size

5.1 Introduction

Chapter 3 introduced the idea that the treatment effect observed in a clinical trial may vary from the true effect because of the two major sources of error – systematic and random error – and emphasized that the random error component can be minimized by randomizing large numbers of patients. The aim of this chapter is to discuss theoretical and practical issues affecting the determination of the ideal sample size for a trial and to describe when and how compromizes from the ideal can be made. While the focus is on randomized trials, we also expand on sample size calculation for the phase II trial designs introduced in Chapter 4. It is beyond the scope of this chapter to detail sample size calculations for all the types of data and circumstances which a researcher may meet. Our aim therefore is to describe ways to determine the appropriate 'input factors' – in particular the size of difference a trial is designed to target – with only brief reference to sample size formulae. We refer readers to published books and software for more detailed options.

Although there is some truth in the statement that any randomized evidence is better than none – in other words that doing a smaller than ideal trial is better than treating patients haphazardly – it is important to be aware of the consequences. A common misconception is to assume that sample size only determines precision, i.e. the width of the confidence interval, and not accuracy or 'closeness' to the true treatment effect. It is important to note that an estimate of treatment effect from a small trial will not necessarily be close to the 'true' treatment effect with the sole disadvantage that it is estimated with uncertainty leading to wide confidence intervals. There will certainly be more uncertainty compared with a larger trial, but in addition there is an increased risk that the estimate will be inaccurate, purely through the play of chance. Note that this does not mean the estimate is biased – repeating many similarly small but properly randomized trials would produce results which, on average, estimate the true underlying effect.

The principle is perhaps best illustrated by considering a sequence of coin tosses. Suppose you were ignorant of the properties of a coin, and wished to estimate the probability that a coin, when tossed, will fall as heads. Clearly this can be estimated by the proportion of tosses that result in heads. Suppose the first toss falls as tails – at this stage your estimate of the probability of heads is 0. The next toss will update your estimate to be 0 still if it falls as tails, or 0.5 if it falls as heads. After three tosses your estimate may be 0, 0.33 or 0.66. As the number of tosses accumulate, your estimate will move closer to the true value of 0.5.

The first estimate is unbiased but, as we know, very far from the truth. An experiment such as this with two possible outcomes is known as a binomial experiment and we know from experience how chance can influence such an experiment, just as we know that as we repeat the tosses of a coin, re-estimating the probability of heads after each one, the estimate will gradually come closer to the truth. In clinical practice of course we are in a position where we never know 'the truth', but an unbiased trial will tend, as the number of patients increases, to give an estimate which comes closer and closer to the truth. This point emphasizes why confidence intervals (CI), which are always important in interpreting the results of a clinical trial, are particularly important for small trials – they define a range with quantified properties. One can say (roughly) that there is a 95 per cent chance that the true effect lies in the range defined by a 95 per cent CI. The interpretation of a single estimate is much more difficult.

Sequential versus fixed designs

The sample size calculations shown in this chapter assume a sample size is to be 'fixed' in advance. An alternative approach, known as sequential analysis, does not fix the sample size in advance, but accrues and analyses patients until sufficiently strong evidence in favour of the experimental or control arms (or against such a difference) emerges. In a fully sequential design, analysis takes place after each patient's response to treatment is known. This is thus most appropriate when the outcome measure can be assessed shortly after the patient enters the trial. Where this is the case, such a procedure can lead to trials being completed more quickly, compared with a fixed sample size design, if larger than expected differences occur. Perhaps because these two conditions rarely apply in cancer trials, fully sequential designs are rarely used. We therefore do not discuss them further here, but recommend a text book [1] for further details. An adaptation of this approach is much more widely used in oncology. In this, a sample size is determined according to the methods described in this chapter, but several interim analyses take place before the sample size is reached. This allows the potential for trials to be stopped early if convincing evidence for either treatment emerges. Schemes for determining the strength of evidence that must be demonstrated at an interim analysis to justify stopping are discussed in Section 9.5.

5.2   Outcome measures

In most trials there are several measures of treatment efficacy or impact of potential interest, and it may be appropriate that all are recorded. Examples commonly used in cancer trials are shown below. It is important to note that all of these examples can potentially be considered as 'time-to-event' data with patients not having the event being censored at the date last seen. This may be useful to remember when attempting to assess the impact of a treatment in a setting where prolongation of a particular state (e.g. complete response) may be as important, or more realistic, than a long-term increase or decrease in the proportion of patients achieving that state.

Choice of primary outcome measure

In any one trial several outcome measures may be of interest, and indeed the decision about whether or not to use a treatment may well entail balancing its impact across a

Outcome measure	Examples of associated time-to-event measure
Death	Survival time
Response (tumour shrinkage)	Duration of response
Recurrence of disease	Time to recurrence
Relief of symptoms	Time to relief of symptoms/without symptoms
Quality of life 'scores'	Time to improvement/deterioration in scores
Toxicity	Time with/without toxicity

number of outcome measures. However, it is generally necessary to focus on one, the primary outcome measure, for the purposes of sample size calculation. As a general rule, outcome measures in trials conducted early in the development of a treatment are usually tumour-based, i.e. they are chosen because they demonstrate measurable treatment impact – tumour shrinkage for example. A good response on these outcome measures, however, may not be of any noticeable benefit to the patient. A characteristic of phase III trials is that the primary outcome measures are those which clearly have the potential to have an impact on the patient, survival time being an obvious example.

In a definitive phase III trial the primary outcome measure would usually be the one which is most important in determining whether or not a treatment would be used outside of the trial, and this would often be survival time. A survival benefit alone may not be a sufficient condition to support the new treatment, but it is often essential to know the size of any benefit before considering other factors. Early randomized trials of a new treatment may use earlier intermediate outcome measures such as relapse or progression [2] which, in this situation, carry three main advantages. Firstly, the events are observed earlier than death, and so patients need not be followed-up so long for the purposes of the trial (though continued follow-up for long-term outcomes will often be valuable). Secondly, there will generally be more relapses or progressions than deaths – and as we will see later, it is the number of events rather than the number of patients which determines the size and power of a trial. Thirdly, as the majority of patients will receive no further treatment until relapse, the impact of treatment allocation can be assessed without the complicating factor of additional treatments before the event of interest. The disadvantage of such outcome measures is that one often does not know if a treatment's impact on the intermediate outcome measure, such as progression rate, will necessarily translate into differences in survival. An outcome measure can only be termed a *surrogate* outcome, and used in a definitive trial instead of survival, if there is good evidence that the impact of treatment on the intermediate outcome is predictive of the impact of the treatment on survival. One strict definition of surrogacy [3] is that the impact of treatment on the intermediate outcome entirely explains its impact on the definitive outcome measure. This is rare in practice, and the best one can hope for is a high degree of correlation. In this respect, it is worth noting that response is a poor surrogate for survival for several cancers. For example, using data from a meta-analysis in advanced colorectal cancer, Buyse *et al.* [4] demonstrate that although an increase in tumour response rate translates into an increase in overall survival for patients with advanced colorectal cancer, knowledge that a treatment has benefits on tumour response does not allow accurate prediction of the ultimate benefit on survival.

Despite numerous potential surrogate outcomes, and despite the potential for high correlations between the surrogate outcome and survival, there are many difficulties associated with the use of surrogates [5]. Therefore, survival will often be the outcome measure of choice for a definitive randomized trial. One reason for this is that trials are often comparing treatment policies, and if for example a combination of a new, perhaps rather toxic, adjuvant therapy with a standard treatment for relapse produces similar survival to a standard adjuvant therapy with the new treatment reserved for those patients who relapse, a prolongation of relapse-free time may not be sufficient to justify using the new treatment for all patients in the adjuvant setting. For example, the EORTC/MRC trial of immediate versus deferred radiotherapy for low grade glioma [6] found that immediate radiotherapy improved progression-free survival, but not overall survival compared with deferred radiotherapy. Proponents of deferred radiotherapy can use this trial to argue that reserving radiotherapy until absolutely necessary has spared many patients the side effects of the treatment without compromising their overall chance of cure.

Whichever outcome measure is chosen, it must be possible to assess the primary outcome measure objectively and consistently on every patient randomized if an unbiased estimate of the treatment effect is to be obtained. If it is really not possible to distinguish a single primary outcome measure, then one should ideally determine the sample size necessary to detect realistic and clinically relevant differences with respect to each outcome measure, and choose as the overall trial sample size the largest number required. This ensures that the trial is adequately powered for all the important outcome measures. An important point to remember though, is that carrying out multiple significance tests across a number of outcome measures increases the chance of one or more of these being 'significant' purely by chance; this can be compensated for by demanding a more extreme level of statistical significance (see also Section 9.5).

The importance of choosing the 'right' outcome measure to power a study is well illustrated with respect to equivalence, or non-inferiority trials. These trials hope to demonstrate that an experimental treatment, which is not expected to have superior efficacy, brings potential benefits such as reduced toxicity which all patients would benefit from, and which would outweigh small differences in efficacy. In this situation it is a common mistake simply to assume that the experimental treatment will have little impact on efficacy, and to base sample size on an outcome measure such as toxicity in which large differences are anticipated. Such a trial will be too small to detect important differences in efficacy that might well outweigh even substantial differences in toxicity. It will often be necessary to plan the trial to be big enough to detect the differences in efficacy that would be considered unacceptable whatever the differences in toxicity.

5.3 Basic considerations

In determining sample size, it is helpful to consider the problem in terms of hypothesis testing, even though the aim of the trial should be to provide an estimate of the treatment effect and not just to enable us to state whether the effect is 'statistically significant' or not.

If we consider a clinical trial comparing treatment A with treatment B with respect to survival, then the 'null hypothesis' (often referred to as H_0) is first defined. Typically,

Table 5.1 Types of error

True effect	Conclusion from trial	
	A = B	A ≠ B
A = B	✓	Type I error
A ≠ B	Type II error	✓

this states that there is no difference in the main outcome measure (OM) between A and B ($OM_A = OM_B$, that is the result you hope not to see).

The 'alternative' hypothesis (H_1) defines the result you hope to see which might be: There is a difference ($OM_A - OM_B = d$, where $d \neq 0$).

Here d, which is a measure of treatment effect, is often known as the effect size. The aim of careful sample size calculation is to ensure that the impact of random error is small in relation to the effect size you wish to detect. Random error itself can act to mask or enhance the true treatment effect, as illustrated in Table 5.1. It is, however, possible to control both type I and type II errors, and the setting of acceptable limits for these is part of the process of calculating the sample size for a given trial.

5.3.1 What size of type I error is acceptable?

To help determine the size of type I error that is acceptable (i.e. the probability of wrongly concluding that there is a difference between treatments when in fact none exists) consider what strength of evidence against the null hypothesis of no treatment difference you would want to see before rejecting it. This quantity is often denoted by α and goes under several synonyms:

- the significance level,
- test size,
- probability of a false-positive result.

At the end of the trial, one would reject the null hypothesis of no treatment difference, and conclude that there is likely to be a genuine difference between treatments, if the p-value from the formal test to compare treatments is less than α. This value is frequently set at 0.05 or 5 per cent but this is arbitrary and the consequences of wrongly concluding there is a difference should be considered for each trial being designed, bearing in mind its impact on sample size, and the significance level set accordingly. Fig. 5.1 shows the impact on sample size of changing the significance level.

As discussed in Chapter 9, p-values alone are an insufficient basis for drawing conclusions from a trial, and while levels must be specified in order to determine sample size, the conclusions should not alter radically if the p-value is very slightly above or below the pre-set significance level.

One-sided or two-sided test?

A related issue which causes some confusion is that of whether one should use a 'one-sided test' (essentially, is A better than B?) or a 'two-sided test' (do A and B differ?).

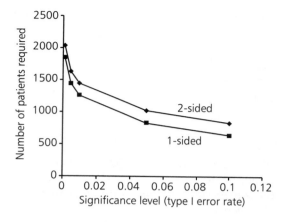

Fig. 5.1 Number of patients required for decreasing type I error levels. *Note*: Example from a 2-arm trial, anticipated 5-year survival rate in group 1=50%, in group 2=60%, 90% power assumed.

A two-sided test is intended for use when it is plausible that the treatment difference could favour either treatment. This is often the case for new cancer therapies which, despite being introduced with the hope of being able to improve outcome over standard treatment, may turn out to have a detrimental effect. Designing a trial with the intention to use a two-sided test allows one to interpret any result simply as evidence for or against either treatment. A one-sided test is intended for use when it is implausible that one treatment (let us say the experimental treatment) could be worse than the control arm with respect to the primary outcome measure. If the actual result favours the existing treatment, one would under these circumstances have to attribute this purely to chance, and conclude only that the experimental treatment was no better than the control. Thus, while many cancer trials are designed, conceptually, with one-sided alternative hypotheses (for example that the experimental treatment improves 5-year survival by 10 per cent), it is often appropriate to design them with a 2-sided test in mind, because an adverse effect of the experimental treatment cannot be ruled out. The results are then straightforward to interpret (and, as most trials use 2-sided tests, to compare with other trials). A trial designed for a two-sided test allows one to draw one of three conclusions: A is better than B, A is worse than B or A and B are not substantially different. A one-sided design and test enables one to draw one of two conclusions; A is better than B or A is not better than B. This choice may be justifiable; non-inferiority trials are often a case in point where it is sufficient to be able to say that A is no worse (by a specified amount) than B. However, one-sided tests are often viewed with suspicion that comes largely from their frequent misuse. Suppose a trial was designed with a two-sided alternative hypothesis; results favour the experimental treatment, but the (2-sided) logrank test on the primary outcome measure gives a p-value of 0.10. Had the trial been designed with a one-sided formulation, the equivalent p-value would be 0.05, which suggests much stronger evidence of benefit to the experimental treatment. If the decision to use a one-sided test is only made *after* observing a trend favouring the experimental treatment this is clearly biased. It is the frequency with which this is done (particularly when the two-sided p-value lies in the range 0.06–0.10) which gives the one-sided test a bad name, and causes many trials which quote a one-sided test result to be viewed with suspicion.

These arguments alone may in fact be considered justification for using 2-sided tests unless the arguments against are compelling.

5.3.2 What size of type II error is acceptable?

Here the question is, how certain do you want to be of detecting a specified treatment difference if it really exists? By 'detecting a difference' we mean finding that in the trial analysis, the difference between treatments is associated with a p-value at or below the chosen type I error rate.

This quantity, often denoted by β, is also known as the probability of a false-negative result, that is the probability of wrongly concluding that there is no difference between treatments. In fact the quantity $1 - \beta$ is used more widely. This is the probability of detecting a targeted difference between treatments, if it really exists, and is known more commonly as the power of a study. Clearly one wants this to be high, as close as possible to 100 per cent; as usual the actual level chosen must take into account the impact that increasing the power has on sample size. This is illustrated in Fig. 5.2. Power of at least 80 per cent, but more usually 90 per cent, is generally considered acceptable, meaning that if there is a true difference between treatments of the size targeted, you would find this to be statistically significant in 80 per cent (90 per cent) of trials. As for type I errors, the consequences of a wrong decision need to be considered for the specific trial, and should influence the actual level chosen. For example in an efficacy trial, the consequence of low power is an increased risk of concluding there is no benefit to the experimental treatment, and therefore of remaining with the current best control. However, in a non-inferiority or equivalence trial in which the experimental treatment is not expected to improve the primary outcome but must be no more than a specified amount worse, the consequence of low power is different. Here there is an increased risk of concluding the experimental treatment is approximately equivalent (if p-values alone are, wrongly, used to judge equivalence) therefore recommending the experimental treatment when in fact it is inferior. It is particularly important therefore to retain high power ($\geq$90 per cent) in an equivalence or non-inferiority trial.

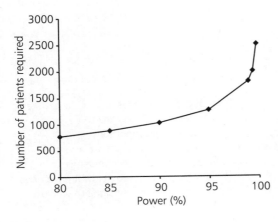

Fig. 5.2 Number of patients required for different power levels.
Note: Example from a 2-arm trial, anticipated 5-year survival rate in group 1 = 50 per cent, in group 2 = 60 per cent, two-sided 5 per cent significance level assumed.

5.3.3   What do you expect of the control arm?

It is important to have an idea of the outcome anticipated in the control group as this forms the baseline from which improvements will be judged, and of course affects the sample size. This is illustrated in Fig. 5.3, which shows the number of patients required in a survival study to detect an 'absolute' difference of 10 per cent according to different control group rates. It is important to distinguish between absolute and relative differences. Given a baseline survival rate of 50 per cent, an absolute difference of 10 per cent, for example, means an increase in survival from 50 to 60 per cent, while a relative or proportionate 10 per cent improvement means an increase from 50 to 55 per cent.

For proportions and time-to-event outcomes, the precision with which the control group rates need to be estimated is least for rates in the region of 50 per cent and greatest for very low and very high rates since, as shown in Fig. 5.3, the slopes are greatest at the extremes. However, the number of events, and hence the number of patients, required to detect an absolute difference of a given magnitude is highest when the baseline rate is in the region of 50 per cent. This is because it is the *relative* difference in event rates that is important (and not the absolute difference). For example, an absolute increase from 50 to 55 per cent is a relative increase of 10 per cent, while an absolute increase from 10 to 15 per cent is a 50 per cent relative increase. For simple proportions, the event rate and non-event rate can be reversed, thus the number of patients required to detect an absolute increase from 10 to 20 per cent is identical to the number required to detect an absolute increase from 80 to 90 per cent; this is because the standard error of a proportion, P, estimated in a group of N patients is $\sqrt{[P(1-P)/N]}$. However, for time to event outcomes, additional information is contained in the time to event; thus in general the number of patients required to detect a given absolute increase in survival proportions is slightly fewer than the number required to detect the same absolute increase in simple proportions when the event rate is high (see Fig. 5.3). However, as

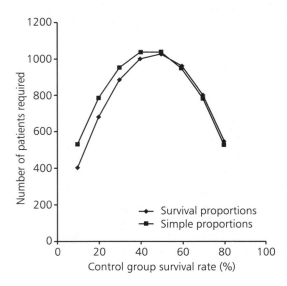

Fig. 5.3 Number of patients required to detect an absolute 10 per cent increase in proportions.
Note: Example from a 2-arm trial, absolute difference to detect = 10 per cent, 90 per cent power and 2-sided 5 per cent significance level.

the additional information is effectively added only by the patients with an event, it is important to distinguish between the event rate and the non-event rate with time-to-event data and, as shown in Fig. 5.3, the number of patients required to detect a given absolute increase is not perfectly symmetrical about the 50 per cent rate. More patients are required to detect an increase from 80 to 90 per cent event-free than to detect an increase from 10 to 20 per cent event-free, since in the latter case many more patients have events and thus contribute the additional information.

The best source of data for the control group outcome is a previous trial using the same eligibility criteria. If this is not available, bear in mind that patients in trials tend to have better survival than those not in trials, that selection criteria will almost inevitably identify patients with a better prognosis than basic registry data would suggest, and wherever possible err on the side of caution by tending towards a rate closer to 50 per cent.

5.3.4 What size of difference between treatments is important?

This is perhaps the key question to be addressed in sample size calculations but also the one for which there are fewest rules and generally accepted guidelines. It is necessary to consider two aspects:

(1) the size of difference that might reasonably be expected with the experimental treatment,

(2) the smallest difference thought clinically worthwhile.

Both are difficult to quantify; the 'expected' difference is always unknown (or you would not be doing the trial), while the 'clinically worthwhile' difference requires a complex assessment of the pros and cons of an experimental treatment to be balanced and con-densed into a single figure, and one which may well change during the course of a trial as experience is gained. It is, though, necessary to consider both issues. In general, one should aim to detect the smallest difference (1 or 2); however, if 1 is much smaller than 2, perhaps the trial should not be done?

In the 1970s and early 1980s many cancer trials focused more on (1) – but overestimated enormously, typically looking for differences of 20 per cent or more in long-term survival rates. As yet, we are aware of no systematic review of randomized trials in solid tumours that has shown an absolute survival improvement of more than 10 per cent. While this does not mean that future treatments will not prove more successful, it does suggest scepticism is valuable; the targeted size of difference to detect has the greatest impact of all on the required sample size, as Fig. 5.4 illustrates.

In fact, as a rule of thumb, an inverse square law applies such that as the size of difference you wish to detect halves, the number of patients required to detect it (with the same error rates) increases four-fold. Thus, in the example above, a trial aiming to detect a 20 per cent absolute difference requires only around 250 patients, while one aiming to detect a 10 per cent difference would require around 1000, with 4000 for a 5 per cent difference.

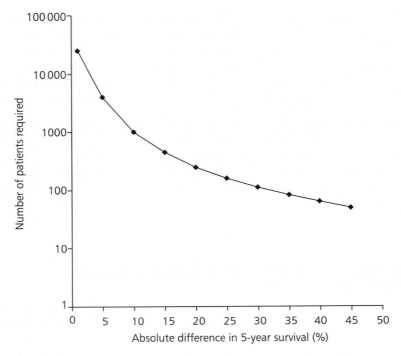

Fig. 5.4 Number of patients required to detect different treatment effect sizes.
Note: Assumes control group survival rate of 50 per cent, 90 per cent power and 5 per cent significance level (2-sided).

General factors affecting the choice of effect size to detect

For a definitive phase III trial, it may be important to consider the potential public health impact of a treatment. Important factors to consider include:

- How common is the disease?
- How widely applicable is the treatment?
- What level of toxicity is expected?

In common diseases, simple treatments that are widely applicable with few side effects (such as aspirin after myocardial infarction) need not demonstrate large survival benefits before being accepted. Even in cancer, improving survival by 5 per cent in common tumours such as lung, colon and prostate cancer would save or prolong many thousands of lives. For example, there are 20,000 deaths from colorectal cancer in the UK every year; a 5 per cent survival improvement may save or prolong 1000 lives a year. However, the following points need to be born in mind:

- Before a large-scale public health trial can be conducted, a lot of people will need to be persuaded that the treatment is safe, and of potential benefit – this can usually only be done through smaller trials.

- More complicated, toxic, specialist treatments will have to demonstrate that any benefit in terms of survival is large enough to outweigh the increased toxicity and perhaps decreased quality of life – so the trial may not need to be extremely large.

In other words, large, moderate and small trials all have a place and will continue to be conducted. Freedman [7] discusses this issue further.

Determining the size of difference to detect in a specific trial

Sometimes the targeted difference to detect can be guided by previous trials or meta-analysis. Where such data are not available, it is common to make decisions based on round-table discussions. However, it may often be useful to supplement this informal process with a more formal one, especially, for example, where one is considering a new treatment, or one for which there may be a difficult balance between benefits and 'costs.' Here, a more structured way of determining the appropriate difference may be useful. We have found formal questionnaires, completed by clinicians involved in the disease in question, to be a very useful means of addressing this issue.

The questionnaires described below are based on those developed by Freedman and Spiegelhalter [8]. They comprise two sections, the first identifying the expected differences in survival, the second attempting to elicit the clinically important differences as well as the factors which affect these values. In describing these questionnaires, the CHART bronchus trial [9] is used as an example. This was a randomized trial comparing conventional radiotherapy with Continuous, Hyperfractionated, Accelerated RadioTherapy (CHART) in the treatment of inoperable non-small cell lung cancer. Conventional radiotherapy was delivered in thirty fractions of 2 Gy, given once a day, Monday to Friday only, over six weeks. CHART was given to a total dose of 54 Gy, given in thirty-six fractions of 1.5 Gy, with three fractions given at 8-hour intervals for twelve consecutive days including weekends. This approach would, it was hoped, improve survival by minimizing the opportunity for tumour repopulation between fractions, and also reduce late morbidity. However, the timings make CHART difficult and expensive to organize and acute morbidity may be more severe.

A. Expected difference questionnaire

What difference between treatments do you think a trial such as this, with several thousand patients, would show? Here clinicians are being asked not to predict the results of the planned trial, but those of a very large and impeccably conducted trial addressing the same question. When asked this question in a structured way, individual clinicians will rarely give a point estimate, it is much more natural to give different weights to various differences. The questionnaire asks the clinician to distribute 100 per cent across various differences as shown in Fig. 5.5.

In the hypothetical example, the clinician is somewhat cautious, giving most weight to there being a modest benefit to the experimental treatment, for example a 25 per cent chance of there being a 0–5 per cent absolute improvement and a 30 per cent chance of there being a 5–10 per cent absolute improvement. She also considers that there is only a 15 per cent chance that the experimental treatment will produce an absolute improvement of more than 10 per cent. The clinician also has some concerns (5 per cent probability) that it could actually be as much as 10–15 per cent worse than control treatment.

Absolute difference between arms (per cent)	Control treatment (C) better					Experimental treatment (E) better					Total
	20+	15–20	10–15	5–10	0–5	0–5	5–10	10–15	15–20	20+	
Hypothetical example	0	0	5	10	15	25	30	10	5	0	100
Your entry											100

Fig. 5.5 Example of 'expected difference' questionnaire.

Ask as many relevant individuals as possible to complete these questionnaires to provide a representative spread of clinical opinion. An overall distribution of anticipated results can be obtained by averaging the percentages allocated to each of the effect-size categories; often this will form a symmetrical distribution of which the mean or median is a reasonable guess at the typical likely difference. Figure 5.6 shows the summary distribution of responses to the question posed with respect to the CHART bronchus trial; here the median difference was approximately 10 per cent.

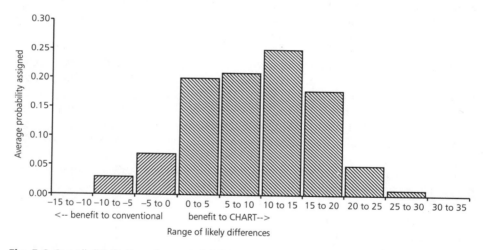

Fig. 5.6 Overall distribution of expected differences – CHART bronchus trial.

B. Worthwhile difference questionnaire

Here a different question is posed; ignoring what differences may be likely, we aim to elucidate the types of differences that, if observed, would be likely to change that clinician's practice. Using the CHART bronchus trial as an example again, we ask the following questions:

Suppose the result of the trial is known with absolute certainty. What is the largest difference in 2-year survival that would lead you to continue with conventional radio-therapy (CRT) as standard treatment? What is the smallest difference that would lead you to adopt CHART?

The clinician is then asked to mark these two points on a diagram, as shown in Fig. 5.7, beginning with a hypothetical example.

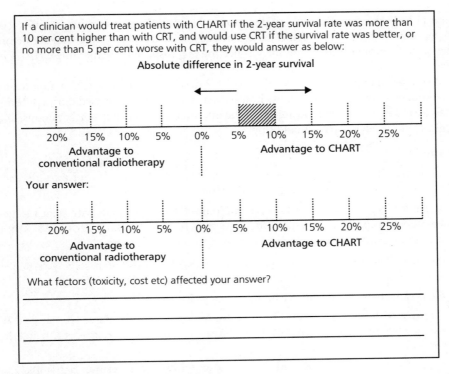

If a clinician would treat patients with CHART if the 2-year survival rate was more than 10 per cent higher than with CRT, and would use CRT if the survival rate was better, or no more than 5 per cent worse with CRT, they would answer as below:

Absolute difference in 2-year survival

20% 15% 10% 5% 0% 5% 10% 15% 20% 25%

Advantage to
conventional radiotherapy

Advantage to CHART

Your answer:

20% 15% 10% 5% 0% 5% 10% 15% 20% 25%

Advantage to
conventional radiotherapy

Advantage to CHART

What factors (toxicity, cost etc) affected your answer?

Fig. 5.7 'Worthwhile difference' questionnaire.

While some clinicians will give a single decision point, most will indicate two. Between these points is what is known as the 'range of equivalence.' Outside this range the clinician is reasonably certain that s/he would consider one or other treatment as standard. Within the range the decision is not so clear-cut and would probably depend on balancing a number of factors.

'Worthwhile' differences can be summarized by taking the average left-hand side end, and the average right-hand side end of the ranges of equivalence to produce a single range. In the CHART bronchus trial, the average range was 11–14 per cent. However, it can also be useful (see example 1 below) to view the ranges individually.

How do you use the answers to both questionnaires?

The ideal trial will be designed to detect reliably the smallest difference identified by these summaries. However, discussion of the questionnaire results with potential collaborators should inform the decision as compromises will often have to be made; these are discussed towards the end of this chapter. Even so, using such an approach has a number of benefits. The questionnaires involve the potential participants much more closely in the determination of sample size, a process which often does not get as much thought as it deserves. Equally importantly, they enable the person determining the sample size to understand the degree of clinical uncertainty prevalent and where appropriate, build this into the sample size calculation. In the CHART example above, the median 'expected difference' was 10 per cent, the average range of equivalence ranged from 11 to 14 per cent; the trial was designed to detect an absolute increase in survival of 10 per cent. In this case, the clinicians demanded a substantial benefit to CHART before they would consider using it routinely, reflecting the 'costs' of implementing CHART in practice.

These questionnaires can be useful not only in designing trials, but also in monitoring their progress. Reference [10] shows how data such as these can be used during interim analyses to help determine the impact of the interim results on clinicians' opinions, and hence to guide when a trial should stop.

Examples

To illustrate some of the issues that can arise in determining the appropriate difference a trial should target, we consider two further trials as case studies.

Example 1: Design of TE18. TE18 was a randomized trial in patients with stage I testicular seminoma conducted by the MRC Testicular Tumour Working Party [11]. At the time of its design, the following pertinent information was known:

- the disease is rare; approximately 500 men are diagnosed with stage I testicular seminoma every year in the UK (approximately 1 per 100,000 population);
- the average patient age is approximately thirty-seven years;
- if untreated following surgery (orchidectomy) alone, approximately 20 per cent of patients will have a recurrence of their disease, with the most common site being the abdominal lymph nodes;
- treatment of recurrence depends on the extent of disease at relapse, but is likely to need several months of chemotherapy;
- currently, we are not able to predict reliably which patients will relapse, and follow-up is intensive and prolonged (up to ten years) in order that relapses are detected at an early stage;
- only one randomized trial had ever been attempted.

For these reasons, to prevent recurrence, standard treatment in the UK and much of Europe was radiotherapy for all patients following surgery. Concerning radiotherapy, the following additional points of relevance were known:

- the 'standard' dose has evolved over time, and differs across Europe – in the UK a dose of 30 Gy given in fifteen treatment fractions over three weeks was fairly standard;
- this is very effective – around 97 per cent of patients will be relapse-free at three years;
- it is also associated with some morbidity – nausea/vomiting and diarrhoea during treatment, peptic ulceration in some patients, prolonged lethargy which can delay return to work for several months, reduced fertility – sperm counts can be reduced to minimal levels for up to two years after treatment and may never recover – and finally a small but definite risk of treatment-induced second cancers.

A policy of adjuvant treatment for all, though effective, would therefore mean that around 80 per cent of patients receive unnecessary treatment, as they were never destined to relapse. This implies that minimizing treatment (and thus side effects) without compromising efficacy is a worthwhile target for a randomized trial. A dose of 20 Gy in ten fractions was chosen as the comparison – a dose that was considered low enough to impact on morbidity, but for which there was reasonable (though non-randomized) data to suggest it may be 'safe' with respect to relapse rates.

The question to address was, would a small increase in relapse rates be an acceptable trade-off for all patients having fewer side effects? To ascertain clinical opinion the questionnaire described above was employed to identify what differences in relapse rate would lead potential participants in the trial (and 'consumers' of the results) to switch from one treatment to another. The results of the questionnaires are shown in Fig. 5.8. Here, points lying to the left of the left-hand side arrows indicate the point at which each clinician would definitely use 30 Gy as standard treatment; points to the right of the right-hand side arrows indicate the point at which each clinician would definitely use 20 Gy. In between are the individual ranges of equivalence. This is an equivalence, or more specifically a non-inferiority trial, where the aim was to show that the difference in relapse rates associated with these two schedules lay within an 'acceptable range.' The data shown in Fig. 5.8 were used to deduce what was an acceptable range. It was hoped that the trial result would show a confidence interval centered close to zero (no difference) and with sufficient patients to ensure, ideally, that the whole confidence interval would lie to the right of the majority of right-hand side arrows (so all plausible differences would still lead clinicians to use 20 Gy). Such an outcome is represented by confidence interval A in Fig. 5.8. This though required several thousand patients, an impossible target for a disease this rare. A reasonable fall-back position is a confidence interval lying to the right of the majority of the left-hand side arrows – so all plausible differences are less than that which would lead clinicians to use 30 Gy as standard (confidence interval B).

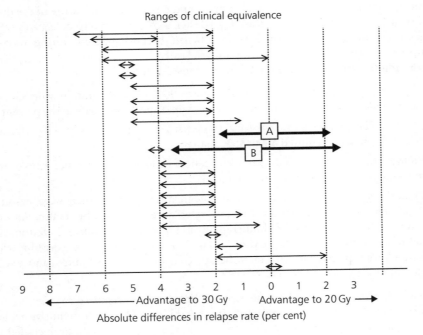

Ranges of clinical equivalence

Advantage to 30 Gy   Advantage to 20 Gy

Absolute differences in relapse rate (per cent)

Fig. 5.8 Proposed stage I seminoma trial.

These considerations led to the need to exclude differences of 3–4 per cent, which in turn required a sample size of between 600 and 1000 patients. This was the aim of the trial.

Example 2: Design of AXIS (Adjuvant Xray and 5FU Infusion Study). In contrast, AXIS was a trial in colorectal cancer, which is second in incidence only to lung cancer in the UK. It was designed in the late 1980s when many trials of adjuvant radiotherapy and of chemotherapy had been performed, but few trials had involved more than a few hundred patients and results were conflicting.

As previous, relevant trials were available, the likely treatment effect in AXIS was estimated by a meta-analysis of previous trials of radiotherapy, and of different chemotherapy regimens [12]. From these the following was concluded:

- Portal vein infusion of fluorouracil (PVI) appeared promising (estimated absolute survival improvement 10–15 per cent) but many previous trials were flawed in their analysis and may have over-estimated the treatment effect. In addition, only 1500 patients had been treated in randomized trials.
- PVI involves one week of chemotherapy given when patients would usually remain in hospital recovering from surgery – it is fairly easy and cheap to administer and the incidence of serious side effects appeared very low. It was therefore potentially a widely applicable treatment and one for which small survival benefits could be very important.
- PVI could be given to both colon and rectal cancer patients.

Based on the results of the previous trials, therefore, the 'likely' difference was large, if flaws in previous trials were ignored, but the size of difference that could be considered clinically worthwhile was much smaller at around 5 per cent. The nature of the disease and treatment meant that it was feasible to design a trial powered to detect this smaller difference; if unequivocal evidence of larger benefit became apparent during the course of the trial, it would be possible to stop the trial early.

For radiotherapy, there were the following considerations.

- There was much more data on radiotherapy (~9000 patients), but the schedules used varied widely and many would be considered inadequate or unsafe in the present day.
- The overall estimate of absolute survival benefit was approximately 4–5 per cent. To detect this reliably required 4000–6000 patients.
- Radiotherapy can be given only to rectal cancer patients; the incidence ratio of colon to rectal cancer is approximately 60 : 40.
- Radiotherapy was already becoming routine treatment because there were reasonably strong data to suggest that local relapse rates were decreased by its use. Although it was not clear if deferred radiotherapy would be any less effective than immediate radiotherapy with respect to survival, it was clear that the number of surgeons willing to randomize patients to a no-radiotherapy control group was limited, and a 4000+ patient target was not felt to be feasible.

Instead therefore, the overall sample size was based on that required for the PVI comparison, namely 4000 patients, with the aim that this should provide definitive evidence for or against the treatment. A radiotherapy randomization would be included in a factorial design for rectal cancer patients; as we could not produce definitive evidence from this trial alone, the aim was to randomize a minimum of 1000 patients (sufficient to detect a 10 per cent survival improvement) thereby contributing a reasonably substantial amount of additional data to the worldwide evidence, and with the aim of contributing to a formal meta-analysis at the end of the trial.

5.3.5 Allocation ratios

Most trials allocate equal numbers of patients to each treatment group, and for a given number of patients, maximum statistical power is (generally) obtained by allocating approximately equal numbers of patients to each treatment group.

However, power is only slightly reduced by unequal allocations such as 3:2 and even 2:1 (e.g. two of every three patients randomized will be allocated the experimental treatment), as illustrated in Fig. 5.9. Why might you take advantage of this? There are a number of situations in which allocation ratios other than 1:1 can enhance a trial, as the examples below illustrate.

Restrictions on the number of patients who can be treated in one arm of the trial

This situation can arise when one of the treatments is in short supply, perhaps a drug is only being made available for use in the trial, and the company supplying the drug impose a restriction on the number of patients they will provide free treatment for. This was the situation at an early stage of the ICON3 trial in advanced ovarian cancer, which compared platinum-based therapy with paclitaxel plus carboplatin [13]. At the launch of the trial, paclitaxel was not widely available in the UK and Europe outside a trial setting. Initially, the company funding the trial would only provide free paclitaxel for 200 patients. Allocating equal numbers of patients to the two arms would give a total of only 400 patients which was insufficient to detect even quite large differences in survival. The trial was therefore designed with a 1:2 allocation to paclitaxel and control, enabling 600 patients to be entered into the trial, increasing the power for the comparison. In this

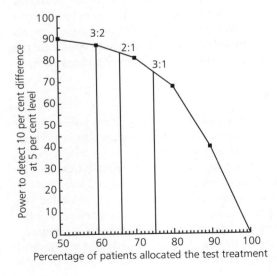

Fig. 5.9 Power according to allocation ratio; control group survival=50 per cent, test group survival=60 per cent.

case, it would theoretically be possible to use an even more extreme ratio, because adding extra patients would always increase the power relative to the smaller size trial. However, in practice there were concerns about the willingness of patients to accept randomization into such a trial, knowing that their chances of being allocated paclitaxel were not 1 : 1 or even 1 : 2 but in fact very much less.

Rare disease

With uncommon diseases, randomized trials are difficult, and inevitably smaller than might be considered ideal. In introducing an experimental treatment in this kind of setting, knowing that there may only be one chance to conduct a randomized trial, unequal randomization can be valuable. For example, in the late 1980s discussions took place about a randomized trial of chemotherapy for primary cerebral lymphoma. Standard treatment for these patients was surgery and radiotherapy and there was considerable experience with this approach. The question of interest was whether adding chemotherapy could improve survival, but there was little experience with the particular chemotherapy regimen of interest in this setting. Here, the total number of patients was limited by the rarity of the disease. However, a 2 : 1 allocation to chemotherapy was employed. This only slightly reduced the overall power of the comparison compared with a 1 : 1 randomization in the same number of patients, but enabled more experience to be gained with the experimental treatment, more data on toxicity, and to obtain a more precise estimate of the survival rates associated with this treatment [14].

Practical considerations

This is perhaps the most common type of situation in which even quite small alterations to the allocation ratio can make participation in the trial much easier, the resulting increase in accrual more than compensating for the slight loss in power associated with moving the allocation ratio away from equality. One example involved the trials of continuous, hyperfractionated accelerated radiotherapy (CHART) in head and neck, and also lung cancer described earlier in this chapter [9]. As CHART is given in multiple daily fractions, without breaks for weekends, patients are treated outside of normal hours and this therefore incurs additional staff costs. It is clearly more cost effective to have several patients ready to treat in succession. In the MRC CHART trials, 3 : 2 randomization was used to increase the number of patients allocated CHART, and therefore increase the chance that participating centres would have several patients to treat simultaneously.

5.4   Calculating sample sizes

Having determined the appropriate error rates, baseline results and target difference to detect, you have all the basic information you need to calculate a sample size, or perhaps more usually to consult appropriate tables or software packages (or statisticians) to do the calculation for you. Readers who are happy to omit the technical details can jump to Section 5.7, which gives some guidance on the use of tables and software and some pitfalls to avoid. It is though useful to have an understanding of the underlying principles for the most common types of outcome measure. We therefore review the basic principles for three common types of data: continuous (normally distributed), binary (i.e. simple proportions) and survival data. In fact, the underlying basis of most sample size calculations (including that for some non-randomized phase II trials) is perhaps best illustrated in the case of continuous data. Section 5.4.1 therefore explains the background in some detail, and sample size issues for phase II studies are described in Section 5.4.5.

5.4.1 Continuous data

The Normal distribution

It is common in statistics to make use of probability distributions; these are distributions (shapes) which are specified by a mathematical formula incorporating one or more 'parameters.' Because they are defined mathematically, we know how they behave under different values of the parameters. If we can assume real data are a sample from a distribution which follows, at least approximately, a known theoretical form, then we can infer certain facts about it and indeed we can calculate how likely it is that a given value could have come from that distribution. The most commonly used probability distribution is the Normal or Gaussian distribution which follows the well known bell-shaped curve which is often seen with 'real' data. Technically, the familiar Normal curve is a frequency curve or 'probability density function' (PDF) centred, on the x-axis, around the mean and with the height representing the 'probability density.' The total area under any PDF is always set to equal one, therefore the area under the curve (AUC) to one side of a given x-axis value can be interpreted as the probability of observing a result at least as extreme as that value.

The shape of the Normal curve (Fig. 5.10) is determined entirely by its two parameters, the mean (m) and the standard deviation (SD). Whatever the actual values of the mean and standard deviation, approximately 68 per cent of the area under a Normal curve will lie within the x-axis range defined by the mean $\pm$ one SD, and approximately 95 per cent will lie within the mean $\pm$ 2SD.

The distance of any point on the x-axis from the mean is known as the standard Normal deviate; effectively this is a variable with mean zero and standard deviation one. The Normal distribution with mean zero and SD 1 is called the Standard Normal distribution, and written as $N \sim (0, 1)$. Any normally distributed variable can be transformed into one with a standard Normal distribution by subtracting the mean and dividing by the standard deviation. This is the basis of many hypothesis tests and hence of sample size

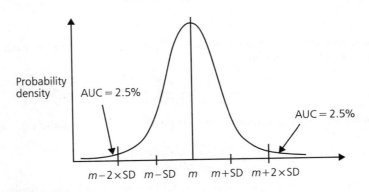

Fig. 5.10 The Normal distribution.

calculations too, as it gives a common reference point whatever the original distribution of the variable. Tables of the Normal distribution are actually of the standard Normal distribution and will tell you, for a given Z (x-axis) value, the proportion of the AUC which lies to one side of the value (these are 1-tailed or 1-sided p-values) or the proportion of the AUC which lies outside the range defined by $\pm Z$ (these are 2-tailed or 2-sided p-values).

The theory underlying sample size calculations using the Normal distribution

Suppose we wish to design a trial in which the main outcome measure is the difference in means of a particular variable in a group receiving standard therapy and a group receiving an experimental therapy. We will assume there will be n patients in each group, that the significance level has been set to be α (one-sided for simplicity) and the power $1 - \beta$. We will also assume that the SD of the distributions from which the two means are calculated is approximately the same, S, hence the SD of the means is $S/\sqrt{n}$. This quantity is referred to as the Standard Error of the mean (SE).

Under the null hypothesis of no difference (H_0), the difference in means ($d = m_1 - m_2$) is assumed to follow a Normal distribution with mean zero and standard deviation

$$S = \text{SD}(m_1 - m_2) = \sqrt{[2 \times (S/\sqrt{n})^2]} = \sqrt{2} \times S/\sqrt{n}.$$

Under the alternative hypothesis (H_1), the difference d is assumed to follow a Normal distribution with mean δ and standard deviation, $\sqrt{2} \times S/\sqrt{n}$, as under the null hypothesis.

To determine the sample size which satisfies both error constraints, we need to find the critical value, D, such that:

$$\text{under } H_0, \qquad p(d < D) = 1 - \alpha,$$
$$\text{under } H_1, \qquad p(d > D) = 1 - \beta.$$

That is,

$$(D - 0)/(\sqrt{2} \times S/\sqrt{n}) = Z_{1-\alpha} \quad \text{therefore } D = Z_{1-\alpha} \times (\sqrt{2} \times S/\sqrt{n}),$$
$$(D - \delta)/(\sqrt{2} \times S/\sqrt{n}) = -Z_{1-\beta} \quad \text{therefore } D \text{ also } = \delta - (Z_{1-\beta} \times (\sqrt{2} \times S/\sqrt{n})).$$

Hence: $Z_{1-\alpha} \times (\sqrt{2} \times S/\sqrt{n}) = \delta - (Z_{1-\beta} \times (\sqrt{2} \times S/\sqrt{n}))$.

This can be rearranged to give the number of patients, n, required in each group to satisfy the defined error rates as

$$n = \frac{2(Z_{1-\alpha} + Z_{1-\beta})^2}{(\delta^2/S^2)}. \tag{5.1}$$

For a 2-sided test, a slight approximation is involved, but the equation can simply be written as

$$n = \frac{2(Z_{1-\alpha/2} + Z_{1-\beta})^2}{(\delta^2/S^2)}. \tag{5.2}$$

The quantity $(Z_{1-\alpha/2} + Z_{1-\beta})^2$ is fundamental to many sample size calculations, and the most commonly used values are given in Table 5.2. In general, in this chapter we

Table 5.2 Value of $(Z_{1-\alpha/2} + Z_{1-\beta})^{2\dagger}$

Significance level (α)		Power ($1 - \beta$)			
2-sided	**1-sided**	**0.80**	**0.85**	**0.90**	**0.95**
0.01	0.005	11.679	13.048	14.879	17.814
0.02	0.01	10.036	11.308	13.017	15.770
0.05	0.025	7.849	8.978	10.507	12.995
0.1	0.05	6.183	7.189	8.564	10.822

$\dagger$ $(Z_{1-\alpha} + Z_{1-\beta})^2$ for one-sided tests.

present sample size formulae in the simplest terms, which will often mean that slight approximations are involved. These should therefore be used only as a rough guide to sample size, and more complete tables or software should be used for final calculations.

Comparing means – an example

Suppose we wish to design a study in which the aim is to compare glomerular filtration rate (GFR) in two groups of ovarian cancer patients, one receiving carboplatin-based chemotherapy and one receiving cisplatin-based therapy. The GFR follows an approximate Normal distribution, and so it would be appropriate to summarize the GFR by the group means, and to compare the groups using a two-sample t-test (see also Section 9.3.3). Assume the GFR in the carboplatin group is 100 ml/min one year after start of chemotherapy. We wish to determine the sample size needed to detect a decrease in GFR of 10 ml/min in the cisplatin group at the same time point. From equation 5.2, we need not only an estimate of the difference in GFR, but also an estimate of the standard deviation in each group (here assumed to be the same). This can be taken from previous data or, as an approximate rule, one can divide the range of possible values of a Normally distributed variable by four to get an estimate of the SD, as 95 per cent of the values are contained in the range mean ±2SD.

Alternatively, it is sometimes easier to think not of the differences of the means and the SD, but of the ratio of the difference in means to the SD. For example, you may wish to detect a difference that is equivalent to half a SD. As the denominator in equation 5.2 is the square of the ratio of the difference in means to the SD, either approach can be taken. In this case, let us assume we are interested in determining whether cisplatin-based therapy decreases GFR at one year by half a SD with 90 per cent power and a 2-sided significance level of 5 per cent. The ratio (δ^2/S^2) then is equal to 0.5^2 and from equation 5.2 and Table 5.2 we see that the number of patients required in each group is $(2 \times 10.507)/0.25 = 84$.

Strictly, when using the two-sample t-test to compare the groups, we need to make an adjustment to equation 5.2 adding an extra term as below as:

$$n = \frac{2(Z_{1-\alpha/2} + Z_{1-\beta})^2}{(\delta^2/S^2)} + \frac{(Z_{1-\alpha/2})^2}{4}. \tag{5.3}$$

This makes a very small difference (for a 5 per cent significance level the additional term is approximately equal to 1) but one which is proportionately bigger for very small studies than for very large studies. It helps us to account for the fact that small samples are less likely to follow a true Normal distribution.

5.4.2 Binary data

Examples of binary data include anything with a yes/no outcome such as response, hence binary data from a group of patients will provide an estimate of the proportion responding. There are several ways in which proportions can be compared. A simple significance test is to use the Pearson chi-square test on data displayed in a contingency table (see Section 9.3.1); alternative methods which lead more naturally to estimates and confidence intervals as well as tests of significance are to compare differences in proportions, or the ratios of proportions (relative risk) or, where appropriate, the odds ratio (the ratio of success to failure in one group divided by the ratio of success to failure in the other).

For the purposes of sample size calculation, we will consider the situation where proportions are to be compared. We define α, β as before and here δ is the difference in proportions, for example $p_2 - p_1$.

An approximate formula for the number of patients required in each group (assuming equal numbers are to be randomized to each group) can be given in a similar form to that for continuous data, namely:

$$N = \frac{(Z_{1-\alpha/2} + Z_{1-\beta})^2 (p_1(1 - p_1) + p_2(1 - p_2))}{\delta^2}. \tag{5.4}$$

Comparing proportions – an example

A randomized trial in advanced colorectal cancer was designed to compare response rates in patients allocated fluorouracil and leucovorin (FUFA), with or without interferon α (IFN). The response rate for FUFA was expected to be approximately 30 per cent, and the study was powered to detect a 20 per cent absolute increase (to 50 per cent) through the use of IFN with 80 per cent power and a 2-sided significance level of 5 per cent. Using equation 5.4 and Table 5.2, the number of patients required in each group was $\{7.849 \times [(0.3 \times 0.7) + (0.5 \times 0.5)]\}/0.2^2 = 91$, i.e. a total sample size of approximately 182 patients.

5.4.3 Survival data

Survival data – or more generally, time-to-event data – in two or more groups will most often be compared using the logrank test (see Section 9.3.4). The method for sample size calculation given here makes certain assumptions and approximations, as have the earlier methods, in particular it assumes 'proportional hazards.' This is discussed further in Chapter 9, but briefly, the hazard is the risk of experiencing an event at a given instant in time. The hazard ratio (HR) is the ratio of this risk in one group divided by the risk in the comparison group. Thus a hazard ratio of 0.8 indicates that the risk of the event in the treatment group is 0.8 of the risk in the control group at a given point in time (i.e. the risk is 20 per cent lower). If we assume proportional hazards, then we assume the hazard ratio is constant over time.

With α and β defined as before, and again assuming equal numbers of patients being allocated to each treatment group, the total number of events (E) needed is given by

$$E = (Z_{1-\alpha/2} + Z_{1-\beta})^2 [(1 + HR)/(1 - HR)]^2. \tag{5.5}$$

In this situation, the proportion of patients who are event-free at a given time in the treatment group (P_2) and control group (P_1) are related to the hazard ratio as follows:

$$HR = \log_e(P_2)/\log_e(P_1). \tag{5.6}$$

Thus, it is only necessary to have estimates of the survival proportions rather than the HR, and indeed most sample size tables offer this option.

The total number of patients (N) required can be derived from this, and is given by

$$N = 2E/(1 - P_2 - P_1). \tag{5.7}$$

It is important to note that these formulae assume that the trial analysis will take place at a minimum time T after the last patient has entered the trial, and also assume that any information obtained after this time is not used in the analysis. Consequently, it slightly over-estimates the total number of patients required, but in general such conservatism is no bad thing. Alternative methods (e.g. [15]) allow one to incorporate estimates of the accrual rate into the sample size calculation hence permitting estimation of the total duration of the trial (accrual and follow-up) required before the required number of events is likely to be observed.

In general, one would of course wish to carry out the definitive analysis of the trial when the majority of events have occurred. The survival rates used to calculate the sample size should be taken from this time T, and should therefore be chosen such that the event rate after this time is low. Graphically, this is generally the point at which survival curves 'level off.'

Comparing survival rates – an example

The AXIS colorectal cancer trial described earlier included a comparison of surgery alone versus surgery followed by portal vein infusion of fluorouracil. A survival rate of 50 per cent at five years after surgery was anticipated in the control group, and a 5 per cent increase in survival through the addition of fluorouracil was the targeted difference. A two-sided significance level of 5 per cent was used, with power of 90 per cent.

Using equation 5.6, the HR corresponding to survival rates of 50% and 55% is

$$\log_e(0.55)/\log_e(0.50) = 0.86.$$

Using equation 5.5, and Table 5.2, the TOTAL number of events to be observed is

$$10.507 \times [(1 + 0.86)/(1 - 0.86)]^2 = 1928.$$

Using equation 5.7, the approximate TOTAL number of patients required is

$$2 \times 1928/(2 - 0.55 - 0.5) = 4060.$$

5.4.4 Non-compliers and drop-outs

It can be useful and important to take account of the fact that some patients may either fail to receive their allocated treatment (non-compliers) or become unassessable for the outcome measure of interest (drop-outs). The impact of these two factors can be very different.

Drop-outs (best avoided by careful choice of outcome measure – see Section 5.2) do not contribute to the outcome assessment, and need to be replaced by an equal number of patients who will contribute, in order for the final analysis to retain the power of the original design. If a drop-out rate R is anticipated, and sample size calculations, assuming no drop-out, suggest a total of N patients, the required sample size is simply $N^* = N/(1 - R)$. Thus for example if a 10 per cent drop-out rate is assumed in a trial of 200 patients, you would aim to enter $200/(1 - 0.1) = 222$ patients. Strictly, this is an approximation, as it assumes that drop-out is unrelated to prognosis. A patient at above average risk of the event of interest is more 'informative' than a patient with a below average risk of the event. Thus if higher risk patients are more likely to drop-out this will slightly underestimate the required sample size, if lower risk patients are more likely to drop-out, it will slightly overestimate the required sample size.

A very different issue arises when patients withdraw from treatment but remain assessable for the primary outcome measure. It will generally be appropriate to analyse patients according to their allocated treatment group, whether or not they received their allocated treatment (i.e. intention to treat analysis – see Section 9.4.1). In this situation, simply 'replacing' the non-compliers does not suffice, and the sample size actually needs to be increased by a similar means to that described in Section 4.3.2. The exact form of the calculation will depend on the treatment actually received by non-compliers (the calculation in Section 4.3.2 assumes cross over to the 'other' treatment), the likely response to that treatment and, as above, on assumptions about the prognosis of the non-compliant patients. Because of the unpredictable nature of many of these assumptions, it is rare to see the impact of non-compliance formally assessed in trial sample size calculations, but common to see sample sizes adjusted as for drop-out. This is at least tending in the right direction, but as demonstrated in Section 4.3.2, a 10 per cent withdrawal rate may require a compensatory increase in sample size of over 50 per cent. Therefore where non-compliance rates are likely to be non-negligible, it can be important to consider, and attempt to take account of, the potential impact on sample size.

5.4.5 Phase II trials

In Chapter 4, three widely used phase II trial designs were described. Here we explain the background to the sample size calculations necessary to use these designs.

Fleming's single stage design [16]

Here we assume that for any experimental treatment, there will be a level of response, p_1, below which the treatment would not be considered for further study, and a higher level, p_2, above which the treatment would certainly warrant further investigation. The sample size is determined by the need to minimize the probability of concluding that the response rate is greater than p_1 when that is false (α) and to minimize the probability (β) of concluding that the response rate is less than p_2 when that too is false. This is analogous to the comparison of proportions described in Section 5.4.2, but here we consider one of the proportions effectively to be fixed. As we do not need to allow for uncertainty in the estimation of one of the proportions, the sample size is considerably smaller (approximately one quarter) than the sample size for comparing two parallel groups.

$$N = \frac{\{Z_{1-\alpha}\sqrt{[P_1(1 - P_1)]} + Z_{1-\beta}\sqrt{[P_2(1 - P_2)]}\}^2}{(P_2 - P_1)^2}. \tag{5.8}$$

An example of a trial designed in this way is given in Box 5.1.

Gehan's two-stage design [17]

In the first stage, a minimum useful level of efficacy (p_m) is determined, for example a 25 per cent response rate, and a maximum acceptable probability (α) of rejecting the treatment if it is truly as, or more, effective than p_m, for example 5 per cent. The probability of seeing n_1 consecutive failures given a true response rate p, where p is greater than or equal to (p_m) is $(1 - p_m)^{n_1}$. The number of patients studied in the first stage is therefore the value of n_1 which satisfies $(1 - P_m)^{n_1} < \alpha$. For example, if the true response rate p is 0.25, then the probability of eleven consecutive failures is $(1 - 0.25)^{11} = 0.04$. Therefore, if you observed eleven consecutive failures, then the trial could stop at this point with the conclusion that the treatment is unlikely (a four in 100 chance) to be associated with a response rate of 25 per cent or more. If any responses are seen, the study continues to the second stage, in which the aim is to estimate the response rate with a specified precision.

The sample size for the second phase depends on two things; the true response rate P – which is estimated from the response rate in the 1st stage of the study – and the desired precision, ε (defined by the standard error of the overall study response rate) which must be specified.

Box 5.1 A phase II trial in high risk stage I non-seminomatous germ cell tumours (NSGCT) using Fleming's single stage design

Patients with high risk stage I NSGCT have a 40% risk of relapse within two years of diagnosis if receiving no post-surgical adjuvant treatment. Most high risk patients receive adjuvant chemotherapy, although for 60% of patients this is unnecessary. Interest surrounded the ability of an alternative scanning method, PET scanning, to identify a group of patients (those with a negative PET scan) with a sufficiently low risk of relapse that they could be spared adjuvant chemotherapy. Because of the expense, it is necessary to demonstrate that a PET scan provides a high level of discrimination between groups with a high (PET positive) and low (PET negative) risk of relapse. Amongst the PET −ve patients it was felt that a relapse-free rate of less than 80% would not provide sufficient discrimination, but that a relapse-free rate of 90% or more would. Using Fleming's single stage design, $p_1 = 0.8$ and $p_2 = 0.9$. Setting α to be 0.05 (so $Z_{1-\alpha} = 1.6449$) and β to be 0.1 (so $Z_{1-\beta} = 1.2816$) 109 PET −ve patients are required.

Suppose

ε = standard error of response rate r (the overall study response rate),

$r_1(r_2)$ = number of responses in the 1st (2nd) stage, and

n_1 (n_2) = number of patients in the 1st (2nd) stage,

Then

$$\varepsilon = \sqrt{[r(1 - r)/(n_1 + n_2)]} \quad \text{where } r = (r_1 + r_2)/(n_1 + n_2).$$

This can be rearranged to calculate n_2:

$$n_2[r(1 - r)/\varepsilon^2] - n_1.$$

However, after the first stage we will know only r_1 and thus the overall response rate r must be estimated. r_1/n_1 could be used, but to add a degree of conservatism, Gehan recommended using instead the upper 75 per cent confidence limit r_1/n_1. This can be calculated approximately as:

$$r_1/n_1 + Z_{0.75} \times \text{SE}(r_1/n_1); \quad \text{where } Z_{0.75} = 0.6745 \quad \text{and}$$

$$\text{SE}(r_1/n_1) = \sqrt{\{[r_1/n_1(1 - r_1/n_1)]/n_1\}}.$$

Therefore the overall sample size depends critically on the response rate seen in the first stage of the study; the closer it is to 0.5, the larger the sample size necessary in the second stage to achieve the same precision. An example of a trial designed using Gehan's method is shown in Box 5.2.

Box 5.2 A phase II trial using Gehan's two-stage design

A phase II trial in recurrent malignant glioma aimed to assess the activity of human lymphoblastoid interferon [18]. The minimum useful response rate was considered to be 20%. The minimum number of failures (n) satisfying $(1 - 0.2)^n < 0.05$ is 14. Therefore, the first stage of the trial aimed to include fourteen patients, and would stop after the first stage if no responses were seen, concluding that the probability that the true response rate was at least 20% was less than 5%.

The aim in the second stage was to estimate the response rate with a standard error of no more than 10% (i.e. $\varepsilon = 0.1$). The upper 75% confidence limit is calculated for a range of response rates in the first stage thus, for example:

If, say, five relapses were seen in the first fourteen patients (a response rate of 35.7%), the upper 75% confidence limit would be given by

$$0.357 + 0.6745 \times \sqrt{[0.357 \times (1 - 0.357)/14]} = 0.4435.$$

Therefore,

$$n_2 = [0.4435 \times (1 - 0.4435)/(0.10)^2] - 14 = 10.7 \text{ (round up to 11)}.$$

Therefore, if five responses were seen in the first fourteen patients, an additional eleven patients would be needed to estimate the overall response rate with a standard error of no more than 10%.

The optimal/minimax Simon Design [19]

This design allows either the number of patients in the 1st stage, or the total number of patients to be minimized if the treatment has an inadequate response rate, subject to specification of the error rates. The former is known as the optimal design, the latter as the minimax design. As for the Fleming single-stage design, this requires specification of an unacceptable level of activity (p_1) and an activity level above which there would be interest in taking the treatment forward for further testing (p_2).

The sample size formulae for this design are not straightforward, and therefore we refer readers to tables such as those by Machin *et al.* [20] for further details. An example of how the Simon design was used in the design of a randomized phase II/III trial in metastatic germ cell cancer is shown in Box 5.3.

Box 5.3   Use of a two-stage optimal Simon design in a randomized phase II/III trial

Standard chemotherapy for metastatic germ cell cancer is the BEP (bleomycin, etoposide, cisplatin) combination. A phase I study suggested high activity levels if the drug paclitaxel was added to this regimen [21]. As this was a relatively rare group of patients, an efficient design was chosen to enable a combined phase II/III design to be carried out. Patients were to be randomized between BEP and paclitaxel-BEP (T-BEP) in several stages. The number of patients in the first two stages was determined using an optimal Simon two-stage design with complete response (CR) rate as the primary outcome measure. The expected CR rate with BEP in this group of patients was 65% (P_1). The minimum activity level of interest for T-BEP was 80% (P_2). With $\alpha = 0.1$ and $\beta = 0.05$, the first step required forty-two patients in the T-BEP arm (an equal number were to be randomized to the BEP arm). If fewer than twenty-nine patients on T-BEP achieve a CR, the trial would stop. Otherwise it would continue until there were eighty-two patients on the T-BEP arm (again randomizing an equal number to BEP). If fewer than fifty-nine patients on T-BEP achieve a CR, the trial would stop. Otherwise, it would continue as a phase III trial to which all the patients randomized so far would also contribute. The primary outcome measure of the phase III trial would be progression-free survival, and it would be powered to detect a 10% increase in progression-free survival.

5.5   The perfect and the practicable

Although careful thought, and a good deal of 'science,' must go into deliberations about sample size, it must be recognized that the final choice of sample size almost always involves compromise between what is ideal and what is practicable.

Therefore, it is important to try to anticipate the likely accrual rates and hence the time the trial will need to run if your ideal sample size is to be achieved.

Sources of information, in decreasing order of value include:

- rate of patient accrual in previous trials in the same disease,
- survey of potential participants,
- estimate of approximate number of eligible patients from national incidence rates.

It must be borne in mind that the latter 2 sources tend to over-estimate the number of patients available and should be considered extremely conservatively. While data on the number of patients with a given diagnosis seen annually might be reliable, it is often difficult to determine what proportion would satisfy the eligibility criteria, what proportion would consent to enter a study and what proportion might be lost through time pressures or other factors meaning they are never approached about the trial.

Estimating the rate of accrual is only one part of the equation. The total time to consider is that from the launch of the trial to the first publication of mature results. It is therefore important to consider the trial outcome measures, and to bear in mind that if the primary outcome measure is survival time, a period of follow-up will generally be required after entry of the last patient before the trial can be analysed definitively. As previously noted, this is because the important factor in survival studies is not the number of patients but the number of events.

Is this timeframe reasonable?

Some helpful points to consider are the following:

- How common is the condition? Remember that in the last forty years only a small proportion of cancer trials have accrued more than 5 per cent of the incident population (diseases treated in specialist centres are an exception).
- How long will enthusiasm for the trial continue – are other treatments 'in the pipeline'? If the trial is asking a fundamental question, or new treatments are at a very early stage of development, a long accrual time may not be a problem. If the answer is likely to be as important at the end of the trial as when you started, it is worth persevering.

What if the accrual period seems unreasonably long?

There are some options that should be considered before the trial is abandoned.

- Can the accrual rate be increased without altering the design of the study?
  Consider whether the number of participating centres can be increased either nationally or internationally, if not by participating in the same, centrally organized, trial then perhaps through running parallel trials with a formal agreement to combine the data for the primary analysis.
- Can the number of potentially eligible patients be increased?
  This implies considering whether any of the eligibility criteria (relating to both patients and perhaps clinicians) can be relaxed in such a way as to increase the number of patients who would potentially be suitable for inclusion in the trial without compromising its aims. Section 4.2.3 discusses the essential features of eligibility criteria.

◆ Can any of the 'inputs' to the sample size calculation be reconsidered?
This is perhaps the least attractive option. If the size of difference the trial is powered to detect is the result of careful assessment and broad discussion, then it is hard to see how this component could be changed. However, if the error rates had been chosen to be particularly stringent, there may be scope to relax these somewhat, accepting lower power for a more rapidly completed trial for example. For survival studies, remember that there are two ways to get a given number of events; a large trial with short follow-up or a smaller trial with longer follow-up. However, one must consider if, for this disease and these treatments, early results will necessarily reflect those which would emerge with longer follow-up.

If the answer to these 3 questions is no, should the trial be abandoned? If the only option appears to be a smaller trial than is ideal – is it worth doing? One can argue that any randomized evidence is better than haphazardly treating patients, but to embark on a trial which has no hope of providing useful information is wasteful of effort and resources, and unfair to patients who consent to be in a trial which they believe will truly help future patients if not themselves.

As a general rule, however, the trial may be worth pursuing provided:

◆ It will contribute new information, or add substantially to existing data.

◆ The limitations of the study resulting from its size are made clear in both the protocol and publications.

◆ It is registered so that, even if it is never published, the trial can be identified and perhaps used in systematic reviews and meta-analyses.

5.6 Changing sample sizes mid-trial

No matter how carefully a target difference to detect is determined, and the sample size calculated, it may be the case that changes need to be considered once the trial is in progress. There are two main reasons for this, summarized in Box 5.4. Firstly, clear

---

Box 5.4 Possible factors motivating a change in sample size mid-trial

Changing input factors

◆ Changes in the anticipated control group outcome

◆ Changes in the anticipated treatment compliance rates

◆ Changing opinions as to the appropriate differences to target

Increasing accrual rates

May allow a larger sample size in order to:

◆ Increase power to detect the same target difference

◆ Permit smaller target differences to be detected reliably

changes to one or more of the 'input' factors; these may result from a lack of good data to design the trial originally, or emerging data from other sources. Secondly, substantially higher accrual rates which make larger trials feasible.

As discussed elsewhere in this chapter, all the possible changes to the 'input factors' have the potential to change the necessary sample size. It is therefore useful to assess periodically how well the original assumptions made with respect to these factors are holding up. Importantly, all can be assessed without revealing comparative outcome data. In general, there are few problems with adjusting sample sizes provided the decision is independent of the current trial results. Decisions which are conditional on, or even marginally influenced by, the current data can be problematic. Thus, although it might seem appropriate to seek the advice of the trial's independent data monitoring and ethics committee (DMEC, see Section 8.10), if one exists, it will generally be better for the decision to be made by an independent group. For example, a DMEC may be reluctant to recommend a major increase to a trial's sample size (with the practical and funding implications that may have) if they are aware that the results are tending to suggest early closure is likely. The DMEC must however be made aware of any changes to the trial design and must, at their next meeting, perform their usual functions and make their usual recommendations with reference to the amended design.

A slightly different issue is raised when accrual rates are better than anticipated, and make larger trials feasible. As discussed in Section 5.5, compromises are often necessary in determining the size of trial to be conducted, and it is not unusual for a trial to be launched which has lower than ideal power for the size of difference which is likely and/or clinically important. If the sample size is increased under these circumstances, it is important that it is done with a specific target in mind, not simply because 'more patients are always better.' Thus for example, it is simple to calculate how many additional patients would be required to provide 90 per cent power rather than 80 per cent power to detect the same treatment difference, and to set a revised sample size in the light of this. Equally, it is possible to recalculate the sample size based on wishing to detect a smaller difference than originally specified. However, in this case it is important that such a change is discussed, and that the decision is made because a smaller difference is genuinely of clinical interest, not simply because it is 'do-able.' It is much more straightforward to make this kind of decision if the original trial protocol details the range of treatment differences which are clinically relevant, even if for practical reasons the trial is planned with a sample size which is less than that required to detect the smallest of these. Again, it is important that decisions about changing sample size in these circumstances are made independently of the accumulating data, but that the DMEC are informed and can advise on the continuation of the trial in the light of these changes at their subsequent meetings.

5.7 Sample size tables and software

Many papers, books and statistical packages present tables, nomograms or software for calculating sample sizes for the most common types of data; for example Machin et al. [20] present sample size formulae and tables for a range of common trial designs and outcome measures. Software is to be preferred for final calculations, particularly for very low or high event rates, since tables cannot cover every eventuality although they are fine for a quick check to get a ball park figure and give an immediate impression of the impact of changing some of the 'input factors.' The widespread availability of sample size software is on the whole a good thing, but anyone inexperienced in its use can make some potentially serious mistakes. Thus, rather than give a summary of the availability of software in what is a rapidly moving field, we describe some features to be aware of and some of the most common pitfalls; these are most evident for time-to-event data.

General potential pitfalls

1. Does your table/software generate the number of patients required in total (assuming a 2-arm trial) or does it give the number per arm? For example, Freedman [22] provided the first tables for calculating sample sizes when two event-free curves are to be compared using the logrank test. These indicate the *total* number of patients required in a 2-arm study. Machin *et al.* [20] in their book of tables for sample size calculations include their versions of these tables, but have chosen to give the number of patients required *per arm*. Without care, you may derive a sample size that is half, or double the actual number of patients required.

2. Do you need to provide actual anticipated results in each group (under the alternative hypothesis), or the control group result and the estimated difference? Using the same examples above, Freedman's tables are displayed in a cross-tabulated form, with the control group event-free rate (p_1) defining the rows, and the difference anticipated between this and the experimental arm rate i.e. $p_1 - p_2$ defining the columns. Others show p_2 across the columns. Mix the two up, and instead of finding, correctly, that to detect a survival increase from 20 per cent in one group to 30 per cent in the other requires around 500 patients, you may derive the figure eighty-five patients, the number required to detect a 30 per cent increase from 20 to 50 per cent.

3. Many packages allow one to specify a withdrawal rate, but it is important to note exactly what is meant by the term. In Section 5.4.4 we distinguish between what we refer to as non-compliance and drop-out, but either may be referred to by others as withdrawal. In particular, the sample size adjustment made by most sample size packages to account for withdrawal is actually as we describe in Section 5.4.4 for drop-out, i.e. it assumes withdrawals are not assessable for the outcome measure of interest and simply need to be replaced by an equal number of assessable patients. As noted in Section 5.4.4, adjustment for patients who withdraw from treatment but remain assessable for the outcome measure of interest requires a different approach.

Potential pitfalls specific to time-to-event data

1. There are two specific pitfalls when considering time-to-event data. Firstly, remember that almost invariably you will be required to enter the *event-free* rate, e.g. survival rate, and not the *event rate*, e.g. death rate since the logrank test is based on comparing event-free rates. This too can have a major impact on the estimated sample size, particular when the control group has a very high or very low event rate. Suppose you wished to determine the sample size necessary to detect a 10 per cent improvement in local recurrence rate, reducing it from 20 to 10 per cent. Entering these figures into standard packages for sample size calculation will generate a figure of 322 patients in total (90 per cent power, 5 per cent significance level). If instead you entered them correctly, as 80 and 90 per cent, the required number is actually 450.

2. The second thing to be aware of is whether the tables or software generate the number of patients required, or the number of events. Clearly these can be very different. It

Box 5.5 Desirable features of sample size software for time-to-event data

◆ Formulae are based on published methods
◆ Will derive both number of events and number of patients required
◆ Allows incorporation of estimates of accrual rates and follow-up periods
◆ Allows for unequal randomization
◆ Allows for differential drop-out and/or withdrawal rates across arms

is important to know both, and the provision of both is a good feature to look for in purchasing books or software. Other important features to look out for in software to calculate sample sizes for time-to-event studies are shown in Box 5.5.

5.8 Conclusions

Determining the appropriate sample size is perhaps the most important design decision for a randomized trial. It is therefore wise to consult a statistician for advice at an early stage, not only to check that software has been used correctly, but also to advise on whether there might be helpful modifications that can be made to the basic design including, for example, unequal randomization. A good statistician – particularly one with experience in the disease area – should also, with the best of intentions, challenge the assumptions that have been made to ensure that the study design is robust to variations in these assumptions.

References

[1] Whitehead, J. (1997) *The Design and Analysis of Sequential Clinical Trials* (2nd edition). John Wiley, Chichester.

[2] Ellenberg, S.S., and Hamiton, J.M. (1989) Surrogate endpoints in clinical trials: cancer. *Statistics in Medicine*, **8**, 405–13.

[3] Prentice, R.L. (1989) Surrogate endpoints in clinical trials: definition and operational criteria. *Statistics in Medicine*, **8**, 431–40.

[4] Buyse, M., Thirion, P., Carlson, R.W., Burzykowski, T., Molenberghs, G., and Piedbois, P. (2000) Relation between tumour response to first-line chemotherapy and survival in advanced colorectal cancer: a meta-analysis. *Lancet*, **356**(9227), 373–8.

[5] Fleming, T.R. (1994) Surrogate markers in AIDS and cancer trials. *Statistics in Medicine*, **13**, 1423–35.

[6] Karim, A.B.M.F., Afra, D., Cornu, P., Bleehen, N.M., Schraub, S., de Witte, O., Darcel, F., Stenning, S., Pierart, M., and Van Glabbeke, M. (2002) A randomized trial on the efficacy of radiotherapy for cerebral low-grade glioma in the adult: EORTC study 22845 with MRC study BR04 an interim analysis. *International Journal of Radiation Oncology Biology Physics*, **52**(2), 316–24.

[7] Freedman, L.S. (1989) The size of clinical trials in cancer-research – what are the current needs. *British Journal of Cancer*, **59**(3), 396–400.

[8] Freedman, L.S., and Speigelhalter, D.J. (1983) The assessment of subjective opinon and its use in relation to stopping rules for clinical trials. *The Statistician*, 32, 153–60.

[9] Saunders, M., Dische, S., Barrett, A., Harvey, A., Gibson, D., and Parmar, M. (1997) Continuous hyperfractionated accelerated radiotherapy (CHART) versus conventional radiotherapy in non-small-cell lung cancer: A randomized multicentre trial. *Lancet*, 350(9072), 161–5.

[10] Parmar, M.K.B., Griffiths, G.O., Spiegelhalter, D.J., Souhami, R.L., Altman, D.G., and der Scheuren, E. (2001) Monitoring of large randomized clinical trials: a new approach with Bayesian methods. *Lancet*, 358(9279), 375–81.

[11] Jones, W.G., Fossa, S.D., Mead, G.M., Roberts, J.T., Sokal, M., Naylor, S., and Stenning, S.P. (2001) A randomized trial of two radiotherapy schedules in the adjuvant treatment of stage I seminoma (MRC TE18). *European Journal of Cancer*, 37(supp 6) abstract 572, S157.

[12] Gray, R., James, R., Mossman, J., and Stenning, S.P. (1991) Guest editorial: AXIS – A suitable case for treatment. *British Journal of Cancer*, 63, 841–5.

[13] The International Collaborative Ovarian Neoplasm (ICON) Group. (2002) Paclitaxel plus carboplatin versus standard chemotherapy with either single-agent carboplatin or cyclophosphamide, doxorubicin, and cisplatin in women with ovarian cancer: the ICON3 randomised trial. *Lancet*, 360, 505–15.

[14] Mead, G.M., Bleehen, N.M., Gregor, A., Bullimore, J., Rampling, R., Roberts, J.T., Glaser, M., Lantos, P., Ironside, J.W., Moss, T.H., Brada, M., Whaley, J.B., and Stenning S.P. For the MRC Brain Tumour Working Party. (2000) A Medical Research Council randomized trial in patients with primary cerebral non-Hodgkin lymphoma. *Cancer*, 89(6), 1359–70.

[15] Shih, J.H. (1995) Sample size calculation for complex clinical trials with survival endpoints. *Controlled Clinical Trials*, 16(6), 395–407.

[16] Fleming, T.R. (1982) One sample multiple testing procedure for Phase II clinical trials. *Biometrics*, 38, 143–51.

[17] Gehan, E.A. (1961) The determination of the number of patients required in a preliminary and follow-up trial of a new chemotherapeutic agent. *Journal of Chronic Diseases*, 13, 346–53.

[18] Priestman, T.J., Bleehen, N.M., Rampling, R., Stenning, S.P., Nethersall, A.J., and Scott, J. (1993) A phase II evaluation of human lymphoblastoid interferon (Wellferon) in relapsed high grade malignant glioma. *Clinical Oncology*, 5, 165–8.

[19] Simon, R. (1989) Optimal two-stage designs for phase II clinical trials. *Controlled Clinical Trials*, 10, 1–10.

[20] Machin, D., Campbell, M., Fayers, P., and Pinol, A. (1997) *Sample Size Tables for Clinical Studies* (2nd edition). Blackwell Science Ltd, Oxford, UK.

[21] De Wit, R., Louwerens, M., Mulder de, P.H.M., and Schornagel, J. (1998) A dose finding study of paclitaxel added to fixed doses of BEP in patients with adverse prognosis germ cell carcinoma of unknown primary (CUP). *Proceedings of the American Society of Clinical Oncology*, 17, 322.

[22] Freedman, L.S. (1982) Tables of the number of patients required in clinical trials using the logrank test. *Statistics in Medicine*, 1, 121–9.

Chapter 6

Quality of life in clinical trials

6.1 Introduction

In recent years, progress in extending survival in most common cancers has mainly been achieved in small incremental steps. In this situation, other outcomes such as progression-free survival, response rates, toxicity, treatment-related deaths, cost, and particularly quality of life (QL), can help determine whether new treatments should, or should not, be pursued. There is therefore an increasing demand that cancer treatments be assessed in the wider framework of the balance between all the benefits and risks so that patients and their clinicians can make individual informed decisions.

As a consequence, from being a somewhat neglected area, QL has become a widely researched area and it could be argued that, at least in the context of clinical trials, it has become somewhat overused. The increase in interest can be gauged from the fact that the average number of papers per year with 'Quality of Life' in their title in the 1970s was sixteen, in the 1980s it rose to eighty-five, and in the 1990s there were over 400. It seems that it is now almost obligatory to include an assessment of QL into every new clinical trial. Indeed the pressure is so strong from all parties, including patients, ethics committees, sponsors, and journal editors, that it may sometimes appear difficult and potentially risky to leave it out, even though the trial may not demand it. A decision not to include QL in a trial can all too easily be interpreted as 'we don't care about patients' QL.' However, the result appears to be that many trials simply bolt on an assessment of QL, without considering whether it has the potential to influence decisions. This results in the collection of huge quantities of largely irrelevant data, the use of considerable resource, overburdening of patients, and a trawl through the data for data-dependent results. Consequently, although QL has often been used as supporting evidence for or against a regimen, in only a small proportion of the trials in which QL has been collected has it played the major role in interpreting the results of a trial.

Investigators therefore need to consider carefully the basis for including QL in their trial, and specifically whether including QL is important for the outcome of the trial. In this chapter we place a lot of emphasis on the importance of defining a QL hypothesis. Such a hypothesis can be generated by clinicians, nurses, patients, or combinations of these groups. A pre-specified hypothesis provides a focus for what aspects of QL, if any, should be measured in a trial.

It could be argued that QL is not particularly relevant in many cancer trials, given the evidence that most patients will accept any reasonable toxicity and a consequent reduction in their quality of life for an increased chance of cure. Indeed Slevin *et al.* [1] showed that patients would accept an intensive treatment (with a considerable number of side-effects and drawbacks such as nausea, vomiting, hair loss, frequent use of needles and drips, 3–4 days per month in hospital, decreased sexual interest and possible infertility) if there was even a 1 per cent chance of cure. However, when cure is not possible, a decision often needs to be made about giving treatment which may result in a longer survival but poorer QL, or reducing or stopping treatment which may result in a shorter survival but better QL. In reality things are seldom so clear cut, but the American Society of Clinical Oncology (ASCO) guidelines adopted in 1995 stated that 'treatment can be recommended in metastatic cancer even without an improvement in survival, if it improves quality of life' [2].

We propose that, in order for QL to truly take its place as an important outcome, trial designers need to focus on the key questions, collect good data, and agree on standard methods of analysing and presenting the data. The recent upsurge of interest in QL does not necessarily mean that rigorous methods for design and analysis are widely available or applied. For instance, Schumacher *et al.* [3] reviewed reports of clinical trials that had 'Quality of Life' in the title, keyword or abstract. They found that only about a third included a detailed QL evaluation with a validated instrument, and that over 40 per cent appeared to use the term QL merely as a 'catch-phrase.'

Nevertheless, several general and cancer-specific questionnaires have now been painstakingly developed and validated and can be considered as 'standard.' However, for many of the issues associated with fully integrating QL into randomized clinical trials, such as improving compliance, standardizing analyses, and interpreting the QL scores obtained, many questions remain.

The aim of this chapter is to give some guidance as to the appropriate use of QL in cancer clinical trials with particular emphasis on practical issues.

6.2   The rationale behind the assessment of QL in randomized clinical trials in cancer

6.2.1   What is quality of life?

The first recorded use of the phrase 'Quality of Life' was in the 1920s, but it is only in the last thirty years that this phrase has become widely used. However, a clear definition of the term is still elusive.

Everyone is instinctively aware of his or her own level of QL, but it is a vague concept, which is highly individual. The World Health Organization has defined good QL as the absence of disease [4], but this is a one-sided definition that concentrates solely on the negative, and ignores the positive aspects. Calman [5] defined QL as 'the difference between the hopes and expectations of the individual and that individual's present experience.' Perhaps one ideal state of QL therefore might be considered to be an absence of disease plus physical, social, and psychological well being. Whatever definition is used, it is clear that QL is highly personal, and that its key components (lifestyle, relationships, job satisfaction, health, housing, etc.) and the relative importance of these components will differ between individuals. Certainly overall QL can rarely be extrapolated from a single component. Thus we should be wary of statements such as '. . . the quality of patients' lives has improved markedly as evidenced by the rapid reduction and eventual elimination of transfusion requirements and serious infections . . .' [6].

The ultimate aim of cancer treatments is to eradicate, or at least control, the disease and thus extend and improve life. When we measure QL in cancer trials we need to know about both the positive and negative effects of treatment. In general we are interested in 'health-related QL,' the aspects or domains that are likely to be changed by treatment, and also the impact and consequences of treatment and disease on a person's life. Although during cancer treatment an individual's overall QL might improve if, for instance, they win the lottery, this is not something that we expect to be directly related to treatment. Thus the assessment of QL in cancer treatment is usually shorthand for the assessment of health-related QL, and in a sufficiently large randomized trial, 'noise' such as that created by non-treatment-related effects, which may be substantial, should on average be equally distributed between treatment groups.

Health-related QL is complex and, as with overall QL, a single definition of the term remains elusive, although clearly it covers the impact of disease and treatment on physical status (symptoms and toxicity), psychological status (well-being, distress, self-esteem), functional status (self-care, shopping, work) and social functioning (relationships).

The aim of most randomized trials is to provide patients and clinicians with information to make informed treatment decisions, bearing in mind the individually different weighting that patients may attribute to the components of QL. It is therefore important to assess and track changes on all the pre-defined key domains and/or symptoms in order to build up a picture of the relative advantages and disadvantages of each treatment in a way which will be more helpful to future patients.

An example of the value an assessment of QL can add was in a randomized trial of cisplatin and vinblastine plus either hydrazine sulphate (HS) or a placebo for patients with advanced non-small cell lung cancer. Herndon *et al.* [7] reported similar results in terms of survival, response and weight gain. Although patients in the HS group experienced significantly more severe neuropathy this was only one of eighty types of toxicity recorded, and it was therefore felt that this alone did not provide a clear indication of which treatment was better. However, QL analyses revealed worse physical functioning, fatigue, lung-cancer-specific and cancer-specific symptoms for patients in the HS group, and the authors concluded that the QL assessment provided a unique viewpoint from which to compare the treatments.

6.2.2 Why measure QL?

In a survey of oncologists and surgeons specializing in breast cancer, Saunders and Fallowfield [8] found that although they were familiar with some QL measures, most did not routinely use them and believed that QL could be assessed adequately without formal instruments. This suggests that many clinicians appear to believe that it is possible to assess the risks and benefits of treatment in an informal unstructured way. Comments made by the specialists surveyed included the statement that using QL questionnaires was too time consuming, did not add enough to justify the time, and increased patient anxiety.

But how good are clinicians at predicting the QL of their patients? In a situation where an aggressive treatment is being compared with a less-aggressive treatment, many people might predict that the aggressive treatment would cause greater side effects that would outweigh improvements in symptoms and result in a poorer QL. However, when QL has been assessed in a number of such trials, counter-intuitive results have been observed, suggesting that what is predicted by clinicians and researchers is not necessarily what is experienced by patients.

For example, in patients with metastatic breast cancer, chemotherapy is often given every three weeks until disease progression is evident (on average for six months). Such continuous treatment can place an enormous burden on patients. In 1987 Coates *et al.* [9] conducted a randomized trial comparing standard continuous chemotherapy versus intermittent therapy. Patients randomized to intermittent therapy received three cycles of chemotherapy, then stopped and only re-started when there was evidence of disease progression. The expectation was that patients on the intermittent policy would experience an improved QL in the period between completion of three cycles and progression. Patients completed questionnaires covering five aspects of QL and one for overall QL. Comparing the change between the score at the end of three cycles to the average score at each assessment up until progression, showed that all QL outcomes favoured continuous treatment. Thus, in this instance, it is likely that the palliative benefits of the continuous chemotherapy outweighed any side-effects and/or provided a level of reassurance for the patient.

Also in metastatic breast cancer, Tannock *et al.* [10] compared a high-dose chemotherapy regimen with one using half-dose chemotherapy, both given at 3-weekly cycles indefinitely. A subset of forty-nine patients completed questionnaires covering thirty-four aspects of QL. Although the scales confirmed greater toxicity in the high-dose arm, they also showed a trend towards improvement in general health and some disease-related indices with this regimen. Similar counter-intuitive results were seen in trials of planned treatment for small cell lung cancer compared to treatment 'as required,' [11] and, in the same disease, immediate treatment compared to selective palliative treatment [12].

Although several of these trials can be criticized on a number of counts such as small sample sizes, much missing data, and methods of analysis, a number of other studies have also suggested unexpected results (see Ref. [13]). All these results emphasize that it is not always easy to predict the likely impact of treatment on QL.

6.2.3 Who should assess quality of life?

The options for collecting QL lie between the patient themselves and a proxy (the doctor, nurse, or the so-called significant other (spouse, son, daughter, sibling, partner, etc.)) and a number of studies have investigated the differences obtained if the same questions are asked of the patients and a proxy.

Although two studies showed that there was about a 70 per cent complete agreement between patients and proxies in terms of recording the severity of a symptom [14,15], most of the disagreement was a result of proxies consistently under-estimating the severity of symptoms [16]. However, patient/proxy comparisons can only be made on patients who are capable of completing QL forms, whereas the real questions are whether proxies can substitute for patients (a) throughout the trial, or (b) when patients are unable to complete forms (for example if they have cognitive impairment, communication deficiencies, are experiencing severe symptoms, or find the forms physically or emotionally too burdensome).

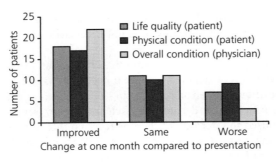

Fig. 6.1 Changes in overall life quality and physical condition related by the patients together with changes in MRC grade for general condition rated by their physicians over one month following radiotherapy (adapted from Regan et al., [18]).

Sprangers and Aaronson [17] reviewed the role of proxies and summarized it as follows:

- health care providers (doctors, nurses, etc.) and significant others (spouses, siblings, etc.) tend to under-estimate (down-grade) the patient's QL,
- health care providers tend to evaluate the patient's QL with a similar level of (in)accuracy as significant others,
- health care providers tend to under-estimate the pain severity of their patients,
- proxy ratings appear to be more accurate when the information sought is concrete and observable (for example physical symptoms rather than psychological distress).

Thus on the surface the role of proxies appears minimal. Nevertheless, although doctors appear to be poor judges of QL, they do seem able to identify improvement or deterioration over time (Fig. 6.1) [18]. Similarly, although Sneeuw et al. [16] showed statistically significant differences between patients and proxies for mean scores in nine of the 15 EORTC QLQ-C30 domains (proxies nearly always reporting worse functioning or increased severity of symptoms), they also showed that data from patients and proxies were equally responsive to change over time. Therefore, if proxies are used throughout the trial to assess QL, similar between-treatment differences can often be observed.

6.2.4 Conditions for patient-completed questionnaires

There may be certain situations where not using proxies would result in insufficient or very incomplete data. An example might be a trial in patients with brain tumours where patients who are deteriorating may become too confused, or otherwise impaired, to complete questionnaires, but the collection of data at this stage in their disease is likely to be very important. This is probably the strongest justification for asking a proxy (for example the spouse or other close relative or friend) to complete questionnaires on behalf of the patient. However, studies have suggested that the magnitude of disagreement between patients and proxies increases with the level of impairment reported by the patient, thus when the need for proxies is most salient, the most unreliable ratings are likely to be obtained. Therefore a better option would be for the patient and the proxy to complete questionnaires in parallel for as long as possible. This would give both a between-treatment comparison based on proxy and patient recording, permit an estimation of the difference between patient and proxy recording, and it might be possible to extrapolate the patient's recording forward when only the proxy was completing the forms [19].

In summary therefore, if proxies are to be used this must be part of the trial design as it is important that proxies are used throughout the trial and not only if and when the patient becomes incapable of completing, or unwilling to complete, the questionnaires themselves.

Thus, although the ideal may be to obtain the patient's own recording of their QL, there may be many practical difficulties, aspects of which may need to be considered before starting the trial.

6.2.5 Response shift

It is useful to address what is actually being measured when discussing changes in QL. As discussed above, Calman [5] defined QL as the difference between expectations and current experience. Thus a small gap between expectations and experience would relate to good QL, and a large gap to poor QL. To improve QL one needs to reduce the gap. However, there are two ways of doing this. Current experience can be improved, by giving a therapy to improve how a person is feeling, or alternatively expectation can be reduced. This does not necessarily mean denying hope but making expectations more realistic. For instance, with increasing age come changes in priorities and goals and although physical activity may decrease, social, emotional and intellectual aspects may improve. Thus, if expectations regarding physical activity are reduced, overall QL may improve even with declining physical health.

Such changes in patients' expectations (in effect, changes in patients' internal standards) may explain the remarkable finding that many studies show that cancer patients do not report themselves to be more anxious, depressed or unhappy than the non-cancer general population. Indeed, Cassileth et al. [20] found that the mean score on the Mental Health Index of the General Well-being Scale for melanoma patients was actually slightly better than for the general public. Another study by the same group [21] noted that patients who had been living with their illness had better mental health scores than those newly diagnosed and explained this as an adaptation or adjustment to their illness. Such findings may be at odds with the external view of doctors, nurses and patients' friends and families.

Changes in patients' internal standards are not solely related to cancer. An extraordinary study by Brickman et al. [22] compared the happiness levels of paralysed victims of road accidents with lottery winners. Although differences were observed the authors state that the accident victims did not appear nearly as unhappy as might have been thought. This adds to previous literature suggesting that poorer, blind or disabled people are not unhappier than the general population [23–27].

Patients who report fewer symptoms or better QL than perhaps might have been expected by external observers are deemed to have under-reported their QL. In cancer, under-reporting may be due to defence mechanisms (denial), adaptation to a changed situation, or social comparison (favourably comparing oneself with others in the same situation), and this generally will result in minimizing the reported change. However, this is not always the case, as when patients improve over time, they can sometimes exaggerate the change, as looking back they consider they were in a worse state. Equally, in the study by Brickman [22], it is particularly interesting that when questioned about 'past happiness' the accident victims rated themselves as being significantly happier in the past, compared to the control group. This therefore may indicate a response shift (i.e. as a result of their accident they have changed their internalized standards).

Response shift, adaptation, and under-reporting are difficult to measure, and the main method of investigating this phenomenon has been the use of the 'thentest' [28], comparing patients' responses at the time with how they recall feeling (for example, comparing QL responses made pre-treatment with a questionnaire given out post-treatment but asking about pre-treatment QL). However, the ability of patients to recall accurately casts doubt on the validity of such methods.

Nevertheless, we have to be very aware that patients' self-reporting, although undoubtedly the best measure of QL available, may not always be as informative as it might initially appear. This is particularly true if we are trying to make statements about changes in QL over time on a particular treatment. Although we need to be aware of response shift, it is less of an issue in randomized trials where the primary comparison is across groups, and can usually be considered as additional 'noise.'

6.3   Implementation of QL into trials

If QL is to make a serious contribution to the evaluation of treatments, scientifically acceptable studies are required [29]. It is vital that all aspects of QL are considered in detail before including the assessment of QL in a trial. The sorts of questions that need to be addressed include: Is it appropriate to include any QL questions in the trial? What QL hypothesis do we need to test? Which questionnaires should we use? When should the questionnaires be administered? What analyses are planned? How will the QL data fit in with the clinical data and how will they be presented?

These are not easy questions, and a number of cancer trials groups such as the European Organization for Research and Treatment of Cancer (EORTC), National Cancer Institute of Canada (NCIC) and the Radiotherapy Oncology Group (RTOG) in the USA have set up QL subcommittees to oversee the systematic inclusion and implementation of QL in their trials.

When such in-house expertise is not available, external expert advice should always be sought as early as possible in the design of a trial to consider all aspects of QL implementation. Indeed it is important that when QL is a key component of a trial, QL expertise is available throughout the trial to advise on monitoring and compliance.

6.3.1   Which trials should include a QL assessment?

Whenever a trial is planned, consideration should be given as to whether it is appropriate or not to include an assessment of QL (see Fig. 6.2). Situations where some aspect of QL assessment may be important are randomized trials in which:

- survival is expected to be similar, but the treatment modalities and/or other aspects such as toxicity, are expected to be very different in the treatment groups under study,
- a small survival benefit is expected with the experimental treatment which may be associated with increased toxicity,
- slightly worse survival is expected with the experimental treatment which may be balanced by substantially less toxicity or greater patient acceptability,
- palliation is the primary outcome measure.

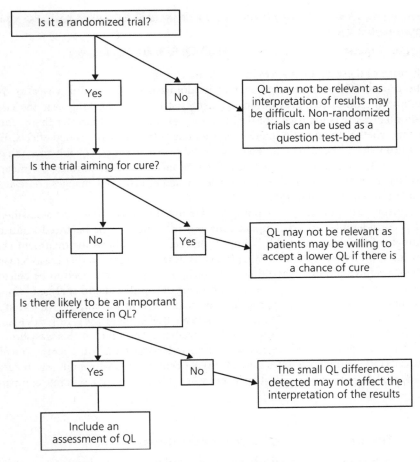

Fig. 6.2 A suggested algorithm for deciding which trials might need QL assessment.

However, these scenarios cover most randomized cancer trials. Indeed, as long ago as 1985, Brinkley, in a BMJ editorial [30], stated 'any evaluation of palliative treatment, especially when included in clinical trials, should always include an assessment of the side-effects and of the general effects on the patients' life'. In addition, a couple of years later, Slevin *et al.* [31] stated 'the question is no longer whether QL should be measured, but what is the most reliable and practical method of obtaining these data.'

A much more pertinent question is perhaps 'What trials do not need QL?' and organizations such as the UK MRC now require justification in trial proposals as to why QL should, or should not, be included [32]. Perhaps the only clear situations in randomized trials where some assessment of QL might not need to be considered is where:

● the survival benefit with a new treatment is expected to be very large,

● both survival and QL are expected to improve,

- patients are likely to accept a chance of cure no matter how much toxicity is increased and/or QL decreased,
- standard therapies are being used in which QL is well documented.

Sadly none of these circumstances in cancer are common.

The case for QL measurement in non-randomized studies is much weaker. Non-randomized studies can provide an excellent test-bed for checking that the correct questionnaires are being used, for deciding the best times to administer them, and for checking whether the questionnaire covers all relevant treatment-related effects. However, the potential biases in patient selection, and response-shift, probably mean that QL should not be used as an outcome measure in non-randomized studies as a means of assessing treatment effect as it may be unclear whether observed changes are related to treatment or patient adaptation.

The theory and practice of including QL are not the same thing. The assessment of QL has considerable resource implications and these need to be balanced against the usefulness of the data and its likely impact on recommendations for treatment choice following completion of the trial [33]. The considerable burden on the research team in terms of resource required should not be overlooked as QL data need to be collected, collated, processed, checked, queried, and missing data pursued and analysed [32].

Whenever it is considered appropriate to include QL in a trial, it is vital that it is seen to be an integral part of the trial and not an afterthought [34]. In particular, the assessment of QL should be written into the protocol. The value of this was shown by Scott *et al.* [35] who reported that in trials conducted by the Radiation Therapy Oncology Group (RTOG) compliance rates were 60–90 per cent in trials where QL was integrated into the trial design, and only 20–40 per cent where QL was run as a separate companion trial.

6.3.2 The importance of setting hypotheses

The easiest way of determining whether it is appropriate to include QL in a trial is to discuss with all relevant parties the likely impact of the treatments on QL and to form a hypothesis about the likely differences to be observed. Such a hypothesis needs to be clinically important, and should relate to the difference that would not only be perceptible by patients but considered sufficient to affect the choice of treatment. Setting the hypothesis for the QL evaluation is as important as setting the principal hypothesis for the trial. If the hypothesis is well framed, this can facilitate the design of the whole of the QL component of the trial, from the choice of questionnaire, to the timing of administration, the sample size required, and the analyses to be performed. Failure to define a hypothesis will mean that the QL aspects of the trial will lack focus, and any results may be open to the accusation of data trawling.

How do we set about defining a hypothesis? The key is deciding what the treatments under study are expected to achieve and how this will impact on QL. For example, a new treatment may be expected to relieve pain better, or may be expected to be more acceptable to patients, or alternatively it may be expected to cause nausea. To find the key, refer to the literature, survey clinicians and/or talk to patients who have had the treatment. A phase II pilot or feasibility study may be the ideal place to clarify these issues.

Groenvold and Fayers [36] suggested that a survey of experienced clinical staff may identify aspects that new treatments should affect. They surveyed doctors and nurses as a method of defining key QL areas in a trial of a combination chemotherapy regimen. Each respondent was asked to predict for each of the subscales and items on all the QL questionnaires to be used, which symptoms would occur more in the combination chemotherapy group, which in the no-treatment group, or those where there would be no difference. Thus, QL hypotheses could be formed around the main predicted differences in treatments.

6.3.3 Identifying key symptoms

The QL assessment typically generates huge amounts of data, and it is therefore important to identify a primary QL outcome, and a few secondary outcomes. Although further analyses are always possible, if they have not been pre-defined they should always be considered as hypothesis generating.

Sometimes a new treatment is specifically aimed at one symptom, and the primary QL outcome can relate to this. For instance, Sur *et al.* [37] tested the effect of sucalfate to palliate radiation oesophagitis, and Marty *et al.* [38] assessed granisetron as an antiemetic in cytostatic-induced emesis. In these situations it is clear that the severity of the key symptom before, possibly during, and after treatment needed to be assessed. In addition it may be useful to assess the effect of these changes on other aspects of patients' lives. For instance, if oesophagitis improves, how does this affect appetite or social functioning?

It may also be important not to focus only on the possible positive aspects of a treatment. Treatment-related adverse effects may also be relevant. For example, in a trial of two thoracic radiotherapy regimens for lung cancer, the key QL outcome might be the duration and severity of dysphagia. In an MRC Lung Cancer Working Party trial [39], patients with non-small cell lung cancer were asked to complete a daily diary card, and the proportion of patients reporting moderate or severe dysphagia was plotted. This suggested that in terms of dysphagia, the shorter radiotherapy schedule (17 Gy in 2f) affected fewer patients and was transient, whereas the longer radiotherapy schedule affected more patients for longer (Fig. 6.3).

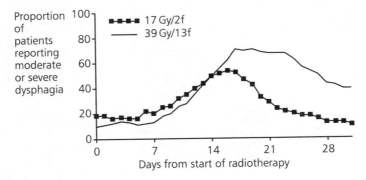

Fig. 6.3 Proportion of patients reporting moderate or severe dyspagia on a daily diary card (adapted from MRC Lung Cancer Working Party, [39]).

Sometimes more than one symptom may be important. For instance, patients may present with a complex mixture of symptoms which the treatment should palliate. In this situation a combination score or an algorithm may be considered. In a trial assessing the value of mitoxantrone and prednisone in twenty-seven patients with hormonally resistant prostate cancer, Moore *et al.* [40] pre-defined a palliative response as: a decrease in analgesic score by ≥50 per cent or a decrease in 'present pain intensity' by ≥2 points without an increase in analgesic score. In this phase II study nine patients were considered 'palliated' using this trial-specific definition, compared with only one who showed a traditional partial response. In an MRC Lung Cancer Working Party trial [41] comparing oral chemotherapy versus standard intravenous chemotherapy in patients with small cell lung cancer, QL was considered to be a primary outcome. In order to be considered 'equivalent' the oral treatment was required 'to achieve at least equivalent palliation of major symptoms (cough, pain, anorexia and shortness of breath) at three months from randomization.' The four scores for these symptoms were added together to get a score at baseline and at three months. Palliation was defined as a reduction in the sum of the scores from baseline to three months (indicating an improvement).

When planning a trial it is crucial to decide what change in QL would represent worthwhile benefit. Burris and Storniolo [42], in a trial of two chemotherapy treatments for pancreatic cancer, created an algorithm (Fig. 6.4) to define worthwhile benefit and to divide their patients into QL responders and non-responders. The algorithm combined pain scores and performance status (PS), with weight change as a tiebreaker if pain and PS were stable. So far, few other groups have used this approach, even though there

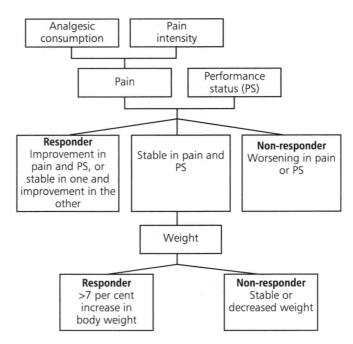

Fig. 6.4 An algorithm to define clinical benefit in a trial of pancreatic cancer (adapted from Burris and Storniolo, [42]).

would be strong arguments for using it in future trials of pancreatic cancer, and for developing standard algorithms for other cancers. Such an approach would also permit cross-trial comparisons.

Before formulating a QL hypothesis, a systematic search of the literature should be performed. This should reveal if any work in that relevant area could be used, as it is generally better to repeat and develop ideas rather than unnecessarily start from the beginning again. However, as so little work has been performed in the field of developing relevant QL hypotheses, the choice of key symptoms or the development of an algorithm will often be unique to the trial.

It would seem that with careful background work in most trials a hypothesis can be formed which directs the QL assessment. This does not mean that other outcomes should be ignored (this situation is analogous to powering a trial for duration of survival but still evaluating response and toxicity), but it does mean that the focus can be on the key QL issues.

6.3.4 Identifying key timepoints

In a paper exploring alternative methods of defining and analysing palliation, Stephens *et al.* [43] demonstrated the impact of assessment timepoint on outcome. Using data from a trial of 4-drug versus 2-drug chemotherapy in SCLC they showed an advantage in terms of palliation of cough in favour of the 4-drug (4D) regimen at one and three months, but in favour of the 2-drug (2D) regimen at two months (Table 6.1).

This finding emphasizes the difficulty of identifying a single key timepoint when designing the trial and how information from a pilot study might have been useful. Although a frequently suggested approach is to choose the timepoint at which the greatest difference is likely to be seen, this seems to be illogical and it may be more logical to provide a more complete summary and choose enough timepoints to give the full picture of advantages and disadvantages. This is analogous to comparing the whole survival curves, not just the point at which differences are greatest. The selection of the primary outcome measure, which is necessary for sample size calculation, is therefore difficult, and rather than choosing a single timepoint, an alternative method, such as looking for the maximum or minimum score over a set time period, or time to an event, might be preferable.

Table 6.1 Improvement in severity of cough at different timepoints (Stephens *et al.*, [43]).

Time from randomization	Number and percent of patients with an improvement Regimen		*p* value
	4D	2D	
1 month	40/64 (62%)	31/76 (41%)	0.02
2 months	18/36 (50%)	30/50 (60%)	0.5
3 months	16/25 (64%)	12/32 (38%)	0.09

Even if to help get a sample size for the QL comparison of the trial we concentrate on a single key timepoint, it is usually important in practice is to administer questionnaires at regular intervals before, during and after treatment, to obtain a more complete picture.

Most standard questionnaires use a time frame of three weeks, i.e. they ask the patient 'how have you been feeling over the last three weeks?' It has been found that this is the longest period over which patients can recall accurately. This has important repercussions on how often questionnaires are completed. Thus, if the first post-treatment questionnaire is administered many weeks or months after treatment, it is unlikely that an accurate record of any transient treatment side effects will be obtained.

The actual timing of questionnaire administration will depend on the hypothesis. However the following guidelines should be noted.

- A baseline questionnaire is essential. Ideally in a randomized trial this should be administered after the patient consents to be in the trial but before the actual treatment is known. In this way all possible bias in terms of patients being pleased or anxious about their allocated treatment can be avoided.

- Most randomized trials are based on the concept of intention to treat (i.e. what happens to patients if a policy of giving a particular treatment is applied). QL should follow this same concept. The most logical assessment points are therefore at set timepoints from randomization. In this way all patients can be accommodated, even though patients may be at different points in their treatment, or indeed withdraw from treatment.

- Completion of questionnaires at times related to treatment or treatment-related events may seem most logical but may cause difficulties in analyses, because, for instance, the duration of treatment can vary from patient to patient, and indeed some patients may not receive treatment. In this way differences between treatments are confounded by differences in times of assessment.

- When choosing timepoints it is important to enable valid comparisons to be made. If, for instance, treatment A is given at 3-week intervals and treatment B at 4-week intervals, it would not be logical to assess QL at eight weeks as patients on treatment A would be between treatments and those on treatment B would be at the time of treatment. It would be much more logical to choose twelve weeks when both groups of patients were at equivalent points in their treatment course.

Thus, although choosing the timepoints to administer QL will depend on the hypothesis, some common sense needs to be applied as, for instance, it would not be justifiable to ask patients to attend clinic purely to complete QL questionnaires and/or to synchronize QL completion between treatments [32].

6.3.5 How many patients are required?

Although in the vast majority of cancer trials it will be most appropriate to have duration of survival as the primary outcome measure and perform power calculations for this outcome measure, it is nevertheless important and useful to calculate a required sample size for the QL aspect.

For example, the primary aim of the QL aspect of a lung cancer trial might be to compare the difference in the proportion of patients who have relief from their cough at three months. If the standard treatment is expected to give 50 per cent of patients relief, then to reliably detect an increase in this proportion to 75 per cent with the new treatment would require a total of 154 patients (seventy-seven per arm).

However, this sample size assumes that all patients will be assessable. In many advanced cancers, attrition due to death, even at three months, may have reduced the trial population by 10 or 15 per cent. In addition, the above scenario requires complete information on all patients and indeed all patients to start with a cough otherwise how could relief be assessed? The framing of the hypothesis is again important, as, for example, Stephens *et al.* [43] have suggested redefining 'palliation' as not just improvement, but also prevention (for asymptomatic patients), and control (for patients with minimal symptoms). In this way all patients could be included in the analysis. Nevertheless, the calculated QL sample size must be adjusted by adding in a realistic proportion of patients to account for deaths, ineligibility, and non-compliance. For instance, in a multicentre trial looking at palliation in poor performance non-small cell lung cancer patients it may be prudent to increase the sample substantially. Obviously this number depends on the timing of the primary QL outcome, the expected attrition and likely compliance.

There may be situations within a large trial where it is only necessary that a subset of patients complete QL questionnaires. This may be because the trial is powered to detect a small difference in duration of survival, but a larger difference in QL. Any decision to assess only a subset of patients must be based on carefully worked out hypotheses and sample size, and it is usually important to ensure that the patients in the subset are representative of the whole group (if you wish to draw conclusions relevant to the whole group), although occasionally a specific subset of patients may be selected for study. However, generally there are a number of options that could be applied when deciding how to acquire a subset sample.

- Collect QL data on all patients until the subset sample size is achieved. This is probably the best option. It should ensure no bias in the sample, assuming that over time the characteristics of patients entering the trial remain approximately the same, and that there is no substantial learning curve in the management of patients.
- Limit the collection of QL data to a few centres. Although this may ensure good compliance (one would naturally choose the centres with most enthusiasm for QL), it is often extremely difficult to predict the number of patients who will be entered from each centre, or whether good compliance can be maintained if, for instance, a key staff member in the local centre leaves. However, it is unlikely that a subset based on centres would be unrepresentative of the whole population, in the way that, for example, a subset based on performance status would be.
- Have QL as an option either for centres or patients. This is the least attractive option. Giving patients the option will almost inevitably result in an unrepresentative sample, as those patients who choose to complete QL may well be the youngest and/or fittest. Experience shows that giving centres the option will almost inevitably cause problems, as many centres, given an option to reduce their administrative burden, will opt out.

6.4 Choosing the questionnaire

Given the decision to include QL in the trial and to collect information from patients at certain timepoints, the question arises of the best way to collect this information.

The usual answer is to use one of the standard questionnaires that have been rigorously developed and validated over the last few years.

The development of a questionnaire is complicated and time consuming. Most of the standard questionnaires cover the domains and items that will be of interest in a clinical trial and therefore in the vast majority of cases there would be no justification for embarking on the development of a new questionnaire. However, some patients may have atypical symptoms, and some new treatments may result in uncommon side effects. If it is felt important to collect such information on the QL form, then it is always more advisable to add extra questions to a standard form than to start afresh.

It is important to remember that questionnaires developed in one context may not be effective in another. The questionnaires referred to in this chapter were all developed for use in clinical trials, they were therefore not designed for the assessment of individual patients in a clinical situation, or for other objectives such as resource allocation.

6.4.1 Single global question and psychometrics

It may seem that the only question you need to ask patients is simply 'How is your QL?' and then measure improvements or deterioration. Indeed there are single question 'performance status' scales [44], such as the Karnovsky [45], Eastern Co-operative Oncology Group (ECOG) [46] or World Health Organization (WHO) performance status [47]. However, these cannot be classed as QL scales because, as discussed above, QL is a complex concept and they only address one of the many aspects of QL.

Although superficially attractive, simply asking a single question about QL makes it impossible to disentangle what components of QL are associated with any changes over time or differences between treatments observed. It is perhaps not surprising that when comparisons are made between health-related questions and overall QL there is rarely good correlation, suggesting of course that health is only one aspect of QL.

From the point of view of analysis and interpretation it would appear superficially helpful to reduce QL to a single score so that the QL of two treatments could be readily compared. Consequently, there is a temptation to combine all the answers from a questionnaire into a single score but there are numerous reasons why this is not an appropriate approach, and perhaps could be compared to reporting toxicity but not specifying what type. As stated earlier, the patient's health is only one element of overall QL and it will be influenced by numerous other aspects of daily life. Simply adding together all the scores from a QL questionnaire does not represent overall QL. Not only would one need information on all the factors that make up QL, but also the patients' individual weighting for each factor.

McHorney *et al.* [48] compared the validity and relative precision of four methods of measuring general health. Although the questionnaire with the most items was considered more reliable, defined more distinct levels of health and better represented the content of health perceptions, this was, of course, at the expense of considerable extra patient and staff time and energy. Shorter questionnaires were not significantly less reliable than the long questionnaires but in turn were much better than single item forms, which failed to detect individual patient changes.

Nevertheless, many questionnaires respond to the demand for a single QL score by supplementing more specific questions with a single question along the lines of 'How would you rate your overall QL?' This is certainly preferable to an aggregated score, but its limitations (as discussed above) must be kept in mind.

Questionnaires have been developed by a number of groups, usually by a long process of surveying patients, compiling lists of questions, and then testing and evolving the questionnaire until they are satisfied with its psychometric (the measurement of human characteristics) properties.

Most of the standard cancer QL questionnaires cover a number of general domains (aspects of QL) and specific symptoms. Usually the scores from a number of questions are combined to give a 'domain' score. The reason for this is that it has repeatedly been shown that in order to get, say, a score of anxiety for a patient, it is much more reliable to ask a series of anxiety-related questions and combine the scores, than simply ask 'what is your level of anxiety'?

Usually subscales are made up of items that are positively correlated. However, there may be problems with the statistical methodology, factor analysis, that often underlie this approach, as described by Fayers and Hand [49] who have attempted to divide symptoms into causal and effect indicators. Thus, increased nausea might cause a decrease in overall QL (i.e. nausea is a causal indicator), whereas poor overall QL might result in depression (i.e. depression is an effect indicator). In addition, some factors, such as insomnia, may be considered as both causal and effect indicators (see Fig. 6.5).

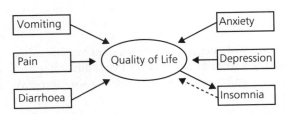

Fig. 6.5 Causal and effect indicators (adapted from Fayers *et al.*, [50]).

This schema may seem obvious and logical, but Fayers *et al.* [50] argue that it could have important implications for the development of questionnaires and especially the formation of subscales. They argue that factor analysis may select both causal and effect indicators to be included in subscales, and that it might make more sense to group together items that make sound clinical sense, such as gastro-intestinal symptoms.

6.4.2 Development of QL questionnaires

Some of the first attempts at measuring QL were LASAs (Linear Analogue Self-assessment Scales) (Fig. 6.6) [51,52].

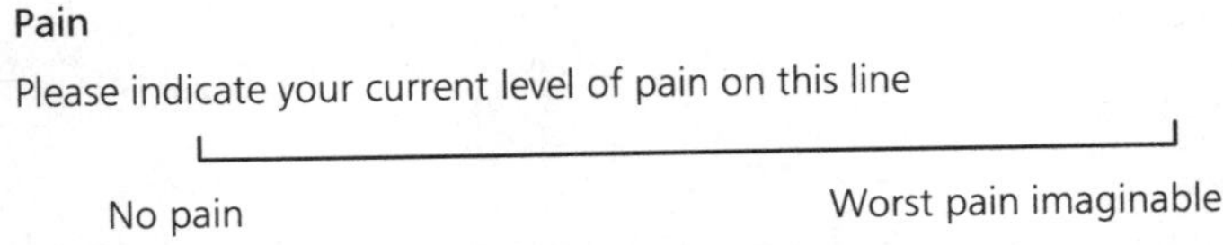

Pain

Please indicate your current level of pain on this line

No pain   Worst pain imaginable

Fig. 6.6 A Linear Analogue Self-assessment Scale (LASA).

On a LASA the patient indicates their current status by putting a mark on the 10-cm horizontal scale (when these scales were drawn vertically they were known as thermometers). The position of the mark is then measured and scored on a 0–100 scale. Advantages of LASAs are that they avoid the necessity to describe categories and that because a large range of scores is obtained, they may be more sensitive than limited answer scales in reflecting within-patient changes [53].

However, the disadvantages are that patients find them difficult to complete because of their unfamiliarity, scoring is time-consuming and scores may be difficult to interpret. For example, what does a score of seventy-five actually represent? The same point on the scale may represent very different things to different patients, and thus they are not appropriate in situations where a range of states is possible, for example acute severe nausea and chronic mild nausea.

Because of these problems, the next step from LASAs was to divide the LASA line into categories (Fig. 6.7).

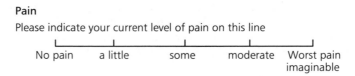

Pain
Please indicate your current level of pain on this line

No pain   a little   some   moderate   Worst pain
                                                imaginable

Fig. 6.7 A LASA scale with categories.

The splitting of the 10-cm line into suggested categories was an attempt to standardize patients' recordings but again interpreting a score of, say, seventy-five is difficult unless it is simply categorized as 'moderate.' The natural extension from this was simply to give the patient a limited choice of answers.

In 1932, Renis Likert invented a measurement method, called the Likert Scales, which were used in attitude surveys. They allowed answers that ranged from 'strongly agree' to 'strongly disagree.' The vast majority of 'standard' QL questionnaires now use these Likert scales (where patients are given a list of answers and tick the one most appropriate to them). Thus, in response to questions about their symptoms, or levels of functioning or psychological distress, patients tick a box indicating, usually, the equivalent of nil, mild, moderate or severe (Fig. 6.8). Although a word like 'moderate' will still mean different things to different people it is still easier to understand and report than a score. For example, it is much more understandable to say 20 per cent of patients had severe nausea, than 20 per cent of patients had a nausea score of >80 per cent.

Pain	None	A little	Moderate	Severe
Please tick the box to indicate your current level of pain	☐	☐	☐	☐

Fig. 6.8 A Likert scale.

When QL is being assessed and compared over a relatively long period, questionnaires can be administered at specific timepoints, often several weeks or months apart. However,

CONFIDENTIAL

Patient Diary Card

This column to be completed once only, before any treatment starts

Date: [   ]

	Week 1						
	Mon	Tue	Wed	Thu	Fri	Sat	Sun

Name . . . .

Hospital Number . . . .

Doctor in Charge . . . .

Next appointment:

Date . . . .

Time . . . .

Loss of appetite . . . . [ ]

Nausea (feeling sick) . . . . [ ]

Vomiting . . . . [ ]

Cough . . . . [ ]

Coughing up blood . . . . [ ]

Chest pain . . . . [ ]

Shortness of breath . . . . [ ]

Difficulty swallowing . . . . [ ]

Please give details of any other health problems here:

Please remember to bring this card with you at your next appointment.

If you can't keep your next appointment then continue to use the spare card, if you have one, and if possible post your completed card to us.

INSTRUCTIONS
Please complete every evening after your last meal, even when you are in hospital, by writing the number of your answer in the appropriate box as follows:
0 – Not at all   2 – Moderately
1 – A little   3 – Very much

Fig. 6.9 A Daily Diary Card (DDC).

on occasions such a schedule of administration will be inappropriate if, for instance, information is required on acute side effects, such as the duration of nausea and vomiting immediately following chemotherapy. To deal with this scenario, daily diary cards have been used to record symptoms that change quickly over time (Fig. 6.9).

The daily diary card (DDC) grew out of the idea that, in chemotherapy for lung cancer, it was felt that the main side effects were known but not their duration or the pattern of severity. Thus, the daily diary card was developed based on previous work in other conditions, such as the assessment of night cough in asthma patients and vaginal bleeding patterns. As patients complete the card each evening it was considered imperative to keep the number of questions to a minimum and for practical reasons to use a four or five point categorical scale. In the first MRC trial to use DDCs the consensus opinion was that the questions should address overall QL, a functional measure (physical activity), the main expected side-effect (nausea and vomiting) and two psychological items (mood and anxiety). These questions were changed in subsequent MRC trials depending on the research question.

Although the psychometric properties of the daily diary card have never been formally assessed, Fayers [54] argues that the data generated by its extensive use can be shown to be sensitive, valid and reliable.

The advantage of a daily diary card is that transient changes, such as nausea and vomiting after chemotherapy, or dysphagia after thoracic radiotherapy, can be monitored in detail. However, the disadvantages are that only a few questions can be asked, patient compliance is difficult to control and patients seem to lose interest very quickly. In addition, concern has been expressed that patients looking back at their history over three or four weeks may find it upsetting if they see themselves deteriorating.

6.4.3 Types of questionnaire

Bjordal and Kaasa [55] compiled a list of criteria that should be considered when choosing a QL instrument for use in a cancer trial. In addition to being cancer specific, completed by patients, brief, and easy to understand and respond to, it is important that it is multi-dimensional and covers physical, functional, psychological and social aspects.

Questionnaires that are now considered standard have undergone a number of rigorous evaluations, to show that they have validity, reliability and responsiveness [29].

- Validity means that the question measures what it is supposed to. There are a number of aspects of validity, namely content, criterion, construct, and discriminative validity.

  - Content validity is an assessment of the relevance and validity of items, i.e. are the questions understood and not ambiguous?

  - Criterion validity is the strength of the relationship between the new instrument and some other criterion measuring the same characteristic (ideally a gold standard).

  - Construct validity is evidence that the instrument is broadly behaving as expected and shows similar (convergent validity) or opposite (divergent validity) relationship with other appropriate measures.

  - Discriminative validity is the ability of the instrument to distinguish groups of people by their responses to the questionnaire and some other criteria (e.g. disease severity).

- Reliability is a measure of random error. It can be assessed by repeated applications of the same test (test–retest reliability) or by analysing the internal consistency of a scale. The latter involves measuring the relationship between a number of questions about the same aspects (i.e. multiple indicators for happiness).

- Responsiveness is the ability of the instrument to detect changes that occur as a result of an intervention. This means that there must be a range of responses to the question, and that not everyone will respond with either the top or bottom category (the so-called ceiling or floor effect).

Two types of questionnaires are likely to be used in cancer trials, those that are generic and those that are cancer-specific. For instance, in a situation such as testicular cancer where cure is common, the aim of QL assessment may be to judge whether the patient has returned to the same QL as the general population, and thus the use of a generic, rather than a cancer-specific, questionnaire might be appropriate. In other situations a cancer-specific questionnaire may be more appropriate.

Generic questionnaires

Generic questionnaires concentrate on such areas as ability to perform daily activities, shopping, caring for oneself, etc. Widely used generic questionnaires include the Medical Outcomes Survey (MOS) Short form (SF36) [56], the Nottingham Health Profile (NHP)[57], the Sickness Impact Profile (SIP) [58] and the McMaster Health Index Questionnaire (MHIQ) [59,60].

The MOS SF36 asks thrity-six questions covering eight health concepts, and has been designed to be self-completed by the patient or administered by a trained interviewer in person or on the telephone.

The NHP is an instrument designed to measure subjective health status in six areas: physical mobility, pain, sleep, emotional reactions, social isolation, and energy. It is composed of a number of statements, which are answered 'yes' or 'no.' Scores in each section are summed and standardized to a 0–100 scale.

The SIP measures behavioural impact of sickness in terms of dysfunction. There are 136 items in twelve categories to which the respondent answers 'yes' or 'no.' It takes an average of 30 minutes to complete. Note that this measures negatives, not levels of positive functioning.

The MHIQ has three scales (physical, social and emotional) and fifty-nine items, some of which are used in more than one scale.

Cancer-specific questionnaires

Cancer-specific questionnaires focus on the symptoms and side effects of specific diseases and/or treatments. Widely used cancer-specific questionnaires include the European Organization for Research and Treatment of Cancer (EORTC) Quality of Life thirty item core questionnaire (QLQ-C30) [61], the Functional Assessment of Cancer Treatment (FACT) [62], the Rotterdam Symptom Checklist (RSCL) [63], the Functional Living Index-Cancer (FLIC) [64] and the Cancer Rehabilitation Evaluation System (CARES) [65].

The EORTC Quality of Life core questionnaire (QLQ-C30) includes thirty questions covering five functional scales (physical, role, cognitive, emotional, and social) three symptom scales, a global QL scale, and a number of single items. Additional modules have been, or are being, developed for bladder, brain, breast, colorectal, gastric, head and neck, lung, oesophageal, ovarian, and pancreatic cancers, as well as leukaemia and myeloma, and to cover aspects such as palliative care, body image, high-dose chemotherapy, and neuropathy.

The FACT-G (FACT General) questionnaire consists of thirty-three core questions covering physical well-being, social/family well-being, relationship with medical staff, emotional well-being and fulfilment/contentment. It does not include symptoms, as these are contained in additional disease-specific questionnaires targeting different disease sites, for instance lung, head and neck, and genitourinary tract.

The RSCL concentrates on physical symptoms and psychological problems. A number of different versions are available, but the original contained thirty items each scored on a 4-point Likert scale, from 'not at all' to 'very much.' Two major subscales can be formed (an 8-item psychological scale, and an 18-item physical scale) but the questionnaire is perhaps lacking in other dimensions of QL – sexual functioning, self care, vocational and social functioning and satisfaction with medical care. However an 'activities of daily living' scale has been added.

The FLIC is a 22-item questionnaire developed to assess vocational, psychological, social and somatic areas of function. Each question takes the form of a visual analogue scale (VAS) and is scored as a whole number between 0 and 7.

The full CARES questionnaire contains 139 items of which the patient completes between ninety-one and 132 items, all scored on a 5-point scale (0–4). It includes global QL, five summary scores (physical, psychosocial, medical intervention, marital, and sexual) and thirty-one specific subscales. A short form version consists of fifty-nine items [66].

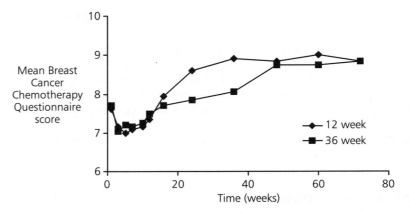

Fig. 6.10 Mean Breast Cancer Chemotherapy Questionnaire (BCQ) score over time (adapted from Levine *et al.*, [67]).

Other relevant questionnaires

A number of more specific questionnaires (not counting the specific modules developed as additions to the EORTC and FACT general questionnaires) have also been developed. For instance, Levine *et al.* [67] developed a questionnaire specifically to assess the outcome of patients with stage II breast cancer undergoing adjuvant chemotherapy. Their paper provides a good example of how questionnaires are developed and how the validity, reproducibility and responsiveness are tested, and Fig. 6.10 shows the responsiveness of their questionnaire to two durations of chemotherapy.

In addition, the Hospital Anxiety and Depression Scale (HADS) [68] has been used in a number of cancer clinical trials. This is because although many instruments have sections covering mental health, most will only detect a 'clinical case' of anxiety or depression and give no information about the nature of the psychiatric disorder. The HADS is a self-assessment mood scale specifically designed for non-psychiatric settings, and focuses on the two most common psychological aspects – anxiety and depression. Most importantly, cut-off points have been calculated for both of the 7-item 4-point scales so that patients can be classed as 'normal,' 'borderline' or 'case' anxiety or depression.

The EuroQol (EQ5D) [69], is a simple questionnaire with a choice of three responses to each of its five questions. It is widely used by health economists because from the responses to these five questions a single utility value can be generated.

6.4.4 Weighting

As mentioned above, the QL is individual and subjective, and although carefully constructed subscales can be formed by combining individual items, there are few current examples where account is made of patient-specific weightings of symptoms or the fact that some patients may consider certain symptoms more important than others. The important symptoms may themselves differ across patients.

Most questionnaires ask whether a patient is experiencing a symptom, or can or cannot perform a function. However, it may appear more relevant to ask whether a patient is concerned by a symptom. For instance, does it matter if a patient has hair loss if he or she is not concerned by it? To get round this, some questionnaires ask 'have you been bothered by . . .' rather than just 'have you had . . .'

With all the unresolved issues regarding the incorporation of QL into trials, incorporating patient-specific weights is probably currently too complex. However, a number of groups have addressed this issue. For example, at the end of each section in the SF36 there is an additional question about how important patients rate this section. Quite how this information is then utilized is unclear at present.

In addition, attempts have been made which allow the patient to define areas of their life which contribute most to overall quality of life. The qualitator for instance [70] asks patients, at each assessment, to choose the most important item from four groups of items. Although this may appear to be more tailored and sensitive to individual patients' concerns, it makes the analysis and presentation of the data collected from such instruments much more complicated and difficult to understand.

6.4.5 Adding trial-specific questions

Despite the detailed development of questionnaires, in most trials there are one or two specific relevant areas, for example, symptoms, side effects, attitudes, which are not included in the standard questionnaires. However, trial-specific questions can nearly always be added at the end of a standard questionnaire. For example, the MRC colorectal group in a trial of three chemotherapy regimens which were given in three very different ways (15-minute infusion every three weeks, 2-day infusion every three weeks, or continuously via a pump) added questions relating to the side-effects (dry or sore mouth and soreness or redness of hands or feet) and attitudes to the regimen (how much has treatment interfered with daily activities). However, it is important to follow the basic principles of question construction outlined above, being careful about the way such questions are worded, and pilot work is usually necessary.

6.4.6 Translations

Many trials are now run multi-nationally, but even in national trials there is an increasing likelihood that a proportion of patients will not speak the native language of the country they are being treated in. Most of the major developers of QL questionnaires have recognized the need to provide their forms in a number of different languages. For example, the EORTC core questionnaire is currently available in thirty-six languages. The process of translating questions from one language into another is time consuming and detailed. It involves forward and backward translation to ensure all the questions have the same psychometric values as the original. Only properly translated questionnaires should be used as it is rarely adequate, or acceptable, to simply translate questionnaires word for word.

6.4.7 Choosing a questionnaire

The key as to which questionnaire should be chosen should be governed by the QL hypothesis to be tested. Once the key QL aspects and timepoints have been fixed the questionnaire can be chosen. The difference between questionnaires often relates to the degree to which they emphasize objective compared with subjective dimensions [71]. It is particularly important that the questionnaire addresses all the components that are important to the patient population and that are susceptible to being affected (either positively or negatively) by the intervention.

Most of the standard questionnaires cover much the same ground, and the choice may then be influenced by continuity (the trials group may have used the questionnaire in the previous trial and are comfortable with it), the need to make comparisons across trials, or the fact that one questionnaire may concentrate in greater detail on the symptoms or side-effects of interest.

Several papers have asked patients to complete more than one questionnaire and have then compared the results. The questionnaires compared in this way include the FACT-G and the EORTC QLQ-C30 [72], the FLIC and the EORTC QLQ-C30 [73] and three lung-cancer-specific questionnaires, the EORTC, FACT, and LCSS [74].

Despite apparently addressing similar domains the studies revealed a number of differences. It was found that only one of the five subscales on the FACT-G was adequately covered by the QLQ-C30, and only three of the eight QLQ-C30 subscales were adequately covered by the FACT-G. The QLQ-C30 does not cover social well being and relationship with the doctor, whereas the FACT-G does not cover cognitive functioning and the LCSS captures the impact of toxicity rather than the detail of side-effects. Although there is general agreement in terms of the domains that questionnaires cover, the actual definitions used appear to differ. Thus social functioning is defined within the FLIC as an 'inclination for companionship with friends and family,' in the EORTC it is defined as 'the impact of disease on social activity and family life.'

Modification of these standard questionnaires is generally not advised and sometimes not permitted, as this would breach copyright. Indeed the questionnaires should be used in exactly the recommended format for the following good reasons:

- the psychometric performances of individual scales and items when used alone are not known,
- only a small proportion of patients find any questions upsetting,
- patients are generally not bothered by questions about symptoms they do not have.

6.5 Practical administration issues

Whilst it is important to put time and effort into getting the design of the QL aspect of a trial correct, it is perhaps even more important that practical administration issues are addressed, to ensure that the quantity and quality of data collected are sufficient to answer the questions posed.

QL data have to be collected prospectively, unlike some clinical data that can often be extracted from patients' notes, and so it is essential that local QL coordinators are identified in each centre, and that they are fully versed on all aspects of QL collection in the trial.

6.5.1 Local QL coordinator

The importance of identifying an individual at each centre to act as a local QL coordinator cannot be overestimated. This person will need to:

- explain to new patients the rationale behind QL questionnaires,
- identify patients when they come into clinic,

* hand out questionnaires,
* make sure patients have somewhere quiet to sit and complete the questionnaire before seeing the clinician,
* collect and check the questionnaire, making sure that any missing items are completed immediately, and return it to the office co-ordinating the trial.

The person responsible for administering questionnaires in the local centre needs to be committed to the importance of collecting QL. Some patients will often be reluctant to complete sometimes long, often difficult, questionnaires that may contain many seemingly irrelevant and sometimes very personal questions. The patient must be convinced that far from being a burden the questionnaire is an essential component of the research. If the rationale is carefully explained to the patients, research has shown that far from patients feeling burdened by the need to complete questionnaires, they actually gain fulfilment from completing them. Indeed the patient themselves can be motivated to remind staff when questionnaires are required.

6.5.2 Administration

The usual standard instructions for completing questionnaires are that they should be completed by the patient, without conferring with a relative or member of staff, whilst waiting in the clinic prior to seeing the doctor.

The advantage of administering questionnaires in the clinic is that the sequence of events and the environment can be controlled. If questionnaires are given to patients to complete at home, there is no control over when the questionnaire is completed, who completes it, whether help was given, whether the questionnaire is posted back, and whether individual items are not answered.

There may be scenarios where posting a questionnaire to the patient's home is the preferable option, for example when data are required at a key timepoint when patients are not due to be seen in clinic. Nevertheless, as with all 'non-standard' QL questionnaire administration, the reasons behind the course of action must be justified in the protocol, and consistency across treatment being compared should be maintained. For example, it is likely to be much better to post every questionnaire to every patient, than to do so on an *ad hoc* basis.

However, the practice of posting questionnaires to patients raises a number of concerns; including the fact that patients may have moved (confidentiality may be breached if the new occupant opens the mail); patients may have died (relatives may be distressed to receive mail for their recently deceased family); patients may be in remission (and be distressed by being reminded of their cancer), and of course it is important to ensure that patients on long-term follow-up have consented to regular follow-ups.

Thus, although posting questionnaires appears an obvious and straightforward option, it may actually require more staff input and result in poorer quality data. Posting questionnaires to patients' homes requires consideration for the patient and their relatives, and if this approach is adopted a recommended routine is that a phone call is made prior to posting to determine that the patient is still alive and willing to complete the form.

Weinberger *et al.* [75] compared telephone, face-to-face and self-administration of the SF36 QL questionnaire. They investigated the relative advantages and disadvantages of each mode of administration, including response rates, expense, interviewer bias, patient burden, anonymity and interpretation of errors. The least effective mode was telephone administration, and although patients expressed a preference for face-to-face administration it provided a more optimistic picture of health than self-administration and of course required more personnel and was less convenient for patients.

6.5.3 How can good compliance be attained and maintained?

The QL data are both multi-dimensional and longitudinal which makes analysis difficult, but the problem is greatly increased if compliance is poor and there is much missing data. When data are 'missing at random,' methods of imputation are possible, but most QL data will be 'not missing at random,' usually due to patients failing to complete forms due to their deteriorating health. Such data cannot normally be imputed, and so every effort should be made to collect as much data as possible.

In QL assessment the strictest definition of compliance is the number of patients who have completed every question of a QL questionnaire at the required timepoint, divided by the number who could have (i.e. were alive at that timepoint). In addition, the definition of 'at the required timepoint' is open to interpretation and most groups now give a time window around the timepoint (e.g. ±7 days) which is considered acceptable. Generally the chosen 'width' of the window will be a reflection of the frequency of form administration, thus if questionnaires are being completed at 3-weekly intervals a window of ±7 days may be appropriate, whereas 6-monthly forms might have a window of ±2 months. Sometimes an asymmetrical window might be used, for instance at baseline where completion should be before randomization, here acceptable times may be −7 to 0 days from randomization.

It is also important to differentiate between questionnaire compliance and individual question (item) compliance (the proportion of items completed on a returned questionnaire).

Questionnaire compliance

Despite differing definitions of questionnaire compliance, many groups have reported similar and disappointingly low levels of compliance in cancer trials. Overall rates are often quoted as being around 70 per cent, but this usually reflects a higher rate at baseline (around 85 per cent) which falls consistently over time. Indeed, long-term compliance rates, at two or more years, can often be as low as 25 per cent [14,76–79].

When good compliance rates have been achieved it has usually been as a result of a well-planned administrative operation. Thus:

- Earl *et al.* [11] reported an overall compliance rate of 87 per cent in the use of daily diary cards (438 cards completed out of a possible 506) and this was attributed to the fact that QL was carried out in only one centre with a research nurse assigned solely for this purpose.

- Langendijk *et al.* [80] attributed their 90 per cent compliance to the appointment of a specific individual (not the treating clinician) to collect QL data, and to limiting the frequency of administration.

- Wisloff *et al.* [81] achieved an overall compliance rate of over 83 per cent in their trial of patients with multiple myeloma using the EORTC QLQ-C30. They attribute this to the fact that patients confirmed their willingness to take part by mailing the completed baseline form to the study secretariat and that all subsequent communication relating to QL took place between the patient and the secretariat.

Some of the best rates of QL compliance have been reported by the National Cancer Institute of Canada who reported a compliance rate of 95 per cent in three breast cancer trials [82]. However they acknowledge that it remains unclear whether similar success can be obtained with different questionnaires, in different types of trials, in different institutions, and during long-term follow-up. To achieve this impressive level, the NCIC used a level of resource that may not be available for all trials. In one study nurses called the patients at home on the appropriate day to remind them to complete the questionnaire and specific measures were instituted prior to trial activation to ensure maximum compliance in the completion and return of QL questionnaires. These included:

◆ QL assessment was incorporated as a specific trial objective,

◆ rationale for QL data collection was included in the protocol,

◆ specific instructions for administration of questionnaires were included in the protocol,

◆ data collection forms were modified to remind data managers to administer questionnaires,

◆ specific reporting schedules were provided,

◆ successful completion of the baseline QL questionnaire was defined as an eligibility criterion,

◆ computer-based reminders were provided in advance of due dates,

◆ pre-trial workshops for nurses and data managers were implemented,

◆ participating centres were given regular feedback on QL via letters and newsletters.

There is no doubt that given careful planning and provided adequate resources are available it is possible to achieve high compliance rates, although of course the patient group may affect what is possible.

The central trials office needs to be effective, efficient and open to new ideas to improve compliance. Ganz et al. [83] have suggested the use of scannable questionnaires to facilitate the rapid and accurate transference of data onto the computer database, and increased use of flow sheets, study calendars, patient tracking cards, training videos and identification or flagging of patient medical records can all help with compliance [84].

Item compliance

Item compliance is generally much less of a problem, although there are some consistent problems surrounding questions about sexual problems, and sometimes poor questionnaire design means that whole pages are missed because patients did not appreciate there were further questions on the back of the form or on another sheet. This emphasises the need for completed questionnaires to be checked before being returned to the data centre.

Patient compliance

Although several groups have noted that poor compliance in multicentre trials is more often related to a lack of commitment in particular centres, poor patient performance status can have a major effect.

In a series of MRC lung cancer trials, QL questionnaires were completed by 92 per cent of the patients whom the clinician assessed as having good performance status, but this fell dramatically to only 31 per cent of those assessed as very poor.

The problem with poor compliance, however, is that its cause is not always obvious. Cox *et al.* [85] suggested that as well as the very sick patients not completing forms, perhaps surprisingly 'those experiencing fewer problems may not be so diligent in returning questionnaires.' Indeed Brorsson *et al.* [86] telephoned non-responders to a mailed-out questionnaire and reported that the vast majority reported considerably better QL than the responders.

Poor compliance in the completion of forms may also result from patients' failure to attend at designated times and patients being perceived as too ill or too distressed to be approached. However, frank refusal is uncommon. It is also of interest that patients can feel very upset if requests for questionnaires to be completed are discontinued. The reason for non-compliance is less likely to be patient refusal, and more likely to be staff reticence about handing questionnaires to patients they perceive to be too sick to complete them.

Centre compliance

Organizational problems within institutions may account for a large part of the failure to collect data. These include:

- lack of staff,
- unavailability of forms,
- priority given to other matters,
- failure to check, collect and return forms,
- staff changes and absences.

A number of studies have investigated the administration of questionnaires. Hopwood *et al.* [87] reported on a survey of centres participating in three trials conducted by the MRC to assess the administration of QL questionnaires. The aim was to see what lessons could be learned regarding the standardization of procedures and improving compliance. Interesting findings included the facts that:

- The baseline questionnaire tended to be given out after and the consultation with the doctor and randomization (and therefore after the patient knew their treatment allocation) but before treatment. Thereafter there was no consistency as to the timing of administration in relation to the consultation with the doctor.

- Forms were often not given out when the patient was perceived as too ill or unsuitable because they had just received bad news. However, the majority of centres reported that patients' reactions to completing questionnaires were favourable, and that patients took them seriously and were impressed with the interest being shown in how they felt. Only one centre mentioned patient refusal as a problem.

- In seventeen of the thrity-six centres surveyed there had been changes in procedures or staff during the course of the trial. The most frequently mentioned staff-related problems were: staff being on holiday or not available for other reasons, staff being unfamiliar with procedures, poor compliance with trial procedures in peripheral clinics, unavailability of questionnaires, and staff forgetting to hand out, check, or collect the questionnaires.
- Many centres were affected by the lack of privacy and quietness for patients completing their forms.

One of the trials had specific funding for dedicated local trials staff, the others had not. The only differences between the specific-funded trial and non-funded trials appeared to be that a variety of staff (doctors, nurses, or radiographers) administered the questionnaires in the non-funded trials, whereas only research nurses did so in the funded trial. Surprisingly, in all other aspects the extra training and resourcing in the funded trial appeared to have no impact on the organizational problems.

Although it is often difficult to find out why QL forms are not completed and returned, questions about QL completion included on the clinical forms can be helpful, especially if the reasons are made explicit, i.e. not just 'patient refused' but the reason why they refused.

6.5.4 Guidelines for protocol writing

It is important that decisions taken regarding the assessment of QL in the trial are pre-planned and written into the trial protocol. Checklists to be followed when drafting a protocol include the following components:

- the rationale for the inclusion of QL assessment,
- the choice of QL instrument, and the timing of administration (including acceptable time windows),
- how to select patients if only a subset are required for the QL assessment,
- guidelines for administration, identifying a named person in each centre, method of data collection (home or clinic), when to hand out the forms, checking forms for completeness, whether help and/or proxy assessments are permitted, and what to do when the patient does not attend,
- adequate information about QL in the patient information sheet,
- statistical considerations (sample size, hypotheses, method of planned analyses, etc.),
- the instrument being included as an appendix.

Guidelines for QL administration

In addition it is useful if, for each trial, guidelines are prepared for local staff, to cover the importance of compliance and of checking completed questionnaires, staff responsibilities, absences and changes, and the role of the trial coordinating office.

An example might include the following points:

- One named member of staff should be made responsible for the administration of QL questionnaires for each trial at each centre, and a named deputy should be available in their absence. The responsible staff member must explain to the patient the importance of QL assessment and how to complete the questionnaires.

- The first questionnaires should be completed before randomization (i.e. before the patient knows which treatment group he has been allocated). On all occasions it is preferable that the form is completed before the patient is seen by the doctor and before each cycle of treatment.

- Unless specified otherwise in the protocol, the patient should complete the questionnaires without conferring with a relative or member of staff.

- Ideally the questionnaires should be checked to ensure that all questions have been answered, and if necessary the patient should be asked to fill in any missing items. However, there may be situations where complete confidentiality is required, and patients may be asked to place the completed form in an envelope for posting directly to the trials office.

- If an assessment is missed because of administrative failure, the patient should be contacted by telephone or letter and asked to complete and return (in a stamped addressed envelope provided) mailed questionnaires as soon as possible. Patients should be encouraged to ask for forms if not given to them.

- If a QL questionnaire is not completed as per the guidelines (for example at home, with help, or after seeing the doctor), this must be indicated on the form.

Patient information sheets

In the vast majority of cancer trials evaluating QL, patient-completed questionnaires are used, so it is important that patients are fully aware of the reasons for collecting QL data. Thus the patient information sheet should include details about the QL aspects of the trial and patients should be made aware of the fact that consent to the trial includes agreement to complete QL questionnaires, although the right of the patient to withdraw at any stage always remains.

It is important that patients feel comfortable about reporting their symptoms and side effects honestly. Patients may answer questions differently (and possibly less honestly) if they believe that the information will be seen by their clinician and/or may influence their treatment [54]. Even completing questionnaires with the help of their partner may affect the answers patients give, and the usual recommendation is that patients are found a quiet space to sit and complete the form, without conferring with staff or relatives, whilst waiting in the clinic to see the doctor.

Patient information sheets should therefore make it very clear what is to be done with the completed QL forms. Ideally, as soon as they have been checked for completeness, they should be sent straight back to the trials centre, but there may be circumstances where they are reviewed by the local nurses and clinicians, or where the data centre reviews the forms and passes information back to the local clinician.

It is usually recommended that completed QL questionnaires or at least sensitive questions are confidential and not made available to nurses or clinicians. In a trial of antihypertensive therapy [88] the responses to items relating to sexual functioning were placed in an envelope and sealed by the patient and mailed directly to the central trials office. In such situations, patients need to be reminded that it is up to them if they wish to discuss any such concerns with the clinician or the nurse. A real dilemma can occur for those collecting the data centrally, if they notice that patients are reporting serious side-effects or psychological problems, and yet this is not reflected in the clinical reports.

Decisions about what to do in these circumstances should be discussed before the trial starts, and guidelines included in the protocol.

Another ethical concern relates to the growing requirement that to be eligible for a trial, patients must be willing and able to complete QL questionnaires. Is it right to exclude a patient from a trial because they are unable to complete the questionnaires (perhaps because they are blind or do not speak English)? This of course depends on what the primary outcome measure is and whether QL is required on all patients or just a sample. One advantage of using standard questionnaires is that many are already translated into a variety of languages.

In many countries, before a trial can start, an ethics committee must approve the protocol and the patient information sheets. When QL is an integral part of a trial the patient information sheets must include specific information for the patient of the reasons for including QL and what will be expected of them.

6.5.5 The future

Newer methods of collecting QL data may be more appealing to patients and may better ensure regular completion, reduce missing items, and eliminate transcription errors from paper to computer. For instance, patients could enter their answers into a personal computer (PC) at home or in the clinic, and hand-held instruments can be programmed to set off an alarm at specific times to remind patients to record their symptom severity. Currently, cost and availability of PCs may be a restricting factor, but it is not too difficult to envisage a scenario in the not too distant future where every patient has their own mobile phone that connects to the Internet. The central trials office could then send a message to every patient on the trial asking them to type in, say, their severity of cough, and get an instant response.

These ideas are already being piloted and their introduction may make an enormous impact on the assessment of patients' QL.

6.6 Conclusions

The assessment of QL can potentially play a key role in choosing between treatments, but to do so requires that much work has gone into the design and conduct of the QL assessment of the trial. The first key to a successful QL component is the pre-defining of a QL hypothesis which will help identify the questionnaire to use, the timepoints to administer it, and the analyses to be conducted (details on the analysis, interpretation and presentation of QL data are included in Chapter 9). The second important factor is to ensure that guidelines and infrastructure are in place to ensure good compliance. Patients need to know about the impact treatments will have on their QL, and it is important that we can supply them with reliable information.

References

[1] Slevin, M.L., Stubbs, L., Plant, H.J., Wilson, P., Gregory, W.M., Armes, P.J., and Downer S.M. (1990) Attitudes to chemotherapy: comparing views of patients with cancer with those of doctors, nurses, and general public. *British Medical Journal*, **300**, 1458–60.

[2] American Society of Clinical Oncology Health Services Research Committee. (1996) Outcomes of cancer treatment for technology assessment and cancer treatment guidelines. *Journal of Clinical Oncology*, **14**, 671–9.

[3] Schumacher, M., Olschewski, M., and Schulgen, G. (1991) Assessment of quality of life in clinical trials. *Statistics in Medicine*, **10**, 1915–30.

[4] World Health Organization. (1948) Constitution of the World Health Organization. Geneva, Switzerland: WHO Basic Documents.

[5] Calman, K.C. (1984) Quality of life in cancer patients – an hypothesis. *Journal of Medical Ethics*, **10**, 124–7.

[6] Thompson, J.A., and Fefer, A. (1987) Interferon in the treatment of hairy cell leukemia. *Cancer*, **59** (suppl 3), 605–9.

[7] Herndon, J.E., Fleishman, S., Kosty, M.P., and Green, A.R. (1997) A longitudinal study of quality of life in advanced non-small cell lung cancer: CALGB 8931. *Controlled Clinical Trials*, **18**, 286–300.

[8] Saunders, C.M., and Fallowfield, L.J. (1996) Survey of the attitudes to and use of quality of life measures by breast cancer specialists in the UK. *The Breast*, **5**, 425–6.

[9] Coates, A., Gebski, V., Bishop, J.F., Jeal, P.N., Woods, R.L., Synder, R., Tattersall, M.H.N., Byrne, M., Harvey, V., Gill, G., Simpson, J., Drummond, R., Browne, J., van Cooten, R., and Forbes, J.F. (1987) Improving the quality of life during chemotherapy for advanced breast cancer. *New England Journal of Medicine*, **317**, 1490–5.

[10] Tannock, I.F., Boyd, N.F., DeBoer, G., Erlichman, C., Fine, S., Larocque, G., Mayers, C., Perrault, D., and Sutherland, H. (1988) A randomized trial of two dose levels of cyclophosphamide, methotrexate, and fluorouracil chemotherapy for patients with metastatic breast cancer. *Journal of Clinical Oncology*, **6**, 1377–87.

[11] Earl, H.M., Rudd, R.M., Spiro, S.G., Ash, C.M., James, L.E., Law, C.S., Tobias, J.S., Harper, P.G., Geddes, D.M., Eraut, D., Partridge, M.R., and Souhami, R.L. (1991) A randomised trial of planned versus as required chemotherapy in small cell lung cancer: a Cancer Research Campaign trial. *British Journal of Cancer*, **64**, 566–72.

[12] Medical Research Council Lung Cancer Working Party. (1989) Survival, adverse reactions and quality of life during combination chemotherapy compared with selective palliative treatment for small-cell lung cancer. *Respiratory Medicine*, **83**, 51–8.

[13] Osoba, D. (1994) Lessons learned from measuring health-related Quality of Life in oncology. *Journal of Clinical Oncology*, **12**, 608–16.

[14] Geddes, D.M., Dones, L., Hill, E., Law, K., Harper, P.G., Spiro, S.G., Tobias, J.F., and Souhami, R.L. (1990) Quality of life during chemotherapy for small cell lung cancer: assessment and use of a daily diary card in a randomized trial. *European Journal of Cancer*, **26**, 484–92.

[15] Stephens, R.J., Hopwood, P., Girling, D.J., and Machin, D. (1997) Randomized trials with quality of life endpoints: are doctors' ratings of patients' physical symptoms interchangeable with patients' self-ratings? *Quality of Life Research*, **6**, 225–36.

[16] Sneeuw, K.C.A., Aaronson, N.K., Sprangers, M.A.G., Detmar, S.B., Wever, L.D.V., and Schornagel, J.H. (1998) Comparison of patient and proxy EORTC QLQ-C30 ratings in assessing the Quality of Life of cancer patients. *Journal of Clinical Epidemiology*, **51**, 617–31.

[17] Sprangers, M.A.G., and Aaronson, N.K. (1992) The role of health care providers and significant others in evaluating the Quality of Life of patients with chronic disease: a review. *Journal of Clinical Epidemiology*, **45**, 743–60.

[18] Regan, J., Yarnold, J., Jones, P.W., and Cooke, N.T. (1991) Palliation and life quality in lung cancer: how good are clinicians at judging treatment outcome? *British Journal of Cancer*, **64**, 396–400.

[19] Sneeuw, K.C.A., Aaronson, N.K., Osoba, D., Muller, M.J., Hsu, M-A., Yung, W.K.A., Brada, M., and Newlands, E.S. (1997) The use of significant others as proxy raters of the Quality of Life of patients with brain cancer. *Medical Care*, **35**, 490–506.

[20] Cassileth, B.R., Lusk, E.J., and Tenaglia, A.N. (1982) A psychological comparison of patients with malignant melonomas and other dermatological diseases. *Journal of the American Academy of Dermatology*, **7**, 742–6.

[21] Cassileth, B.R., Lusk, E.J., Strouse, T.B., Miller, D.S., Brown, L.L., Cross, P.A., and Tenaglia, A.N. (1984) Psychological status in chronic illness: a comparative analysis of six diagnostic groups. *New England Journal of Medicine*, **311**, 506–11.

[22] Brickman, P., Coates, D., and Janoff-Bulman, R. (1978) Lottery winners and accident victims: is happiness relative? *Journal of Personality and Social Psychology*, **36**, 917–27.

[23] Schneider, M. (1975) The quality of life in large American cities: objective and subjective social indicators. *Social Indicators Research*, **1**, 495–509.

[24] Liu, D.C. (1973) The Quality of Life in the United States: 1970. Kansas City, Mo, Midwest Research Institute.

[25] Easterlin, R. (1973) Does money buy happiness? *The Public Interest (Winter)*, **30**, 3–10.

[26] Cameron, P. (1972) Stereotypes about generational fun and happiness vs self-appraised fun and happiness. *The Gerontologist (Summer)*, **12** (2, Pt 1), 120–3.

[27] Cameron, P., Titus, D.G., Kostin, J., and Kostin, M. (1973) The life satisfaction of non-normal persons. *Journal of Counseling and Clinical Psychology*, **41**, 207–14.

[28] Visser, M.R.M., Smets, E.M.A., Sprangers, M.A.G., and de Haes, H.J.C.J.M. (2000) How response shift may affect the measurement of change in fatigue. *Journal of Pain and Symptom Management*, **20**, 12–18.

[29] Fletcher, A. (1995) Quality of life measurement in the evaluation of treatment: proposed guidelines. *British Journal of Clinical Pharmacology*, **39**, 217–22.

[30] Brinkley, D. (1985) Quality of life in cancer trials. *British Medical Journal*, **291**, 685–6.

[31] Slevin, M.L., Plant, H., Lynch, D., Drinkwater, J., and Gregory, W.M. (1988) Who should measure quality of life, the doctor or the patient? *British Journal of Cancer*, **57**, 109–12.

[32] Machin, D. (1996) Assessment of Quality of Life in clinical trials of the British Medical Research Council. *Journal of the National Cancer Institute Monographs*, No 20.

[33] Young, T., de Haes, H., Curran, D., Fayers, P., and Brandenberg, Y. (1999) Guidelines for assessing Quality of Life in EORTC clinical trials. *EORTC*.

[34] Fayers, P.M., Hopwood, P., Harvey, A., Girling, D.J., Machin, D., and Stephens, R. (1997) Quality of Life assessment in clinical trials – Guidelines and a checklist for protocol writers: the UK Medical Research Council Experience. *European Journal of Cancer*, **33**, 20–8.

[35] Scott, C.B., Stetz, J., Bruner, D.W., and Wasserman, T.H. (1994) Radiation Therapy Oncology Group Quality of Life assessment: design, analysis and data management issues. *Quality of Life Research*, **3**, 199–206.

[36] Groenvold, M., and Fayers, P.M. (1998) Testing for differences in multiple Quality of Life dimensions: generating hypotheses from the experience of hospital staff. *Quality of Life Research*, **7**, 479–86.

[37] Sur, R.K., Kochhar, R., and Singh, D.P. (1994) Oral sucralfate in acute radiation oesophagitis. *Acta Oncologica*, **33**, 61–3.

[38] Marty, M. on behalf of the Granisetron Study Group. (1992) A comparison of granisetron as a single agent with conventional combination antiemetic therapies in the treatment of cytostatic-induced emesis. *European Journal of Cancer*, **28A**(suppl 1), S12–6.

[39] Medical Research Council Lung Cancer Working Party. (1996) Randomized trial of palliative two-fraction versus more intensive 13-fraction radiotherapy for patients with inoperable non-small cell lung cancer and good performance status. *Clinical Oncology*, **8**, 167–75.

[40] Moore, M.J., Osoba, D., Murphy, K., Tannock, I.F., Armitage, A., Findlay, B., Coppin, C., Neville, A., Venner, P., and Wilson, J. (1994) Use of palliative endpoints to evaluate the effects of mitoxantrone and low dose prednisone in patients with hormonally resistant prostate cancer. *Journal of Clinical Oncology*, **12**, 689–94.

[41] Medical Research Council Lung Cancer Working Party. (1996) Comparison of oral etoposide and standard intravenous multidrug chemotherapy for small-cell lung cancer: a stopped multicentre randomised trial. *Lancet*, **348**, 563–6.

[42] Burris, H., and Storniolo, A.M. (1997) Assessing clinical benefit in the treatment of pancreas cancer: gemcitabine compared to 5-fluorouracil. *European Journal of Cancer*, 33 (suppl 1), S18–22.

[43] Stephens, R.J., Hopwood, P., and Girling, D.J. (1999) Defining and analysing symptom palliation in cancer clinical trials: a deceptively difficult exercise. *British Journal of Cancer*, 79, 538–44.

[44] Orr, S.T., and Aisner, J. (1986) Performance status assessment among oncology patients: a review. *Cancer Treatment Reports*, 70, 1423–9.

[45] Karnovsky, D.A., and Burchenal, J.H. (1949) The clinical evaluation of chemotherapeutic agents in cancer. In Macleod CM ed. Evaluation of chemotherapeutic agents. New York: Columbia University Press, 191–205.

[46] Zubrod, C.G., Schneiderman, M., Frei, E., Brindley, C., Gold, L.G., and Schnider, B. (1960) Appraisal of methods for the study of chemotherapy of cancer in man: comparative therapeutic trial of nitrogen mustard and triethylene thiophosphoramide. *Journal of Chronic Diseases*, 11, 7–33.

[47] World Health Organization. (1948) WHO handbook for reporting results of cancer treatment. WHO offset publication No 48. World Health Organization.

[48] McHorney, C.A., Ware, J.E., Rogers, W., Raczek, A.E., and Lu, J.F.R. (1992) The validity and relative precision of MOS short- and long-form Health Status Scales and Dartmouth COOP charts. *Medical Care*, 30, MS253–5.

[49] Fayers, P.M., and Hand, D.J. (1997) Factor analysis, causal indicators and Quality of Life. *Quality of Life Research*, 6, 139–50.

[50] Fayers, P.M., Hand, D.J., Bjordal, K., and Groenvold, M. (1997) Causal indicators in Quality of Life research. *Quality of Life Research*, 6, 393–406.

[51] Priestman, T.J., and Baum, M. (1976) Evaluation of quality of life in patients receiving treatment for advanced breast cancer. *Lancet*, I, 899–901.

[52] Boyd, N.F., Selby, P.J., Sutherland, H.J., and Hogg, S. (1988) Measurement of the clinical status of patients with breast cancer: evidence for the validity of self assessment with linear analogue scales. *Journal of Clinical Epidemiology*, 41, 243–50.

[53] Selby, P. (1985) Measurement of the quality of life after cancer treatment. *British Journal of Hospital Medicine*, 33, 266–71.

[54] Fayers, P.M. (1995) MRC Quality of Life studies using a daily diary card – practical lessons learned from cancer trials. *Quality of Life Research*, 4, 343–52.

[55] Bjordal, K., and Kaasa, S. (1992) Psychmetric validation of the EORTC core quality of life questionnaire, 30-item version and a diagnosis-specific module for head and neck cancer patients. *Acta Oncologica*, 31, 311–21.

[56] Ware, J.E., and Sherbourne, C.D. (1992) The MOS 36-item short-form health survey (SF-36). *Medical Care*, 30, 473–83.

[57] Hunt, S.M., McKenna, S.P., McEwen, J., Backett, E.M., Williams, J., and Papp, E. (1980) A quantitative approach to perceived health status: a validation study. *Journal of Epidemiology and Community Health*, 34, 281–6.

[58] Bergner, M., Bobbitt, R.A., Carter, W.B., and Gilson, B.S. (1981) The Sickness Impact Profile: development and final revision of a health status measure. *Medical Care*, 19, 787–805.

[59] Sackett, D.L., Chambers, L.W., MacPherson, A.S., Goldsmith, C.H., and McAuley, R.G. (1977) The development and application of indices of health: general methods and a summary of results. *American Journal of Public Health*, 67, 423–8.

[60] Chambers, L.W., Macdonald, L.A., Tugwell, P., Buchanan, W.W., and Kraag, G. (1982) The McMaster Health Index Questionnaire as a measure of quality of life for patients with rheumatoid disease. *The Journal of Rheumatology*, 5, 780–4.

[61] Aaronson, N.K., Ahmedzai, S., Bergman, B., Bullinger, M., Cull, A., Duez, N.J., Filiberti, A., Flechtner, H., Fleishman, S.B., de Haes, J.C.J.M., Kaasa, S., Klee, M., Osoba, D., Razavi, D., Rofe, P.B., Schraub, S., Sneeuw, K., Sullivan, M., and Takeda, F. (1993) The European Organization for

Research and Treatment of Cancer QLQ-C30: a Quality of Life instrument for use in international clinical trials in oncology. *Journal of the National Cancer Institute*, 85, 365–76.

[62] Cella, D.F., Tulsky, D.S., Gray, G., Sarafian, B., Linn, E., Bonomi, A., Silberman, M., Yellen, S.B., Winicour, P., Brannon, J., Eckberg, K., Lloyd, S., Purl, S., Blendowski, C., Goodman, M., Barnicle, M., Stewart, I., McHale, M., Bonomi, P., Kaplan, E., Taylor, S., Thomas, C.R., and Harris, J. (1993) The functional assessment of cancer therapy scale: development and validation of the general measure. *Journal of Clinical Oncology*, 11, 570–9.

[63] de Haes, J.C.J.M., van Knippenberg, F.C.E., and Neijt, J.P. (1990) Measuring psychological and physical distress in cancer patients: structure and application of the Rotterdam Symptom Checklist. *British Journal of Cancer*, 62, 1034–8.

[64] Schipper, H., Clinch, J., McMurray, A. and Levitt, M. (1984) Measuring the Quality of Life of cancer patients: the functional living index – cancer: development and validation. *Journal of Clinical Oncology*, 2, 472–83.

[65] Schag, C.C., Heinrich, R.L., Aadland, R., and Ganz, P.A. (1990) Assessing problems of cancer patients: psychometric properties of the cancer inventory of problem situations. *Health Psychology*, 9, 83–102.

[66] Schag, C.A.C., Ganz, P.A., and Heinrich, R.L. (1991) Cancer Rehabilitation Evaluation System – Short Form (CARES-SF). *Cancer*, 68, 1406–13.

[67] Levine, M.N., Guyatt, G.H., Gent, M., de Pauw, S., Goodyear, M.D., Hryniuk, W.M., Arnold, A., Findlay, B., Skillings, J.R., Bramwell, V.H., Levin, L., Bush, H., Abu-Zahra, H., and Kotalik, J. (1988) Quality of life in stage II breast cancer: an instrument for clinical trials. *Journal of Clinical Oncology*, 6, 1798–810.

[68] Zigmond, A.S., and Snaith, R.P. (1983) The Hospital Anxiety and Depression scale. *Acta Psychiatrica Scandinavica*, 67, 361–70.

[69] Kind, P. (1996) The EuroQoL instrument: an index of health-related quality of life. In: Spilker, B., Quality of Life and Pharmacoeconomics in Clinical Trials, Philadelphia: Lippincott-Raven.

[70] Fraser, S.C.A., Ramirez, A.J., Ebbs, S.R., Fallowfield, L.J., Dobbs, H.J., Richards, M.A., Bates, T. and Baum, M. (1993) A daily diary for quality of life measurement in advanced breast cancer trials. *British Journal of Cancer*, 67, 341–6.

[71] Testa, M.A., and Simonson, D.C. (1996) Assessment of quality of life outcomes. *New England Journal of Medicine*, 334, 835–40.

[72] Kemmler, G., Holzner, B., Kopp, M., Dunser, M., Margreiter, R., Greil, R., and Sperner-Unterweger, B. (1999) Comparison of two quality of life instruments for cancer patients: the Functional Assessment of Cancer Therapy-General and the European Organization for Research and Treatment of Cancer Quality of Life Questionnaire-C30. *Journal of Clinical Oncology*, 17, 2932–40.

[73] King, M.T., Dobson, A.J., and Harnett, P.R. (1996) A comparison of two quality of life question-naires for cancer clinical trials: the functional living index-cancer (FLIC) and the quality of life questionnaire core module (QLQ-C30). *Journal of Clinical Epidemiology*, 49, 21–9.

[74] Hollen, P.J., and Gralla, R.J. (1996) Comparison of instruments for measuring quality of life in patients with lung cancer. *Seminars in Oncology*, 23, 2(suppl 5), 31–40.

[75] Weinberger, M., Oddone, E.Z., Samsa, G.P., and Landsman, P.B. (1996) Are health-related quality of life measures affected by the mode of administration? *Journal of Clinical Epidemiology*, 49, 135–40.

[76] Ganz, P.A., Haskell, C.M., Figlin, R.A., La Soto, N. and Siau, J. (1988) Estimating the Quality of Life in a clinical trial of patients with metastatic lung cancer using the Karnofsky performance status and the Functional Living Index – Cancer. *Cancer*, 61, 849–56.

[77] Finkelstein, D.M., Cassileth, B.R., Bonomi, P.D., Ruckdeschel, J.C., Ezdinli, E.Z., and Wolter, J.M. (1988) A pilot study of the Functional Living Index-Cancer (FLIC) Scale for the assessment of

quality of life for metastatic lung cancer patients. An Eastern Cooperative Oncology Group study. *American Journal of Clinical Oncology*, 11, 630–3.

[78] Hurny, C., Bernhard, J., Joss, R., Willems, Y., Cavalli, F., Kiser, J., Brunner, K., Favre, S., Alberto, P., Glaus, A., Senn, H., Schatzmann, E., Ganz, P.A., and Metzger, U. (1992) Feasibility of Quality of Life assessment in a randomized phase III trial of small cell lung cancer. *Annals of Oncology*, 3, 825–31.

[79] Giaccone, G., Splinter, T.A.W., Debruyne, C., Kho, G.S., Lianes, P., van Zandwijk, N., Pennucci, M.C., Scagliotti, G., van Meerbeeck, J., van Hoesel, Q., Curran, D., Sahmoud, T., and Postmus, P.E. (1998) Randomized study of paclitaxel-cisplatin versus cisplatin-teniposide in patients with advanced non-small cell lung cancer. *Journal of Clinical Oncology*, 16, 2133–41.

[80] Langendijk, J.A., ten Velde, G.P.M., Aaronson, N.K., de Jong, J.M.A., Muller, M.J., and Wouters, E.F.M. (2000) Quality of life after palliaitve radiotherapy in non-small cell lung cancer: a prospective study. *International Journal of Radiation Oncology Biology and Physics*, 47, 149–55.

[81] Wisloff, F., Eika, S., Hippe, E., Hjorth, M., Homberg, E., Kaasa, S., Palva, I., and Westin, J. (1996) Measurement of health-related quality of life in multiple myeloma. *British Journal of Haematology*, 92, 604–13.

[82] Sadura, A., Pater, J., Osoba, D., Levine, M., Palmer, M., and Bennett, K. (1992) Quality of life assessment: patient compliance with questionnaire completion. *Journal of the National Cancer Institute*, 84, 1023–6.

[83] Ganz, P.A., Moinpour, C.M., Cella, D.F., and Fetting, J.H. (1992) Quality of life assessment in cancer clinical trials: a status report. *Journal of the National Cancer Institute*, 84, 994–5.

[84] Moinpour, C.M., Feigl, P., Metch, B., Hayden, K.A., Meyskens, F.L., and Crowley, J. (1989) Quality of Life endpoints in cancer clinical trials: review and recommendations. *Journal of the National Cancer Institute*, 81, 485–95.

[85] Cox, D.R., Fitzpatrick, R., Fletcher, A.E., Gore, S.M., Spiegelhalter, D.J., and Jones, D.R. (1992) Quality of life assessment: can we keep it simple? *Journal of the Royal Statistical Society*, 155, 353–93.

[86] Brorsson, B., Ifver, J., and Hays, R.D. (1993) The Swedish health-related quality of life survey (SWED-QUAL). *Quality of Life Research*, 2, 33–45.

[87] Hopwood, P., Harvey, A., Davies, J., Stephens, R.J., Girling, D.J., Gibson, D., and Parmar, M.K.B. (1997) Survey of the administration of Quality of Life (QL) questionnaires in three multicentre randomised trials in cancer. *European Journal of Cancer*, 34, 49–57.

[88] Testa, M.A., Hollenberg, N.K., Anderson, R.B., and Williams, G.H. (1991) Assessment of quality of life by patient and spouse during antihypertensive therapy with atenolol and nifedipine gastrointestinal therapeutic system. *American Journal of Hypertension*, 4, 363–73.

Chapter 7

Putting plans into practice

7.1 Introduction

In this chapter, we consider all that needs to be done up to the launch of a trial. We describe the functions and roles that the team responsible for conducting the trial needs to fulfill, a team we denote generically as the trial management group.

Some trials will be planned and conducted by an individual person, others as part of a programme of multi-centre randomized trials by an established trials office. Setting up and conducting a single trial or a programme of trials is, however, a major and specialized activity which should only be undertaken by persons or groups with the necessary expertise and experience, whether or not they constitute an established long-standing group. Individuals conducting the trial should include, or have access to, the necessary statistical, medical, computing and data management expertise. Such expertise is essential and can be provided in a number of ways through the course of the trial. It is important to recognize, however, the need for continuity of personnel and for the non-clinical staff to be conversant with the medical issues. The same expertise should also be available to those running small trials or phase II studies within a single centre. Expert advice on such matters as histopathology, quality of life assessment, and health economics, may also be required.

It is essential that those involved in setting up and conducting trials are experts in their own specialized areas and keep up-to-date on all aspects of their work, including progress in the treatment of the cancers with which they deal and developments in trials methodology and computing software. This could involve attending appropriate training courses, providing in-house training, including relevant higher degrees and diplomas, and participating in specialist conferences and clinical and scientific meetings. The trial coordinators must assign sufficient time and funding to training.

7.2 What needs to be done?

The tasks that need to be undertaken before a trial is activated are shown in Box 7.1. An outline proposal may or may not have to be prepared and costed for the sponsor and other potential funders, but a protocol must always be written, and ethics approval obtained.

Underlying all these tasks is the need to plan and set up the trial in accordance with internationally agreed standards of practice. We therefore describe these first before considering the tasks in detail and who is responsible for fulfilling them.

> **Box 7.1 Tasks that need to be undertaken up to the launch of a trial**
>
> - Set up a trial management group
> - Prepare grant proposals for a sponsor, if required
> - Prepare and distribute trial protocols and forms to potential collaborators
> - Prepare trial-specific operating procedures for trial co-ordinators
> - Obtain ethics approval from Institutional Review Board/Independent Ethics Committees, Multi-centre Research Ethics Committees, or their equivalents

7.3 International standards for conducting trials

Clinical trials should be conducted in accordance with the principles set out in the International Conference on Harmonization's Good Clinical Practice (ICH GCP) Guideline. This guideline defines GCP as: 'A standard for the design, conduct, performance, monitoring, auditing, recording, analyses, and reporting of clinical trials that provides assurance that the data and reported results are credible and accurate, and that the rights, integrity, and confidentiality of trial subjects are protected.' The ICH GCP guideline was developed to provide a unified standard for the European Union, Japan and the US in order to facilitate the mutual acceptance of clinical data by the regulatory authorities in these jurisdictions. It was developed in accordance with the current GCP of the countries involved and of Australia, Canada, the Nordic countries and the World Health Organization. It is primarily concerned, however, with the development of new, investigational, medicinal products. In the UK, the British Medical Research Council, in consultation with the National Health Service Research and Development Programme, has therefore published guidelines, based on the ICH GCP principles but adapting the guideline for more general application, intended to be of use as a practical handbook to any engaged in conducting clinical trials (http://www.mrc.ac.uk/b2/pdf-ctg.pdf) [1].

The list of publications and web sites shown in Box 7.2 should prove useful for reference purposes.

These documents define the individuals and groups involved in conducting trials and list their roles and responsibilities. They also make recommendations on protocol design; statistical matters; trial coordination and monitoring; data collection, verification and handling; and ethical issues. The COREC web site is a useful route to other relevant sites.

7.4 Who does what?

7.4.1 The trial sponsor and trial funders

The trial sponsor is defined in the ICH GCP guideline as: 'An individual, company, institution or organization which takes responsibility for the initiation, management, and/or funding of a clinical trial.' This is the sense in which we use the term here. Other bodies may also, however, provide aspects of funding or support. For example, a

Box 7.2   A selection of publications and web sites relevant to GCP

- International Conference on Harmonization Guideline for Good Clinical Practice. ICH Technical Coordination, London, 1997 [2]
- International Conference on Harmonization web site: http://www.ifpma.org/ich1.html
- MRC Guidelines for Good Clinical Practice in Clinical Trials. Medical Research Council, London, 1998 [1]
- MRC web site: http://www.mrc.ac.uk/b2/pdf-ctg.pdf
- United Kingdom COREC (Central Office for Research Ethics Committees) web site: http://www.corec.org.uk
- United States Food and Drug Administration web site: http://www.fda.gov/oc/ohrt/irbs. Guidance for Institutional Review Boards and Clinical Investigators
- Guidelines for the Ethical Conduct of Medical Research Involving Children. British Paediatric Association, 1992 [3]
- Royal College of Paediatrics and Child Health web site: http://www.rcpch.ac.uk
- Code of Conduct for Clinical Trials. United Kingdom Children's Cancer Study Group (UKCCSG), 1999 [4]

pharmaceutical company may provide drug free or at reduced cost, or may contribute to the funding of a non-industry-led trial, without being the sponsor.

7.4.2   The trial management group

Once the decision has been made that a new trial should be undertaken, a trial management group should be set up to develop and manage the trial (see Box 7.3). This is essential whether it is a small trial run by a single centre or a large multi-centre collaboration. The differences between small and large trials are those of scale and detail, not of principle, but the conduct of a trial should rarely, if ever, be the responsibility of only one person. The trial management group should include the principal investigator(s), together with the expert advisers who carried the idea through the planning and design stages described in previous chapters. Thus, it is typically the protocol development group who become the trial management group.

It is the trial management group who are ultimately responsible for ensuring that a trial is conducted efficiently, completed successfully, and published promptly. However, by agreeing to collaborate in a trial, the expert advisers and collaborating clinicians all accept responsibility for their own contributions. To be successful, a trial requires good communication, close cooperation, and a high level of commitment from all those involved. All concerned with the conduct of a trial must ensure that every effort is made to promote the trial, to conduct it ethically and safely in accordance with

Box 7.3 Membership of the trial management group

- Principal investigator
- Clinical advisers
- One or more expert advisers or independent assessors
- Medical statistician
- Clinical trials manager
- Supporting data management, computing, administrative and secretarial staff

good clinical practice, and to complete it within the planned timescale and budget with enough patients and with data that are correct and as complete as possible so that the results of the trial are reliable. These goals can only be achieved by good trial management.

Many of the responsibilities of the trial management group relate to the period up to launch of the trial. Those involving its launch and subsequent conduct are mentioned briefly in this chapter for ease of reference but are described more fully in Chapter 8.

The trial management group is responsible for preparing any funding proposal that may be needed, overseeing the preparation, printing and distribution of the final protocol and trial documentation, obtaining ethics approval, making any final alterations to the protocol that may be required by the ethics committee (preferably having had the protocol independently and meticulously reviewed for accuracy, comprehensibility and layout), recruiting centres, conducting the trial on a day-to-day basis, undertaking analyses, and ensuring that the results are presented at appropriate scientific meetings and published in peer-reviewed journals.

7.4.3 Principal investigator

It is essential to identify a principal investigator. This is the person ultimately responsible for initiating the trial, organizing and obtaining any funding that may be needed, organizing any relevant industrial support, conducting the trial in collaboration with the other members of the trial management group, and taking the lead in preparing reports for publication. The principal investigator must ensure that all collaborating personnel fully understand the trial, their responsibilities and roles in its conduct, and the procedures involved. Principal investigators are typically clinicians and, as such, provide expert clinical advice to collaborating centres; they will usually have limited time to devote to the conduct of the trial but should nevertheless accept final responsibility for the functions shown in Box 7.4, even if many of these are shared or delegated.

Thus, principal investigators need to take ultimate personal responsibility for the success of the trial; they should randomize as many of their own patients as they can, and encourage others to do the same. They are responsible for ensuring that the trial is run ethically, efficiently and to the highest standards, and should ensure that appropriate independent expert advice, assessment, and monitoring are available. The principal

Box 7.4 Functions of the principal investigator

- Respond promptly to clinical queries raised by collaborating centres. Such queries commonly include the boundaries of eligibility criteria, finer details of treatment (including permissible minor variations from protocol), toxicity, supportive care, and the best ways of explaining the trial to patients

- Look for, and accept, opportunities for promoting the trial and encouraging colleagues to collaborate

- Establish contact with groups undertaking similar trials and exchange information with them on progress

- Present information on the progress of the trial at collaborators' meetings and respond to any queries or problems raised about collaborating in the trial. Any areas of legitimate major concern should be raised with the data monitoring and ethics committee or trial supervisors (see Section 8.10)

- Communicate with patient advocacy groups on the reasons for conducting the trial and on its progress

- Collaborate in preparing regular reports for the trial sponsors and supervisors

- In collaboration with other members of the trial management group, present results at conferences and draft reports for publication

investigator must therefore keep the trial monitors and supervisors (see Section 8.10) informed about the progress of the trial and about any problems that may arise during its conduct.

7.4.4 Clinical advisers

The clinical advisers include the clinicians who suggested the trial (one of whom is likely to be the principal investigator) and so have a personal commitment to it. They should include at least one member for each of the treatment modalities under study. They help write the protocol and promote the trial. They are responsible for clinical aspects at all stages and for answering relevant queries. They may present results at conferences and help draft reports for publication. Ideally, they should have experience in the conduct of trials.

7.4.5 Expert advisers and independent assessors

Most trials require expert advice from an early stage in their development. The advice needed depends on the trial, but it can include, for example, advice on details of chemotherapy dosage and administration, radiotherapy dosage and fractionation, surgical procedures, ways of avoiding and treating adverse effects of treatment, histo-pathological definitions, quality of life assessment, health economics, patient advocacy, microbiology, and pharmacy. Additional advisers may also be needed on such matters as novel radiotherapy or surgical techniques and on new treatment modalities. They should be involved in the trial from the early planning stages. The clinical advisers can provide much of the expertise needed, but many trials require advice from other specialists as well.

Few cancer trials can be conducted on a double-blind basis (see Section 4.8). This may be because the treatments being compared differ too much from each other (radiotherapy versus surgery, for example) or because a blind comparison would be unethical: for example, subjecting patients to dummy invasive procedures. Under these circumstances, it may be important to ensure that some assessments of subjective outcome measures, such as tumour response and disease-free survival, are made blind, that is, by expert advisers unaware of the patient's treatment group. Blind assessment is not necessary if the assessments can be made objectively without being affected by knowledge of the treatment group. The protocol should state who will make any blind assessments.

Consideration should be given to making blind assessments on a random sample of patients if to do so on all would be administratively problematic.

7.4.6 Medical statistician

Trials require medical statistical expertise at all stages of their design and conduct, and this should be available from as early a stage in the trial's development as possible. Such expertise is essential for defining the appropriate trial design, sample size and statistical methods, and for undertaking and interpreting interim analyses for the data monitoring and ethics committee during the intake to the trial, and final analyses for published reports on its completion.

Whenever possible, the same statistician should be responsible for both design and analyses. It is also highly desirable for the statistician to have experience in the relevant disease area.

7.4.7 Clinical trials manager

The clinical trials manager is the person of first contact for all trial-related matters and is usually responsible for much of the drafting of the protocol, for clinical report form design, and instituting randomization procedures, in addition to the day-to-day running of the trial. For a multi-centre trial, duties are likely to include visiting and recruiting centres, setting up databases, managing data, dealing with queries, maintaining mailing lists, organizing meetings, preparing newsletters, and reporting on progress to collaborating centres and the data monitoring and ethics committee. The clinical trials manager is thus the key and essential person responsible for the practicalities of trial management on a day-to-day basis, and it is invaluable to have an experienced person in this role.

For a large or data-intensive trial, it can be useful to appoint a further person or persons who works with the clinical trials manager and may be responsible for data entry, data management, maintaining the database, chasing up overdue data, and for raising queries about data with collaborating centres. Many trials will also require computing (see Section 8.11), administrative and secretarial support.

7.4.8 Collaborating centres

By agreeing to take part in a trial, clinicians undertake to conduct the trial in their own centre in accordance with the protocol and to provide the data required promptly.

7.5 Developing and drafting an outline proposal

Whatever processes are used for assessing proposals for new trials, the group developing an idea will often need to draft an outline proposal for independent assessment before developing a detailed protocol. An outline proposal may be required for presenting to sponsors, potential collaborators, and patient advocacy groups, and will sometimes be needed in applying for funding. The drafting of such a proposal for a new trial must therefore be done with care and thoroughness.

The ways proposals are assessed and prioritized, and decisions reached about whether or not they should be funded, vary between sponsors, but the principle remains that to attract funding from a sponsor and enthusiastic support from the clinical community and patient advocacy groups, the proposal must make a persuasive case for conducting the trial. It must show that the trial is needed to answer important questions, that it is appropriately designed, and that it stands a good chance of answering the questions reliably, of accruing the required number of patients during the planned accrual period, and of leading, ultimately, to improvements in clinical practice.

Groups submitting outline proposals need to bear in mind that their proposals are likely to be judged in comparison with others and that it may not necessarily be possible even for all highly rated proposals to be funded. This emphasizes the need to ensure the relevance and timeliness of proposed new trials, and of making the application clear and compelling, even to a non-specialist reader.

To fulfill these requirements, a proposal should be drawn up as follows. Different sponsors have different formats, but the information required is essentially the same.

7.5.1 Title

Choose a title that is brief but informative so that the design of the trial is clear from its title. For example: *A randomized trial to evaluate the efficacy and toxicity of treatment A compared with treatment B in advanced C cancer* is far more informative than *A study of treatment A in C cancer*. An acronym can be useful for future reference, once participants are familiar with the trial.

7.5.2 The need for the trial

- Indicate how common the disease is in the general population.
- Indicate the sorts of patients affected and what proportion of all patients with the relevant type of cancer they represent; grant applications are often assessed by people without experience in the specific disease area. Indicate also the scientific questions that the trial will answer, the ways in which it is likely to influence routine clinical practice, and how it may inform the planning of future research.
- Give a clear and full account of the issues that gave rise to the proposal for a new trial, explaining why they are important. Make sure that all relevant references are given, briefly summarizing the findings from any relevant previous studies. This will involve conducting a literature search, or preferably a systematic review (see Section 11.5.4), and consulting colleagues and other research groups. The aim should be to justify the need for the trial for external referees and sponsors.

◆ Describe what, if any, other trials studying the same or similar problems are currently being conducted or planned by other groups, making it clear why it would not be feasible to plan a joint or parallel trial with another group or to join an already open trial. This will involve consulting trial registers (see Section 11.5.4) and other research groups on currently open relevant trials.

◆ State the hypothesis to be tested by the trial. This should be a brief but comprehensive statement, for example: *In the treatment of advanced A cancer, regimen B is more effective than the standard regimen C in terms of survival, symptom control, disease progression and quality of life, and/but is less/more toxic.*

◆ State why the trial is needed now. Referees and sponsors, as well as potential collaborators, need to prioritize new research proposals, and need adequate reasons for supporting the trial in comparison with other competing proposals.

◆ If previous randomized trials have addressed the same question, explain why another trial is needed rather than a systematic review and meta-analysis of previous trials (see Chapter 11). If a systematic review has generated the hypothesis to be tested, then give details and explain how it has identified the need for the trial.

7.5.3 The design of the trial

◆ It is often helpful to include a diagram of the design of the trial so that this can be seen at a glance. Fig. 7.1 shows an example of a summary design for a prostate cancer trial.

◆ List the eligibility criteria (see Section 4.2.3). These should define the type of cancer, the acceptable diagnostic evidence, the general characteristics of the patients, and should state the need for informed consent. Patients must be fit for either (or any) of the randomized interventions, and must not have previous or current illnesses likely to interfere with the protocol, the treatments, or the assessments of the outcome measures. Arbitrary restrictions that have no scientific basis, such as age limits, should be avoided. See also Sections 4.2.3 and 7.6.7.

◆ Describe the means of allocating patients to treatments, including, when appropriate, details of the randomization method (see Section 4.7).

◆ Describe the treatment policies to be evaluated and compared. Enough detail should be given for external referees to satisfy themselves that the interventions have the

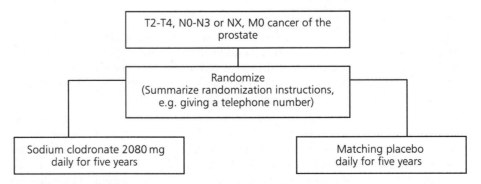

Fig. 7.1 Example of a summary design for a prostate cancer trial.

potential to be effective and are unlikely to be excessively toxic. Drug dosages should be stated and the number of cycles of chemotherapy and the intervals between them. Total doses and fields of radiotherapy should be stated and the number of fractions and the intervals between them. Surgical procedures should be given their standard name or, if necessary, described in detail in an appendix. How toxicity is to be graded should be indicated, and it may be necessary to describe how adverse effects are to be handled, particularly if novel approaches to managing them are to be part of the trial. Indicate which components of treatment are at the clinician's discretion.

- Indicate the frequency and duration of follow-up assessments. It is important to restrict the number of follow-up attendances to the minimum required for trial purposes. For example, it may be necessary for patients to be seen monthly for satisfactory clinical management, but for trial data to be collected only every three or six months. It is good practice, in most cancer trials, to keep patients under follow-up until death, although for long-term survivors only minimal data may be needed. The frequency of follow-up must be the same in all treatment groups.

- List the outcome measures. The primary outcome measure is the one on which estimates of the size of the trial are made (see Section 5.2). It is often duration of survival. The primary outcome measure should be the most important outcome and one that can be unambiguously measured. Secondary outcome measures might include tumour response, adverse effects, disease progression, quality of life, and economic measures. All outcome measures should be justified as being necessary for answering the trial's hypothesis satisfactorily.

- Describe the data that need to be collected. Methods of recording adverse effects should be stated, including relevant laboratory tests; any quality of life instruments should be specified and referenced. Resist the temptation to collect data that are not needed for assessing the specified outcome measures.

- State the number of patients needed, indicating how this was calculated. In a randomized trial this involves estimating the likely outcome rates in the control group and the differences that are clinically worthwhile and can realistically be expected in the experimental groups. Give reasons for the choice of targeted difference to be detected. In equivalence trials, numbers are based upon the size of any differences that are to be excluded. Sample size estimation is fully discussed in Chapter 5.

- State the methods to be used in analysing the main outcome measures. Standard methods should be listed and, if necessary, referenced. State what, if any, subgroup analyses are planned.

- Indicate the expected frequency of confidential interim analyses for the data monitoring and ethics committee, although during the course of the trial the committee may decide that more or less frequent meetings are desirable.

7.5.4 The level of interest the trial is likely to attract

State the anticipated rate of patient accrual. Before a proposal for a multi-centre trial is submitted, it is often useful to conduct a survey among potential centres to find out their level of interest and how many patients they would expect to be able to enter per year. This can be done by sending them a copy of the draft outline proposal, and a brief questionnaire, asking them to state (1) whether they are interested in participating in the trial and, if so, (2) how many patients they would expect to be able to enter per year, and (3) inviting comments. It is important to bear in mind that estimates of patients per year usually reflect numbers of potentially eligible patients seen per year; the numbers fulfilling all eligibility criteria and agreeing to take part are usually substantially fewer. In the light of our own experience, we therefore suggest dividing such estimates by four.

Make it clear in the proposal that the anticipated rate of accrual is based on the results of a survey.

7.5.5 The costs of the trial and the funding requested

It is important to ensure that all applicable monies and claims are sufficient to cover all anticipated costs likely to be incurred as direct results of conducting and participating in the trial. The main items are listed in Box 7.5. If other sources of support, for example

---

Box 7.5 Summary of the costs of a trial

Research costs

- Staff salaries, or proportions of salaries, for e.g. a medical statistician, a clinical trials manager, a data manager, and computing, administrative, and secretarial support
- Recruitment costs for advertizing posts and for training personnel
- Equipment expenses for e.g. personal computer and printer
- Printing costs for protocols, case reports forms and newsletters
- Hire of venue and travel and accommodation expenses for meetings of the trial management group, collaborating clinicians, the data monitoring and ethics committee, and the trial steering committee
- Travel costs for members of the trial management group to visit collaborating centres and for quality assurance visits, if required
- Costs of any expert reviews
- Flagging for notification of deaths or other events, if available, with the appropriate national registry – the Office of National Statistics in the UK
- Costs of reprints of publications
- General office expenses (consumables) to cover e.g. photocopying, faxing, telephoning, and postage
- Per-patient payments to collaborating centres to cover local costs of collaboration, if appropriate

Box 7.5 *(continued)*

Treatment and other costs

- Costs of treatment additional to those of standard routine management outside the trial; when external funding is not available these costs have to be borne by the health care system
- The costs of investigations additional to those of standard routine management outside the trial
- The costs, for centres and patients, of additional attendances for treatment and follow-up required by the trial

from the pharmaceutical industry, are likely to become available, this should be stated in the proposal or in a covering letter.

The periods over which these costs will be incurred need careful consideration. It is essential that statistical expertise is available throughout the total period of the trial, from planning to reporting, and that the clinical trials manager is appointed at an early stage, but it may be possible to stagger the appointments of some other staff. An example of a summary of staff required for the central coordination of a large randomized cancer trial is shown in Box 7.6.

The trial management group is likely to need to meet at least twice per year. Annual meetings of all collaborators, of the data monitoring and ethics committee, and of any trial supervisory committee will probably be desirable. Visits to centres by the trial management group might typically amount to two visits per centre by two members of the group during the course of the trial.

Treatment costs will depend upon the nature of the trial. The costs not only of anti-cancer drugs but also of supportive care need to be considered.

Box 7.6 Summary of staff required for the central coordination of a typical large randomized cancer trial

Staff salaries

- 20 per cent of a medical statistician for the full eight years
- One full-time clinical trials manager for the full eight years
- 50 per cent of a data manager from year two to year eight
- 20 per cent of a trials assistant from year two to year eight
- two full-time-equivalent research nurses for the full eight years

Include costs of recruiting and training staff

7.5.6 The research team

The sponsor will need to be convinced that trial management is likely to be efficient. It is therefore necessary to describe how the trial will be coordinated and by whom.

- List all the team members and proposed investigators who will be conducting the trial, that is, the trial management group.
- Describe the responsibilities of each team member, demonstrating that collectively they cover the required range of disciplines and possess the necessary skills and qualifications.
- Indicate whether the team already has experience in completing large multi-centre trials successfully. In the case of a small group wishing to conduct a local trial, indicate what experience the group has and what advice is readily available to it.
- Provide a list (possibly as an appendix) of all the centres and consultants who have expressed an interest in collaborating, indicating the numbers of patients that these centres expect to be able to randomize each year.

If required by the sponsor, list the members of the supervisory committee, and suggest possible members of an independent data monitoring and ethics committee (if different from the supervisory committee), indicating whether or not they have been approached and agree to fulfill their required functions.

7.6 Preparing the trial protocol

The trial management group should prepare the trial protocol. In the following plan we indicate items of information and the main headings that need to be included and suggest a logical sequence. Groups will have their own styles but the contents are unlikely to differ substantially.

7.6.1 Front cover

Name the sponsor, and other groups providing support, and state the identifying trial number, the full title, the abbreviated title, the International Standard Randomized Controlled Trial Number (ISRCTN) for all randomized trials, and the date and the version number of the protocol. If amendments have been made, state the date of the amended version.

7.6.2 Inside front cover

List the names and addresses, the telephone and fax numbers, and the e-mail addresses of relevant members of the trial management group, indicating their roles, and any relevant laboratories. Give the contact details for registration, randomization and enquiries.

7.6.3 Contents

List the contents and page numbers for easy reference. At the end of this list, we suggest a standard paragraph such as the following to remind collaborators of the nature of the trial. It will, of course, need modification according to individual circumstances.

'This document describes a multi-centre, randomized [sponsor's name] trial in cancer of the [type of cancer] and provides information about the procedures for entering patients into it. It should not be used as an aide-memoire or guide for the treatment of other patients. Every care was taken in its drafting, but corrections or amendments may be necessary. These will be circulated to collaborating centres, but centres entering patients for the first time are asked to contact [the trial coordinator] to ensure that they have the correct version of the protocol.'

7.6.4 Trial outline

Give a one-page diagrammatic summary of the trial, indicating its design (e.g. factorial, open-label, double-blind, etc.) and showing the main eligibility criteria, the timing of

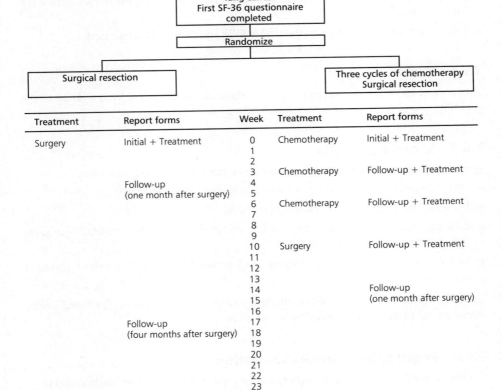

Fig. 7.2 Example of a one-page trial outline from a lung-cancer protocol.

registration or randomization, the treatment regimens in summary form, the sequence of reports, the frequency of follow-up assessments, and the outcome measures. This one-page diagrammatic summary can be a useful reference document for clinical centres that have already entered patients into the trial and are familiar with the procedures. An example is given in Fig. 7.2.

7.6.5   Background

- Give full justification for conducting the trial, indicating its clinical relevance and importance for future management.
- List any other trials addressing the same question, and state why the present trial is needed.
- Justify the trial design and outcome measures and, if necessary, the omission of some outcome measures.
- Ensure that the background to the trial is fully and relevantly referenced.

7.6.6   Aims

Give a short and clear account of the aims of the trial, ensuring that their relation to the eligibility criteria and outcome measures is clear.

7.6.7   Eligibility criteria

- List the eligibility criteria, ensuring that each one is relevant and necessary.
- Avoid arbitrary exclusion criteria such as upper and lower age limits.
- Include the requirements of informed consent.
- Include, where appropriate, completion of baseline patient-completed question-naire(s), e.g. quality of life questionnaires.
- Definitions such as those of staging and performance status are best given in appendices.

Box 7.7 gives an example of the eligibility criteria from a randomized trial in the management of malignant pleural mesothelioma.

7.6.8   Registration and randomization

- Give clear instructions for the procedure for registering or randomizing patients.
- For randomized trials we suggest including at the end of this section a standard statement such as the following, to remind collaborators of the implications of randomizing patients into the trial.

'This trial is a comparison of treatment policies. Once a patient has been random-ized, that patient remains in the trial and all report forms are required. If the patient decides to withdraw from treatment, report forms should continue to be sent giving such information as is available on the patient's progress.'

Box 7.7   Eligibility criteria for a randomized trial in the management of malignant pleural mesothelioma

Inclusion criteria

Patients must fulfill all of the following criteria to be eligible for the trial:

- Microscopically and immunohistochemically confirmed malignant pleural mesothelioma, including epithelial and other histological types, with a maximum time from date of diagnostic biopsy to randomization of three months
- Any symptomatic pleural effusion treated and brought under control by drainage, pleurodesis or pleurectomy
- CT scan to be performed within a month prior to randomization and, whenever possible, after pleurodesis
- Patients who have undergone surgical resection of mesothelioma are eligible provided two CT scans, six weeks apart, show stable or progressive disease
- No previous chemotherapy for mesothelioma
- Patients who have had local radiotherapy to a wound site after an exploratory thoracotomy are eligible
- No other disease or previous malignancy likely to interfere with the protocol treatments or comparisons
- WHO performance status 0–2
- WBC $> 3 \times 10^9$/L, neutrophils $> 1.5 \times 10^9$/L, platelets $> 100 \times 10^9$/L, and no clinical evidence of infection
- Considered medically fit to receive chemotherapy; creatinine clearance > 50 ml/min
- Patient has read the patient information sheet and signed the consent form
- Patient has completed a quality of life questionnaire before being told the treatment allocated

7.6.9   Treatment regimens

- Give a detailed account of all treatment regimens including, where appropriate, recommended hydration and anti-emetic regimens and other procedures for avoiding toxicity.
- Always use generic names for all drugs unless there is a special case for not doing so.
- Nomograms for calculating drug dosages as mg/m^2 body surface area are best given in an appendix.
- Ask relevant expert advisers to comment on the descriptions of the regimens, for example: medical oncologists and oncological pharmacists on chemotherapy

regimens, radiation oncologists on radiotherapy regimens, and surgeons on surgical regimens and procedures.

♦ Recommend procedures for general management during treatment.

7.6.10   Adverse effects of treatment

♦ List the main adverse effects that may be encountered and make recommendations for managing them.

♦ List the types of serious adverse event that should be reported without delay on a Serious Adverse Event form. A serious adverse event is defined in the ICH GCP guideline as follows.

Any untoward medical occurrence that at any dose:

> results in death,
>
> is life-threatening,
>
> requires inpatient hospitalization or prolongation of existing hospitalization,
>
> results in persistent or significant disability/incapacity, or
>
> is a congenital anomaly/birth defect.

Accidental overdose should be included.

7.6.11   Relapse procedures

Indicate the action that should be taken on relapse and death.

7.6.12   Assessments and investigations

♦ List the investigations required before treatment (or before registration or randomization), during treatment, and during subsequent follow-up.

♦ Restrict investigations to those essential for answering the questions posed.

7.6.13   Quality of life assessment

♦ When quality of life outcome measures are included, ensure that staff in local centres responsible for applying quality of life questionnaires are identified, and describe the procedures for training them.

♦ Ensure that centres are supplied with guidelines and patient information sheets [5, 6].

The assessment of quality of life is fully covered in Chapter 6.

7.6.14   Outcome measures

♦ List the primary and secondary outcome measures.

♦ Ensure that each measure is precisely defined and that the required investigations are listed.

♦ Restrict outcome measures to those essential for answering the questions posed by the trial.

7.6.15   Statistical considerations

- State the basis of the sample size calculation in sufficient detail that it could be reproduced by those reading the protocol (see Section 5.3).
- State the number of patients required, the significance level, and the power.
- Indicate over what period it is expected to complete the intake.
- List the responsibilities of the independent data monitoring and ethics committee, and how often it is expected that they will meet to review interim analyses.

Planned analyses should be described in sufficient detail that a statistician new to the trial can clearly see the general approach intended. It is important to outline how any 'non-standard' data, such as quality of life data, are to be analysed. It may be useful to state the details of analysis in a separate analysis protocol which could be made available on request.

7.6.16   Ethical considerations

- State the ethics procedures already completed and those that local investigators must follow before entering patients.
- The details of ethical requirements vary from country to country. For a multi-centre trial, the following statement might be appropriate.

'This trial protocol has been approved by the [appropriate ethics committee]. The patient's consent to participate in the trial must be obtained before entry and after a full explanation has been given of the treatment options, and the manner of treatment allocation. The patient should be given a copy of the patient information sheet and allowed time to discuss this with other staff and with family and friends, if desired, before deciding whether to participate. A patient information sheet and patient consent form are attached. Locally relevant details, such as persons to contact and their telephone numbers, can be added to the leaflet as required. One copy of the completed and signed patient consent form should be given to the patient and another retained in the patient's casenotes.

'The right of a patient to refuse to participate without giving reasons must be respected. After the patient has entered the trial, the clinician must remain free to give alternative treatment to that specified in the protocol at any stage if he or she feels it to be in the patient's best interest, but the reasons for doing so should be recorded and the patient should remain within the trial for the purposes of follow-up and data analysis. Similarly, the patient must remain free to withdraw at any time from protocol treatment without giving reasons and without prejudicing his or her future treatment; as much information as possible relevant to the trial should continue to be collected, particularly on the primary outcome measure.'

- The protocol should require each patient to be given a patient information sheet describing the trial in addition to a verbal explanation from their doctor or a research nurse. It should require each patient to give 'written, informed consent' and to sign and date a consent form, unless this is inappropriate as in emergency situations or trials involving children, for example where the relevant National guidelines should be followed (see also Sections 7.8.2–7.8.4).

7.6.17 Data access and quality assurance

Specify if direct access to source data or documents will be required for trial-related monitoring or audit by, for example, the trial co-ordinators, collaborating pharmaceutical companies, regulatory authorities, or ethics committees. Indicate what monitoring and audit is planned.

7.6.18 Publication

- State how the authorship of major publications will be reported.
- State what acknowledgements will be made, ensuring that all sources of finance and material assistance, such as the provision of free or reduced-cost drug, are acknowledged.

7.6.19 References

- Ensure that all sections of the protocol are adequately referenced with up-to-date references.
- Check that all references are relevant and correct.

7.6.20 Patient information sheet

We discuss general issues relating to the use of patient information sheets in Chapter 2 (see Section 2.3.4), but discuss the main practical aspects of drafting them here.

- State the name of the trial, its purpose, design and duration, and who is conducting and sponsoring it. Indicate why the patient has been invited to take part. State the advantages and possible disadvantages of taking part, indicating whether participants or only future patients are likely to benefit. Describe the treatment regimens and the possible advantages and risks associated with each of them. For randomized trials, explain the randomization process and why it is needed. If a placebo is used, explain why this is necessary. Arrange for the patient information sheet to be translated into all the relevant languages.
- Indicate the standard treatment the patient would be likely to receive if not in the trial.
- Describe what the trial involves, including not only the treatment regimens but also the investigations required.
- Indicate how data are recorded, assuring patients that confidentiality will be preserved.
- Explain that there is no obligation to take part and indicate patients' right to withdraw at any time without giving reasons and without affecting their relationship with hospital staff or their treatment.
- State what, if any, expenses will be reimbursed. Payments made to patients should only be for expenses reasonably incurred and that would not be incurred outside the trial. Payments should never be such as to constitute an inducement to patients to participate against their better judgement.

- State what will happen if new information becomes available during the trial, and what happens when the study stops.
- State how they can obtain further help and advice should they require it, and the complaints and indemnity procedures.
- Use simple non-technical language and short sentences.
- Invite critical comments on the content, wording and comprehensibility of a draft sheet from an independent body such a cancer charity or patient advocacy group.

Standard definitions of randomization, double-blind trial, cross-over trial, and placebo are available; the UK MREC definitions provide a useful model (http://www.corec.org.uk/wordDocs/pis.doc).

In the UK, the Central Office for Research Ethics Committees advises splitting topics into a series of questions and answers on the patient information sheet, and gives examples of possible wordings. The question headings are shown in Box 7.8, and further information can be obtained from their web site (http:www.corec.org.uk).

Box 7.8 Suggested contents for a patient information sheet

- Study title
- Invitation paragraph
- What is the purpose of the study?
- Why have I been chosen?
- Do I have to take part?
- What will happen to me if I take part?
- What do I have to do?
- What is the drug or procedure that is being tested?
- What are the alternatives for diagnosis or treatment?
- What are the side effects of any treatment received when taking part?
- What are the possible disadvantages and risks of taking part?
- What are the possible benefits of taking part?
- What if new information becomes available?
- What happens when the research study stops?
- What if something goes wrong?
- Will my taking part in this study be kept confidential?
- What will happen to the results of the research study?
- Who is organizing and funding the research?
- Who has reviewed the study?
- Contact for further information

7.6.21 Storage of tissue and biological samples

Technical advances, particularly the ability to extract genetic material, have meant that the potential to use stored tissue or biological samples for research is increasing. It is not uncommon for such specimens to be collected from participants in a trial and stored centrally for possible future research [7]. This is not the place to discuss the legal and ethical issues raised by such research, but the implications for participants in a trial must be explained and their consent obtained for storage. Since consent to provide such samples might be refused by someone otherwise consenting to participate in the trial, it will usually be helpful (although not essential) to have a separate consent form. Indeed, having a separate patient information sheet as well may help to avoid confusion.

When a trial includes collection of such samples, the patient information sheet should make the following points, as appropriate.

◆ Description of the samples to be collected; in a cancer trial, these will usually be a single blood sample and a single tissue sample from the tumour.

◆ Patients in the study are being asked to consider donating samples because it will be useful for researchers to have access to samples from a wide cross-section of people with [type of] cancer.

◆ The samples can be obtained at the same time as samples for tests relevant to the study (if this is true – it usually is).

◆ The samples are not required for the present study, but are being collected and stored for future research.

◆ Giving samples is entirely voluntary, and declining to donate them does not affect the main study.

◆ The samples will be sent to a laboratory designated by [the sponsor], and will be kept as part of a store for possible future research; this research could include genetic (DNA) tests and studies of factors that predispose to [type of] cancer or that influence response to treatment.

◆ [The sponsor] will specify the arrangements for access to and control of the use of the collection.

◆ Access to the collection by the commercial sector as well as by academic researchers is not excluded, but no one commercial company will be given exclusive rights of access.

◆ Donors of samples will not be entitled to a share in any profits that might ensue.

◆ Personal information about donors of samples will be stored confidentially and will only be accessible to staff who have a duty of confidentiality to the donors. State if results of tests could have any implications for the patients and their families, and whether they will have access to the results.

◆ All research projects involving the stored samples will have to be approved by an independent ethics committee.

For further guidance, see the Medical Research Council's operational and ethical guidelines on human tissue and biological samples for use in research, available on their website (http://www.mrc.ac.uk).

7.6.22 Patient consent form

- The patient consent form must include the title of the trial and should be signed and dated by the patient and, if required by the local ethics committee, by a witness.
- A recommended consent form is shown in Fig. 7.3. This is based on UK MREC recommendations.
- A recommended consent form for providing tissue or biological samples is shown in Fig. 7.4.

CONSENT FORM
(Form to be on headed paper)

Name of trial:

Centre:

Patient's name or other identifier:

Please initial box

I have read and understand the patient information sheet for the above study [version, dated] and have had the opportunity to ask questions and discuss it with my doctor.

I understand that my participation is voluntary and that I am free to withdraw at any time, without giving any reasons, without my medical care being affected.

I understand that my medical notes may be looked at by responsible individuals where it is relevant to my taking part in research. I give permission for these individuals to have access to my notes but understand that strict confidentiality will be maintained. The purpose is to check that the study is being carried out correctly.

I agree to take part in the above study.

| Name of patient | Date | Signature |

| Name of person obtaining consent | Date | Signature |

One copy should be given to the patient and one should be kept with hospital notes.

Fig. 7.3 A recommended patient consent form.

CONSENT FORM FOR PROVIDING TISSUE OR BIOLOGICAL SAMPLES
(Form to be on headed paper)

Name of trial:

Centre:

Patient's name or other identifier:

Please initial
box

I have read and understand the patient information sheet for the above study [version, dated] and have had the opportunity to ask questions and discuss it with my doctor.

☐

I agree that the samples I have given and the information gathered about me can be looked after and stored on behalf of [the sponsor] for use in future projects, as described in the information sheet. I understand that some of these projects may be carried out by researchers other than [the sponsor], including researchers working for commercial companies.

☐

I understand that I shall not benefit financially if future research leads to the development of a new treatment or medical test.

☐

I agree to donate the samples requested.

☐

Name of patient _____ Date _____ Signature _____

Name of person obtaining consent Date _____ Signature _____

One copy should be given to the patient and one should be kept with hospital notes.

Fig. 7.4 A recommended patient consent form for providing tissue or biological samples for storage with a view to future research.

7.6.23 Trial report forms

Good trial report form design is vital. The layout must be simple and easy to follow. The requirements for good forms are shown in Box 7.9.

♦ Include a copy of all trial report forms and questionnaires in the protocol.

♦ Use self-copying forms when possible, the top copy to be sent to the trials office, the other to be retained in the patient's notes.

♦ In designing the forms, be careful to ensure that the layout and wording are simple, direct and easy to understand so that the forms are easy to complete without ambiguity. Missing items should be obvious at a glance.

♦ Include only such questions as are essential for answering the trial questions.

♦ Wherever possible, use a simple coding style or a box-ticking style; avoid text entries.

♦ Ensure that all questions are worded in such a way that they require an answer.

♦ Ask for date of birth, not age.

Box 7.9   Requirements for good trial report forms

- They identify the trial and the patient
- They include brief and clear instructions for their completion
- They request only data essential for full and unbiased evaluation of the treatments being compared
- They can be completed quickly and accurately
- They are in a format compatible with database and statistical software, allowing rapid and accurate computerization
- They request the name of the person completing the form and the date it was completed

- They state to whom the completed form should be sent

- Ask for height and weight as well as for surface area.
- Collect continuous data in original units used by the collaborating centre and ensure that the units are clearly noted.
- Be consistent with codes within and across forms: e.g. 1 = No; 2 = Yes; 9 = Not known.
- Use standard definitions whenever these are available. The following list of source documents is not intended to be comprehensive, but is widely used.

The National Cancer Institute toxicity criteria definitions (http://ctep.info.nih.gov/CTC3).

The World Health Organization criteria for reporting performance status, toxicity, and tumour response [8].

Revised guidelines (RECIST criteria) for evaluating tumour response [9].

Other performance status scales such as the Karnofsky scale and the ECOG scale [10,11].

The International Union Against Cancer definitions of tumour staging which are up-dated regularly (http://www3.uicc/tnm) [12].

The European Organization for Research and Treatment of Cancer core questionnaire, the QLQ-C30, for recording quality of life in cancer patients [13,14], for which a number of cancer-site-specific modules are available [15,16]. A number of other validated quality of life instruments are available and it is wise to seek the advice of an expert adviser on the most appropriate instruments for a particular trial. The assessment of quality of life is discussed in detail in Chapter 6.

The basic set of forms likely to be required in a trial is shown in Fig. 7.5.

Examples of forms from a multi-group randomized trial of chemotherapy with or without G-CSF in operable osteosarcoma are shown in Figs. 7.6–7.8.

7.7   Trial-specific procedures

Trial-specific procedures for managing the trial and the data should be drawn up by the clinical trials manager, whether the trial is a large multi-centre trial being conducted by a

Type of form	Data collected
Registration/randomization	Patient identification details Eligibility checks Stratification factors
On-study/pre-treatment	Baseline patient characteristics
Treatment	Details of treatment given Treatment modifications Protocol deviations Adverse effects

Follow-up	Details of patient's status (dead/alive)
	Details of disease status (response)
	Events since last assessment
	   Relapse/recurrence
	   Additional treatment
	   Late treatment effects

Other forms may include: histopathological review, details of death.

Fig. 7.5 Basic set of trial report forms.

trials office or a trial conducted within a single institution or by a local group. Although most of the activities they describe relate to the conduct of a trial after its launch, they need to be planned and drafted in parallel with the trial protocol before the launch of the trial and we therefore consider them here. They should give clear instructions so that another clinical trials manager could take over the trial on a temporary or permanent basis.

For multi-centre trials involving more than one trials group, it is important to state which group is the lead group and to list the responsibilities of all the groups.

Trial-specific procedures must be kept up-to-date and revised as and when necessary. Although they can vary substantially from trial to trial, they should usually include the following information.

7.7.1 Trial personnel

List the trial personnel with their responsibilities, addresses, telephone and fax numbers, and e-mail addresses.

7.7.2 Computer database

Describe and define the computer database definitions and procedures, including detailed computer consistency check files and procedures for coding, entering, checking and querying data.

7.7.3 Registration and randomization

Give instructions for registering or randomizing patients and list and define any stratification variables and the questions that need to be answered before a patient can be entered; these relate to eligibility checking and factors required for stratification.

EORTC : 80931
MRC : BO06

Form 1

EOI TRIAL OF CHEMOTHERAPY +/- G-CSF IN OPERABLE OSTEOSARCOMA

REGISTRATION/ON-STUDY FORM

Please complete this form before randomising the patient and send top copy to your data coordinating centre.

Patient's name/ID code: ....

Institution: ....
(*where chemotherapy will be given*)

Initial biopsy hospital: ....

Surgeon: ....
(*definitive surgery*)

Responsible Clinician: ....

Hospital number: ....

Pathologist: ....
(*initial biopsy*)

Pathology ref. no: ....
(*initial specimen*)

1 ☐☐☐☐☐☐ **Date of birth** (D,M,Y)

Sex
2 ☐ 1 = Male
   2 = Female

ELIGIBILITY Please confirm the following by ticking the box ☐

1. Biopsy proven osteosarcoma of long bones of an extremity
2. Untreated non-metastatic disease
3. Age ≤40 years
4. Chemotherapy planned to start within 4 weeks of biopsy
5. Neutrophils ⩾1.5×10^9/l (or WBC ⩾3.5×10^9/l if neutrophils not available) and platelet count >100×10^9/l
6. Glomerular Filtration Rate ⩾60 ml/min 1.73 m²
7. Serum bilirubin <20 μmol/l
8. No history of cardiac malfunction
9. Informed consent should be obtained according to local regulations

Thoracic scan
3 ☐ 1 = Normal
   2 = Equivocal

4 ☐☐☐☐ IU/L **Alkaline phosphatase**

5 ☐☐☐☐ IU/L **LDH**

Location of tumour
6 ☐ 1 = Femur
   2 = Tibia
   3 = Fibula
   4 = Humerus
   5 = Radius
   6 = Ulna

Location on bone
7 ☐ 1 = Proximal
   2 = Mid-shaft
   3 = Distal

Intended surgical procedure at randomisation
8 ☐ 1 = Amputation
   2 = Disarticulation
   3 = Rotation plasty
   4 = Limb salvage

RANDOMISATION

Allocated treatment
9 ☐ 1 = Regimen 1 (CDDP + DOX)
   2 = Regimen 2 (CDDP + DOX + G-CSF)

☐☐☐☐☐☐ **Date of randomisation**
(D,M,Y)

☐☐☐☐☐ **EORTC/MRC patient number**

Signed .... Date ....

Fig. 7.6 Registration/on-study form from an osteosarcoma trial.

EORTC : 80931
MRC : BO06

Form 2

EOI TRIAL OF CHEMOTHERAPY +/- G-CSF IN OPERABLE OSTEOSARCOMA

CHEMOTHERAPY FORM

Please complete this form at the end of each cycle of chemotherapy and send top copy to your data coordinating centre.

Patient's name/ID code: .... □□□□□ **Date of birth** (D,M,Y)

Institution: .... □□□ **EORTC/MRC patient number**

1 □ **Cycle number**

3 □□ cm **Height**

2 □.□□ m² **Surface area**

4 □□ Kg **Weight**

5 □□□□□□ **Date of start of cycle** (D,M,Y)

6 □□□□ mg **CDDP Dose this cycle**

8 □□□ mg **DOX Total dose this cycle**

7 □ **Major reason for delay/reduction**
1 = No delay/reduction
2 = Administrative
3 = Haematological toxicity
4 = Renal toxicity
5 = Ototoxicity
6 = Neurotoxicity
7 = Infection
8 = Other, specify ....

9 □ **Major reason for delay/reduction**
1 = No delay/reduction
2 = Administrative
3 = Haematological toxicity
4 = Renal toxicity
5 = Ototoxicity
6 = Neurotoxicity
7 = Infection
8 = Other, specify ....

FOR G-CSF REGIMEN ONLY

10 □□□□ µg **G-CSF Total dose this cycle**

Was any toxicity attributed to G-CSF
1 = No
11 □ 2 = Yes, specify ....

Laboratory values	Before start of cycle	Day 8 (G-CSF) or Day 10	Day 15 (G-CSF) or Day 22
Date of test (D,M,Y)	12 □□□□□□	23 □□□□□□	27 □□□□□□
WBC x 10⁹/L	13 □□.□	24 □□.□	28 □□.□
Neutrophils x 10⁹/L	14 □□.□	25 □□	29 □□.□
Platelets x 10⁹/L	15 □□□	26 □□□	30 □□□
Renal clearance ml/min/1.73m²	16 □□□		
Alkaline phosphatase IU/L	17 □□□		
LDH IU/L	18 □□□		
Calcium mmol/l	19 □.□□		
Magnesium mmol/l	20 □.□□		
LFT } 1 = Normal 2 = Abnormal	21 □		
Electrolytes	22 □		

Side effects of treatment (*Please use toxicity coding on back of book and specify grade*)

31 □ Nausea/Vomiting

35 □ Neurological

32 □ Oral

36 □ Ototoxicity

33 □ Infection

37 □ Cardiac

34 □ Other, specify ....

Signed .... Date ....

Fig. 7.7 Chemotherapy form from an osteosarcoma trial.

EORTC : 80931
MRC : BO06

Form 4

EOI TRIAL OF CHEMOTHERAPY +/- G-CSF IN OPERABLE OSTEOSARCOMA

FOLLOW-UP FORM

Please complete this form at end of treatment and then 6-monthly thereafter. Send top copy to your data coordinating centre.

Patient's name/ID code: .... ☐☐☐☐☐☐ **Date of birth (D,M,Y)**

Institution: .... ☐☐☐ **EORTC/MRC patient number**

---

1 ☐☐☐☐☐☐ Date of terminating protocol treatment
Date of examination   } *whichever is appropriate*
Date of death

Complete this section only at the end of protocol treatment

2 ☐ **Total number of cycles given**

3 ☐ **Was surgery performed**
1 = No, specify ....
2 = Yes

4 ☐ **Reason for terminating protocol treatment**
1 = Protocol treatment completed
2 = Disease progression (including death due to disease)
3 = Excessive toxicity (including death due to toxicity)
4 = Treatment refusal (reason other than toxicity)
5 = Other, specify

....

5 ☐ **Disease status**
1 = No disease
2 = Local progression
3 = Local recurrence
4 = Distant metastases
5 = Local progression and distant metastases
6 = Local recurrence and distant metastases

6 ☐ **Survival status**
1 = Alive
2 = Dead, due to osteosarcoma
3 = Dead, treatment related death
4 = Dead, other specify

....

7 ☐☐☐☐☐☐ **Date of first recurrence or progression at any site (D,M,Y)**

SITE OF DISTANT METASTASES

8 ☐ **Lung**
1 = None
2 = Suspicious
3 = Definite

9 ☐ **Liver**
1 = None
2 = Suspicious
3 = Definite

10 ☐ **Bone**
1 = None
2 = Suspicious
3 = Definite

11 ☐ **Brain**
1 = None
2 = Suspicious
3 = Definite

12 ☐ **Other, specify** ....
1 = None
2 = Suspicious
3 = Definite

---

13 ☐ **Late surgical complications**
1 = No complications
2 = Infection
3 = Instability
4 = Loosening prosthesis
5 = Device failure
6 = Further surgery
7 = Other, specify (inc. combinations) ....
8 = Not applicable

Signed .... Date ....

Fig. 7.8 Follow-up form from an osteosarcoma trial.

7.7.4 Enrolling new centres

List the documents that need to be sent to new centres and indicate where they can be found. These will include protocols, summary protocols, the completed local ethics committee application form (if required), a quality of life pack (if relevant), a standard letter indicating the responsibilities of clinicians collaborating in the trial, and a centre accreditation checklist.

State whether a centre has to be visited by a member of the trials office team before randomizing patients and, if so, the purpose of the visit.

State whether clinicians' CVs are required and whether clinicians need to be registered with the regulatory authority – the Medicines Control Agency in the UK – before they start randomizing patients. In the UK, CVs are required if the trial involves a new unlicensed drug, or a drug used outside its licensed indications, and is being conducted under a Clinical Trial Certificate Exemption (CTX) held by a company or a Doctors' and Dentists' Exemption (DDX) held by a clinician who is not a consultant or adviser to a company (http://www.open.gov.uk/mca) [17].

Describe the conditions under which centres from abroad can participate.

Indicate whether other bodies, such as trial sponsors, should be given details of new centres. In the UK, the Medicines Control Agency has to be informed of new centres for trials conducted under a CTX or DDX.

7.7.5 Instructions for initial site visits by trial coordinating staff

- List the people who need to be seen. They could include participating clinicians, research nurses, a local data manager, the person responsible for coordinating quality of life assessment, a pharmacist, specialist nursing staff, and the person responsible for administering funding.

- List the documents that need to be taken. These should always include a standard checklist of what needs to be achieved during the visit. Other documents could include pharmacy instructions and record sheets, clinicians' agreement statements for signature, trial manuals containing all trial documentation, quality of life packs, a supply of report forms, and protocol summaries.

- List the documents that need to be collected (or sent by post). These could include the local ethics committee's letter of approval, a copy of the patient information sheet if this has had locally relevant information added to it, signed agreement statements of collaborating clinicians, local laboratory normal ranges for relevant tests, a copy of the laboratory's certificate of accreditation, copies of any outstanding CVs, and details of the bank account into which support funding should be paid.

- State the procedures for reporting serious adverse events.

- Include a copy of all standard documents for the visit, including a visit report form.

7.7.6 Instructions for subsequent monitoring visits

- Describe what source data verification is required and the procedures for undertaking it. These may include identifying a random selection of data for verification, and the procedures for ensuring that the relevant patient notes and facilities for checking data are made available in confidence.

- List the people who need to be seen. These are likely to include collaborating clinicians, a pharmacist, locally involved research staff, and the person responsible for coordinating quality of life assessments.
- List the documents that need to be taken. These include copies of the protocol, copies of reports of all previous visits to the centre, copies of all report forms with outstanding queries, and a list of any problems relating to the data from that centre.
- Include instructions for checking that the centre is complying with the protocol, including the prompt reporting of serious adverse events.
- Emphasize the desirability of sorting out and correcting any data discrepancies or other problems during the visit.
- Include a copy of all standard documents for the visit, including standard letters, a monitoring visit checklist, a source data verification form, and a visit report form.

7.7.7 Standard documents

Trial management is greatly assisted by having standard letters and documents for dealing with routine situations. Include copies of all standard letters and other standard documents in the trial-specific procedures indicating where they can be found. The following are examples of topics covered by standard letters.

- Approaching potentially interested centres not yet involved in the trial.
- Recruiting new centres.
- Confirming patient registrations or randomizations.
- Informing centres of overdue or missing data.

The following are examples of other standard documents.

- One-page protocol summaries.
- Clinicians' agreement statements.
- Quality of life assessment guidelines.
- Procedures for reporting serious adverse events and the associated report forms.
- Site visit checklists and report forms.
- Report forms for the supervising and sponsoring bodies.
- Pharmacy instructions and dispensing records.
- TNM and other staging definitions.

7.7.8 Filing

List all the trial files, making it clear how they are used and what documents should be filed in each.

7.7.9 Finance

State the procedures for administering the grant that is funding the trial, including the provision of progress reports to the sponsor.

7.7.10 Other instructions that may be relevant

The following additional instructions will be relevant for some trials.

- Procedures for ordering drug supplies from a pharmaceutical company.
- Key personnel for liaising with a pharmaceutical company, their position in the company and their role in the trial.
- Guidelines for breaking treatment codes in double-blind trials.
- Procedures and documentation for independent review, e.g. of pathology, staging or tumour response.

7.8 Ethics

It is essential to observe all ethical requirements for the country concerned. All randomized trials require ethics approval. The guidance we give here conforms in general with the functions of Institutional Review Board/Independent Ethics Committees as set out in the ICH GCP Guideline for international use, the NCI Investigators' Handbook (http://ctep.info.nih.gov/handbook/HandBookText), and the COREC system, and is therefore widely applicable.

7.8.1 Ethics committees

It is necessary to obtain ethics approval from the appropriate ethics committees using their standard application forms. The following points should be borne in mind when completing the form.

- Ethics committees include lay members; it is essential to use non-technical language.
- Ensure that all abbreviations are explained.
- Answer all questions; do not rely on referring to the protocol.
- Include sufficient information for a thorough ethics review to be made.

Ethics committees generally expect to receive protocols that have already been subjected to critical scientific evaluation. Thus, if the trial management group have made sure that the scientific case for a trial has been well argued, that the protocol has been appropriately designed and independently evaluated, and if the ethics application form has been correctly completed, the committee is most unlikely to raise major objections. It is not uncommon, however, for them to request minor changes or to ask for clarification on some details.

If, during the conduct of a trial, the protocol has to be modified, the ethics committee must be informed. If major modifications effectively change the trial into a different trial or will affect trial participants, the ethics committee are likely to need to review the protocol.

The UK Central Office for Research Ethics Committees (COREC) web site (http://www.corec.org.uk) is a useful source of information on ethical issues related to clinical trials. It is updated regularly, it reproduces the Declaration of Helsinki, and it provides a valuable statement of compliance with the ICH GCP Guideline.

7.8.2 Patients' consent

The responsibility for obtaining patients' consent to participate in a trial lies with the collaborating clinicians (see Chapter 2). The trial management group is responsible for ensuring that the trial is conducted ethically.

In a few trials, fully informed consent is not possible: for example, trials studying emergency situations. In such trials, the relevant ethics committee should be informed that immediate patient consent is not possible, and that the relevant National guidelines for this situation would be followed.

For consent to be legally valid, the patient must be competent to consent to take part in a trial. Consent must be based on adequate information. It is therefore desirable that all patients entering a trial sign a consent form confirming that the trial has been explained to them and that they have read and understand the patient information sheet. The following points should be considered in obtaining consent.

- Give the patient time to consider how to respond and time to discuss the matter with others.
- Encourage the patient to ask questions.
- Ask the patient to sign and date a consent form.

7.8.3 Obtaining consent from children and adolescents

The age categories used to define children and adolescents vary between regions, but children are commonly defined as being under twelve years of age and adolescents as aged 12–16 years. These categories are to some extent arbitrary, however, and it is the person's level of development and understanding rather than age that is relevant.

As a rule, children and adolescents are legally unable to provide informed consent. They are therefore dependent on their parents or legal guardians to assume responsibility for their participation in a clinical study. Fully informed consent should be obtained from parents or guardians in accordance with regional laws and regulations. All such participants should nevertheless be informed to the fullest extent possible about the study using appropriate language and without inappropriate inducements, and age-specific patient information sheets should be provided for younger and older children. Whenever possible, verbal assent should be obtained from children and adolescents after an age-appropriate explanation of the issues involved and, if they are able to do so, they should sign and date the standard study consent form or a separately designed and appropriately worded assent form.

When appropriate, children and adolescents should be told that they can withdraw from the study if they want to, but there may be circumstances in which, in the opinion of the investigator and parent or guardian, the welfare of the participant would be jeopardized by failure to participate. In such circumstances, the consent of the parent or guardian should be sufficient. In some countries, emancipated or mature minors (defined by local laws) may be legally capable of giving autonomous consent.

To minimize risk in studies involving minors, collaborating clinicians should be properly trained and experienced in studying the paediatric population, including the evaluation and management of potential paediatric adverse events.

7.8.4 Adult patients whose capacity to give consent is impaired

Adult patients' capacity to give consent may be impaired by the nature or severity of their disease, or for other unrelated reasons. When an incapacitated adult is unable to give consent, the responsible clinician should fully inform the subject's legally acceptable representative of all pertinent aspects of the study, including the written information and the acceptability of the study to the relevant ethics committee.

Incapacitated patients can be entered into trials, but researchers should try to obtain consent at whatever level is possible, based on information that is understandable by the individual. When there is doubt about patients' ability to consent, independent assessors or witnesses should be asked to help assess whether consent is valid.

If the consent of such patients cannot be obtained, they should not be entered into the trial, although in some regions, consent can be obtained from legally acceptable representatives. When this is the case, representatives should be given time and opportunity to enquire about details of the study and to decide whether or not to permit participation. Before participation, the representative should sign and date the consent form and the consent procedures should be witnessed by an impartial witness who should also sign and date the consent form. By doing so, the witness attests that the information in the patient information sheet and consent form was accurately explained to and apparently understood by the subject's legally acceptable representative.

7.9 Collaboration between industrial and non-industrial partners

Some trials involve collaboration between industrial and non-industrial partners. Examples are trials involving unlicensed drugs or drugs that although licensed are being used outside the licensed indication, and trials involving new designs of equipment or appliances such as stents or prostheses not yet regarded as standard. In addition, industry may provide partial financial support to trials for which it is not the main sponsor.

A company's support for a trial can involve providing drug free or at reduced cost, contributing towards per-patient payments to collaborating centres and the trials office's administrative costs and salaries, and promoting the trial within the oncological community.

The following principles should be observed in such collaborative trials, and should be agreed by the collaborating bodies and trial sponsor in a formal contract. These principles should be established as early as possible in the course of exploratory discussions. Companies, universities and Government, charitable or other organizations are usually experienced in collaborating with each other and are often well aware of the issues involved.

- Establish the need for collaboration and its purpose and nature. This is best done through the process of initial informal discussions and correspondence between the collaborating bodies, leading to the drafting of a formal contract.

- Accrual into a collaborative trial should not start until the contract has been signed, if the trial is dependent on drug or money from the company or companies involved.

- The body with scientific control of the trial must be unambiguously stated. This includes its planning, its design, its conduct, its analysis and publication of the findings. The non-industrial research group conducting the trial should normally retain scientific control of the trial.

◆ The trial data belong to the group conducting the trial. The contract must state what access, if any, other collaborative bodies, including the industrial partner, will have to the data or the results of the trial. Normally, they will only have access to results when they have been published. If the data monitoring and ethics committee recommends discontinuing the trial or making a major modification to the protocol, and the trial supervisors accept its recommendation, then the industrial and any other collaborating bodies should be informed straight away of the decision and the reasons for it.

◆ Results of analyses and data required by a company for licensing and regulatory purposes will often only be released to the company when the results of the trial have been published or accepted for publication. It is essential to agree in advance what data will be supplied in confidence to the company and the licensing body for licensing and regulatory purposes, and when.

◆ The group conducting the trial are responsible for reporting adverse effects of treatment. They will, however, immediately report serious adverse events to the company if an unlicensed drug is being tested.

◆ The company's support should be stated on the patient information sheet and acknowledged in all publications and presentations of the trial.

In establishing these principles, drawing up a contract and avoiding misunderstanding, the following questions need to be answered.

◆ What is the license status of any drug being provided? Is the drug licensed for the clinical indication to be used in the trial and, if so, will it be administered in accordance with normal clinical practice? Is it licensed but for a different indication or dosage schedule? Is it unlicensed?

◆ What are the arrangements for labelling and delivering supplies of drug to collaborating centres?

◆ Who is the named company contact? Who is the named contact for the group conducting the trial? Correct channels of communication must be established and maintained.

◆ What has already been discussed and provisionally agreed on an informal basis? All relevant correspondence must be copied to all concerned and kept for reference. Also, notes should be made of any discussions or telephone conversations. We recommend writing a letter to all concerned, summarizing what was said.

◆ What have the company agreed to contribute? What have the collaborating investigators agreed to in return?

◆ What has been agreed concerning indemnity, compensation, data release, adverse event reporting, monitoring, and audit?

Informal agreement will usually be reached quite rapidly between the collaborators' representatives. However, formal legal advice to either group can take time to obtain. It is therefore advisable to get contracts drafted as early as possible.

When a trial is investigating an unlicensed drug or a licensed drug but for a new indication, it is particularly important for the industrial and non-industrial partners to agree the level of source data verification and monitoring visits to collaborating centres. These activities may be more extensive than in other trials and may well involve the need to employ and fund additional staff or for industrial and non-industrial staff to work together on these issues. If regulatory approval is required, how this will be obtained must be agreed.

7.10 Collaboration between research groups

Different research groups conducting clinical trials may decide to collaborate in a large national or international trial or in an extended programme of research. Collaboration is highly desirable to achieve rapid rates of intake into trials investigating uncommon cancers, trials requiring large numbers of patients, or if there are reasons why accrual is likely to be slow or difficult. International collaboration has been highly productive, for example, in trials of advanced bladder cancer, osteosarcoma, glioma, stomach cancer, gynaecological cancers, testicular cancer, and lymphoma. Forms of collaboration are indicated in Box 7.10.

In practice, collaboration may take several forms varying in the level of collaboration involved.

- Separate groups agree to run parallel protocols. These protocols may be prepared individually by each group, but are designed to answer the same questions and are therefore similar (and may be identical), although adhering to the style and practices of the separate groups. Each group is responsible for its own data collection and

---

Box 7.10 Possible forms of collaboration between research groups

- Outline proposals are mutually drafted and agreed and are independently reviewed by a single set of referees on behalf of all collaborating groups
- By mutual agreement, one group is designated the lead group for a trial. This group develops the full protocol, in consultation with the other groups, which is then approved, if necessary, and applied by all groups
- All groups obtain ethics committee approval of the protocol according to their national requirements
- The lead group is responsible for data management and analyses, in close consultation with other groups. Randomization may be undertaken by one or each collaborating group
- The lead group provides the other groups with regular reports on accrual, patient characteristics, toxicity and total event rates
- The lead group organizes independent review of confidential interim analyses by a data monitoring and ethics committee, the members of which are agreed by all groups
- The lead group is responsible for preparing reports for publication, but closely consults and collaborates with the other groups and ensures that all groups agree final drafts

management. The groups agree prospectively to undertake joint analyses of their data, even if each component trial is published individually as well. (This is sometimes called a prospective meta-analysis.)

The advantages of this approach are that styles of protocols and forms and basic procedures, including randomization procedures, are familiar to collaborating centres because they are the same as for other trials. Collaborators also continue to relate to their usual coordinating office, often with people well known to them. Potential disadvantages are low levels of communication between groups, and differences in quality control, software, coding and databases and hence difficulties in merging data and conducting joint analyses. This may therefore be an inefficient method of collaboration.

- A trial has already been started by one group, and the same protocol is then adopted by one or more other groups without further independent review. New groups accept the original protocol without modification. The analyses are conducted by the instigating group and the trial is published as a collaborative trial.

- The optimal form of collaboration is full collaboration between groups in all aspects of the trial from design to publication. One group is designated the lead group and is responsible for data management. The other groups then become satellite groups doing minimal work except perhaps for collecting data for onward transmission, undertaking site visits, promoting and publicizing the trial and undertaking randomizations within their group.

When groups collaborate over an extended period in several trials, they may take it in turns to be the lead group. Close communication between collaborating groups is essential. Some groups may exchange minutes of all planning group meetings so that opportunities for running collaborative trials can be identified as soon as they arise.

A disadvantage of this model is that satellite groups can find it difficult to maintain a sense of corporate group identity among their collaborating centres. This is much less of a problem, however, once a programme of collaborative trials has been established, and groups take their turn in being the lead group for a trial.

Because of differences in timing and in style between countries, it can prove difficult to agree a common, identical protocol. It may then be necessary to accept one of the other approaches to collaboration. When this is necessary, every effort should be made to use randomization procedures, protocols and forms that are as similar as possible. Whenever feasible, all forms should be sent to one centre responsible for data management. If data are collected and processed by a number of groups, problems can arise in pooling data for analysis. On the other hand, agreeing to run parallel data management systems or even protocols is sometimes the only practicable way to make collaboration possible.

Whatever the level of collaboration adopted for a trial, the implications for staffing, funding, sponsoring by industry (if relevant), and indemnity need to be thoroughly discussed and agreed.

7.11 Conclusion

If the trial management group and others involved in the trial have followed the procedures described in this chapter, funding, if required, will have been secured, ethics approval obtained, the protocol and other trial documents printed, centres interested in collaborating identified, and patient advocacy groups fully informed and involved. The trial is ready for launching.

References

[1] Medical Research Council (1998) *MRC Guidelines for Good Clinical Practice in Clinical Trials.* Medical Research Council, London.

[2] International Conference on Harmonization (1997) *ICH Guideline for Good Clinical Practice.* ICH Technical Coordination, London.

[3] British Paediatric Association (1992) *Guidelines for the Ethical Conduct of Medical Research Involving Children.* British Paediatric Association, London.

[4] United Kingdom Children's Cancer Study Group (UKCCSG) (1999) Code of conduct for clinical trials. UKCCSG Data Centre, 22–28 Princess Road West, Leicester LE1 6TP, UK.

[5] Fayers, P.M., Hopwood, P., Harvey, A., Girling, D.J., Machin, D., and Stephens, R., on behalf of the MRC Cancer Trials Office (1997) Quality of life assessment in clinical trials – guidelines and a checklist for protocol writers: the U.K. Medical Research Council experience. *European Journal of Cancer*, 33, 20–8.

[6] Hopwood, P., Harvey, A., Davies, J., Stephens, R.J., Girling, D.J., Gibson, D., and Parmar, M.K.B. (1998) Survey of the administration of quality of life (QL) questionnaires in three multicentre randomized trials in cancer. *European Journal of Cancer*, 34, 49–57.

[7] Medical Research Council (2001) *Human Tissue and Biological Samples for use in Research: Operational and Ethical Guidelines.* Medical Research Council, London.

[8] World Health Organization (1979) WHO Handbook for Reporting Results of Cancer Treatment. WHO Offset Publication No. 48. World Health Organization, Geneva.

[9] Therasse, P., Arbuck, S.G., Eisenhauer, E.A., Wanders, J., Kaplan, R.S., Rubinstein, L., Verweij, J., Glabbeke, M. van, Oosterom, T., van, Christian, M.C., and Gwyther. S.G. (2000) New guidelines to evaluate the response to treatment in solid tumors. *Journal of the National Cancer Institute*, 92, 205–16.

[10] Karnofsky, D., and Burchenal, J.H. (1949) The clinical evaluation of chemotherapeutic agents in cancer. In: *Evolution of Chemotherapeutic Agents* (ed. C.M. Macleod). Columbia University Press, New York.

[11] Oken, M.M., Creech, R.H., Tormey, D.C., Horton, J., Davis, T.E., McFadden, E.T., and Carbone, P.P. (1982) Toxicity and response criteria of the Eastern Cooperative Oncology Group. *American Journal of Clinical Oncology*, 5, 649–55.

[12] International Union Against Cancer (1997) TNM classification of malignant tumours, 5th edition (eds. L.H. Sobin, and Ch. Wittekind) John Wiley, New York.

[13] Aaronson, N.K., Ahmedzai, S., Bergman, B., Bullinger, M., Cull, A., Duez, N.J., Filiberti, A., Flechtner, H., Fleishman, S.B., de Haes, J.C.J.M., Kaasa, S., Klee, M., Osoba, D., Razavi, D., Rofe, P.B., Schraubs, S., Sneeuw, K., Sullivan, M., and Takeda, F. for the European Organization for Research and Treatment of Cancer Study Group on Quality of Life. (1993) The European Organization for Research and Treatment of Cancer QLQ-C30: a quality-of-life instrument for use in international clinical trials in oncology. *Journal of the National Cancer Institute*, 85, 365–76.

[14] Fayers, P., Aaronson, N., Bjordal, K., Curran, D., and Groenvold, M. (1999) EORTC QLQ-C30 scoring manual, second edition. Quality of Life Unit, EORTC Data Center, Brussels.

[15] Aaronson, N.K., Bullinger, M., and Ahmedzai, S. (1988) A modular approach to quality-of-life assessment in cancer clinical trials. *Recent Results in Cancer Research*, 111, 231–48.

[16] Sprangers, M.A.G., Cull, A., Bjordal, K., Groenvold, M., and Aaronson, N.K., for the EORTC Study Group on Quality of Life (1993) The European Organization for Research and Treatment of Cancer approach to quality of life assessment: guidelines for developing questionnaire modules. *Quality of Life Research*, 2, 287–95.

[17] Medicines Control Agency (1993) Medicines act 1968: guidance notes on applications for clinical trial exemptions and clinical trial certificates. Medicines Control Agency, London.

Chapter 8

Conducting trials

8.1 Introduction

In this chapter, we describe the launching and conduct of a trial. For a trial to succeed, all those involved should promote and publicize it and do everything they can to maintain impetus and enthusiasm. We consider all aspects of conducting the trial on a day-to-day basis, paying particular attention to the membership, roles and methods of functioning of the committees responsible for independent data monitoring and supervision, and raise issues concerning computing and information technology, data protection, and the prevention of research misconduct.

8.2 What needs to be done?

The operational requirements to be considered in activating and conducting a trial are shown in Box 8.1.

Box 8.1 Operational requirements in activating and conducting a trial

- Launching the trial at a meeting for potential collaborators
- Recruiting centres for a multi-centre trial
- Promoting and publicizing the trial
- Undertaking the day-to-day conduct of the trial and collecting, checking, entering, and managing the data
- Maintaining good rapport with centres collaborating in a multi-centre trial through day-to-day contact and regular collaborators' meetings
- Conferring with patient advocacy groups
- Conducting interim and final analyses
- Preparing trial reports for presentation and publication
- Setting up data monitoring and supervisory committees; organizing their meetings, and preparing reports for them

8.3 Launching the trial and recruiting centres

In a multi-centre trial, once the protocol has been finalized and printed, the funding agreed and any necessary contracts signed, it is highly desirable that the trial management group launch the trial at a meeting to which all potential collaborators are invited. This meeting gives collaborators and members of the trial management group the opportunity to meet each other to publicize the opening of the trial, and to encourage the recruitment of centres. It also enables the trial management group to remind people of the importance of the trial and of key aspects of its design and conduct. All those attending the launch meeting should be encouraged to promote the trial among their colleagues and at relevant meetings, and it can be helpful to provide sets of slides or a PowerPoint presentation describing the trial for this purpose.

Centres that are likely to be interested in collaborating in the trial will have been identified during the planning and preparation of the proposal. It is quite likely that additional centres will also have been identified subsequently. It is highly desirable that the trial management group invite representatives from all these centres to the meeting. Any other potential collaborating centres should also be included.

A general problem with a large multi-centre trial is that collaborators can find it difficult to feel that they own it. A launch meeting can help to engender a sense of corporate endeavour in which the collaborating centres appreciate that their role is essential.

The format for a typical launch meeting is shown in Box 8.2.

The trial management group should then, if appropriate, start visiting centres and recruiting them. It is important to maintain the initial impetus and to recruit centres and establish a good rate of intake as rapidly as possible. A good rate of intake reassures centres that are already collaborating and encourages others to join.

If the trial management group already has a well-established group of centres collaborating in a programme of multi-centre trials, they will not necessarily need to

---

Box 8.2   Format of a typical trial launch meeting

- The principal investigator welcomes everyone to the meeting and introduces the members of the trial management group, indicating the role of each

- The principal investigator reminds people of the importance and timeliness of the trial

- The expert advisers explain their roles

- The medical statistician and clinical trials manager emphasize important aspects of the design of the trial and data management

- The meeting is opened to discussion, comments and queries

- Members of the coordinating staff provide centres with protocols, sets of forms, and publicity material for promoting the trial among their colleagues. These may include sets of slides or a PowerPoint presentation describing the trial

- Where appropriate, members of the coordinating staff start arranging dates for visiting centres to recruit them to the trial

visit all centres before starting a new trial because some will already be familiar with the general procedures and requirements for collaboration, and trial-specific operating procedures can be dealt with by telephone and correspondence. If, however, a centre is new to collaborating in trials or there are trial-specific procedures that require special attention, an appropriate member of the group should visit a centre before it starts randomizing patients. It is the responsibility of the trial management group to ensure that in all collaborating centres all procedures are fully understood and that the local staff responsible for the trial are identified, are conversant with the protocol, and are fully aware of their responsibilities before the first patient is randomized.

By agreeing to take part in a trial, clinicians undertake to conduct the trial in their own centre in accordance with the protocol and to provide the data required. They should pay particular attention to the following issues.

- Adhere to the trial protocol.
- Ensure that the requirements for freely given, fully informed consent are adhered to.
- Arrange for the patients to be assessed at the times stipulated in the protocol.
- Ensure that any patient questionnaires, such as quality of life questionnaires, are completed by patients at the times stipulated and that all questions are answered.
- Ensure that forms are filled in clearly, legibly and completely, and that queries are answered promptly.
- Cooperate in any source data verification that may be required.
- Contact the principal investigators or trials coordinating staff about any queries or concerns.

8.4 Promoting and publicizing the trial

As soon as a trial is open to recruitment, the trial management group should ensure that it is registered with at least one appropriate trial register, irrespective of whether or not national law requires this. Chapter 11 discusses trial registration further and provides website details in Table 11.5. They should also ensure that the trial has been assigned a unique identifying number such as the ISRCTN (see Box 11.1); this will usually be issued by the trial sponsor or funding organization. Copies of the protocol should also be sent to any relevant national cancer charities and patient advocacy groups. The trial sponsor (defined in Section 7.4.1) and trial management group may also want a summary statement to send to the press.

Promoting and publicizing a trial does not end when it has been launched. Indeed, the trial management group should always be on the lookout for opportunities to encourage collaborating centres to enter all consenting eligible patients and appropriate new centres to join. To these ends, a regular programme of promotional activities should be instituted. These might include the following.

- Send out regular newsletters to centres that are already collaborating and others that might be interested in doing so. These should remind people of the purposes and design of the trial and report on the progress of the intake and data collection. Give encouragement where things are going well, and draw attention to any problems, suggesting how they can be dealt with.

- Send a protocol summary to suitable journals to publicize the trial. A number of journals, if approached, may agree to publish brief summary protocols of multi-centre randomized trials, with the aim of encouraging participation.
- Arrange to give presentations at local meetings within centres during centre visits.
- Request facilities, such as poster space or a stand, from the organizers of relevant conferences for promoting the trial and for providing handouts.
- From time to time, contact centres that originally expressed an interest in the trial but have not yet started entering patients. Report to them on the progress of the trial and encourage them to join.

8.5 Day-to-day conduct of the trial and data management

Because obtaining complete and reliable data is crucial to the successful completion of a trial, compliance in the provision of data by centres and accuracy of data entry need to be monitored. If centres send forms to the trial coordinators as soon as they have been completed, and if data management staff conversant with the trial check the information on the forms on arrival, and the data are then entered onto the trial database and subjected to checks, this may be sufficient as a routine method of monitoring for most trials. It is likely, however, that at least for some trials, further monitoring and checking will be desirable. It is, of course, important to ensure that the local centre is contacted about missing or inconsistent data.

8.5.1 Obtaining, recording and checking data

To obtain reliable data, it is helpful to provide collaborating centres with a schedule of dates for treatments, assessments and investigations for each patient on registration or randomization in the trial. A typical example of such a schedule is shown in Fig. 8.1. The importance of collecting, recording and checking data efficiently and accurately cannot be overemphasized. This is most likely to be achieved if the trial management group keep in close contact with all collaborating clinicians and local coordinating staff by telephone, correspondence and visits, and at formal and informal meetings. They must ensure that centres are kept supplied with report forms, that they fully understand them, that they complete them correctly and accurately, and that they answer queries. They should regularly ask for missing or overdue forms to be sent.

There are two components to checking data: checking that the data are recorded correctly onto the report forms by collaborating centres (source data verification), and checking that the data are correctly entered by trial data management staff onto the database.

8.5.2 Source data verification

To assess the accuracy and completeness of data recorded by collaborating centres onto report forms, source data verification is used. Industry-sponsored trials typically use extensive source data verification. It is widely accepted, however, including by the ICH GCP Guideline (see Section 7.3) and the US Food and Drug Administration, that trials

MRC TE08: A Study of CT Scan Frequency in Stage I NSGCT

Patient : ABC

Trial Number: 1234

Date of orchidectomy 15/02/02

Allocated treatment: 5 CT Scan Schedule

Date of birth 01/07/75

Date Registered 10/03/02

Hosp No: 12345678

Follow-up investigations and forms required for this patient and approximate dates:

Date   Investigations/forms

18/03/02 AFP, HCG, LDH, chest X-ray, clinical examination

17/04/02 AFP, HCG, LDH, chest X-ray, clinical examination

17/05/02 AFP, HCG, LDH, CHEST AND ABDOMEN CT SCAN, clinical examination

17/06/02 AFP, HCG, LDH, chest X-ray, clinical examination

17/07/02 AFP, HCG, LDH, chest X-ray, clinical examination

17/08/02 AFP, HCG, LDH, CHEST AND ABDOMEN CT SCAN, clinical examination, TE08/1 form to trials office

16/09/02 AFP, HCG, LDH, chest X-ray, clinical examination

17/10/02 AFP, HCG, LDH, chest X-ray, clinical examination

16/11/02 AFP, HCG, LDH, CHEST AND ABDOMEN CT SCAN, clinical examination

17/12/02 AFP, HCG, LDH, chest X-ray, clinical examination

16/01/03 AFP, HCG, LDH, chest X-ray, clinical examination

15/02/03 AFP, HCG, LDH, CHEST AND ABDOMEN CT SCAN, clinical examination, TE08/2 form to trials office

17/04/03 AFP, HCG, LDH, chest X-ray, clinical examination

17/06/03 AFP, HCG, LDH, chest X-ray, clinical examination

17/08/03 AFP, HCG, LDH, chest X-ray, clinical examination

17/10/03 AFP, HCG, LDH, chest X-ray, clinical examination

17/12/03 AFP, HCG, LDH, chest X-ray, clinical examination

15/02/04 AFP, HCG, LDH, CHEST AND ABDOMEN CT SCAN, clinical examination, TE08/3 form to trials office

17/05/04 AFP, HCG, LDH, chest X-ray, clinical examination

16/08/04 AFP, HCG, LDH, chest X-ray, clinical examination

15/11/04 AFP, HCG, LDH, chest X-ray, clinical examination

14/02/05 AFP, HCG, LDH, chest X-ray, clinical examination, TE08/4 form to trials office

This schedule has been designed to be used as a guide and to help the clinician in charge in forecasting which examinations are needed according to the protocol. It is not an official document relating to the follow-up of this patient and clinical discretion should guide exact timings. IF THE PATIENT RELAPSES IT IS IMPORTANT THAT THE LDH SHOULD BE MEASURED ALONG WITH THE AFP AND HCG and the TE08/5 relapse form should be filled in and sent to the trials unit as soon as possible.

Fig. 8.1 Example of a schedule of dates from a randomized trial in testicular cancer.

Box 8.3   Factors that may influence a decision to use limited or no source data verification

- The existence of a plan other than source data verification to assure data quality
- Trials with a low susceptibility to bias: trials with simple procedures, noncritical eligibility criteria, and readily assessed outcome measures not susceptible to observer bias
- Trials in which sample data can readily be compared against supporting records, such as hospital records
- Trials conducted by groups with established standard operating procedures and a history of implementing such procedures effectively
- The existence of a clear prospectively specified analysis plan

that are not industry-sponsored may employ less stringent procedures and may use no source data verification at all (http://www.fda.gov/cber/guidelines.htm). The extent of source data verification should be based on trial-specific factors such as design, complexity, size, and outcome measures. If little or no source data verification is used in a trial, it is essential to ensure close control, review and speedy checking of case report forms, and close contact with collaborating centres to ensure that procedures are understood and are being followed and all queries efficiently dealt with. Factors that may influence a decision to use limited or no source data verification are shown in Box 8.3.

The trial management group should decide for each trial the level of source data verification, if any, that is needed.

When source data verification is used, information provided on case report forms is compared against patients' hospital records at a visit by members of the trial management group to the centre concerned, or sometimes by an independent body. As a minimum, the following checks should be made for all or, more commonly, a random sample of participants.

- Check patient eligibility.
- Check that informed consent is being obtained.
- Check key baseline data.
- Check data essential for the trial outcome measures.
- Check that important events have been reported.

Inform the centre in plenty of time which patient records or other data will be required for checking.

Some centres may at first find source data verification intrusive, implying, perhaps, that they cannot be trusted to provide reliable data. Explaining the need for checks at all levels, including within the trial coordinating centre, will help to allay any such concerns if it is done sensitively.

8.5.3 Data entry checking

The data management staff should inspect all incoming forms and immediately query obviously suspect data relating to major issues. Information from forms should be entered into the computer database as soon as possible after it has been received from collaborating centres. It must be checked for completeness and consistency, and queries must be dealt with speedily. Local staff are more likely to be able to answer queries rapidly and accurately soon after a patient has been assessed than weeks or months later. Moreover, if a patient has failed to complete a quality of life (or other) questionnaire, this can sometimes be rectified within an acceptable time window if local coordinating staff are notified straight away. If items of data are missing from forms, the reasons for this should always be sought. The rapid handling of forms by data management staff emphasizes to local centre staff the importance of providing complete data efficiently and without delay. Good collaboration between the trial coordinating staff and local centres is essential and well worth time and effort to nurture it.

The level of data entry checking may be a trials group policy, affecting a number of trials, or may be trial-specific, the size and complexity of the trial, the training and experience of the data management staff, and the software and programming support available influencing this level [1]. Different approaches to data-entry checking are adopted by different trials groups. These approaches are complementary and can include automatic consistency checks, double data entry, and checking computer output against information on report forms.

Automatic consistency checks should be installed into the trial database and most trial management software makes this possible. It is possible to set up checks for the patient identifier on all forms, checks to compare data across forms, range checks to ensure that values are within acceptable limits and are in line with previous results from the same patient, and schedule checks to ensure that forms are being completed at the appropriate times. Such checks are designed to provide feedback and to maintain a complete record of problems and queries. Regular cross-tabulation using statistical packages can be performed to help locate possible data errors by highlighting outlying or unlikely values.

All checks must be used with common sense. It is irritating to local staff to have to deal with queries that are simply fussy: a patient's name has been spelt slightly differently on two forms, for example, although all other patient identifiers are correct. On the other hand, if the results of tests relevant to trial outcomes are unclear or ambiguous, or have been given inherently unlikely values; or if the names of drugs or accounts of important procedures are wholly or partially illegible; or if ambiguous abbreviations have been used, clarification is essential. When centres see that queries are relevant and important, they are encouraged to improve on the standard and clarity of their reporting.

However much care is taken in recording data onto the database, errors are bound to occur. There is some variation in practice about the checks that are undertaken to keep errors in the database to a minimum but the level of checking should reflect the importance of the data being checked, data relating to primary outcome measures being the most important.

One method of checking data input is to use double data entry for all forms. Two people independently enter the data and the two sets of data are compared. Any inconsistencies are then checked against the original forms. This is time-consuming and can be an inefficient use of resource. A study of double data entry in which the person initially entering the data did not know that double entry was to be undertaken, showed that the number of differences between the two entries was seventy-five per 10,000 data items (95 per cent confidence interval 63–89), less than 1 per cent. Furthermore, more than 50 per cent of the differences were of a trivial nature (defined as errors that had no impact on analyses). The error rate for the initial entry alone was 1.5 (0.95–2.2) per 10,000 items. Moreover, the error rate for a principal outcome measure or a major error on any other outcome measure was only 2.5 (0.68–6.4) per 10,000 items [2]. Others have reported error rates as low as 0.001 per cent [1]. Although using double data entry can be a valuable method for assessing the level of accuracy of new staff, it may not be a cost-effective use of resource. When the people responsible for entering data are dedicated to the trial and understand the data, errors in data entry are likely to be rare if forms are well designed. Double data entry should be considered, however, if data are entered by inexperienced staff or data clerks, and in assessing the accuracy of staff.

The level of checking data entry should be decided according to the person responsible, the results of previous checks, and the type of data. If data are entered by someone with little understanding of the nature of the data and their implications, the error rate for simple data may be low, but for data requiring some interpretation may be higher. In this situation, data entry should be checked routinely, either by using double data entry or by checking a random sample of data regularly and routinely. The checking should be done by a second person because a single person is more likely to make the same error twice. Where experienced personnel are responsible for data entry, the error rate is likely to be low, and occasional checking at irregular intervals by double data entry of a sample of data by a second person without prior warning, should ensure that standards are being maintained.

In assessing error rates in data entry, emphasis should be focused on errors on a principal outcome measure and major errors on any other outcome measure. The aim must be to keep the rate of major errors very low. Minor errors on secondary outcome measures and errors that have no impact on the analyses are obviously much less important. Even so, the aim should be to keep errors to a minimum.

8.6   Maintaining good collaboration

Establishing and maintaining good collaboration between the trial coordinators and the collaborating centres is essential for a trial to succeed in its objectives. Collaboration can be nurtured through close day-to-day contacts and regular collaborators' meetings.

8.6.1   Day-to-day contact between trial coordinators and collaborating centres

A high standard of data management does much to maintain good collaboration with centres. The clinical trials manager (the person of first contact concerning trial issues) should become well known to all relevant staff in the collaborating centres. Consultant staff in these centres soon learn that data are being recorded and checked efficiently, that any queries from centres are being dealt with speedily, and develop confidence in the management of the trial.

The trial management group should also ensure that both active and potential collaborating centres are kept informed about the progress of the trial. They should keep the intake from all centres under close scrutiny. If the rate of recruitment from a centre falls, then they should try to find out why: there may have been unexpected toxicity, or staff may have left or changed. They may be able to help with the training and encouragement of new staff, for example.

Collaboration in a trial can be greatly assisted if the trial enjoys a high profile among the clinical community. Opportunities can usually be found to promote the trial at many types of meeting, ranging from small local groups to major international conferences, and as a summary protocol in various publications. However, it is essential that no interim results be presented by regimen while the intake is still in progress (see Section 8.8).

In some centres, there will be barriers to participation. This could be so for trials that require close coordination between clinicians from different specialities. Administrative problems can be considerable if, for example, different treatment modalities have to be organized by different staff at different hospitals. Such problems can sometimes be partially solved by discussing them with all the involved staff at a local meeting. The views of local specialists must be respected, however, and if one or more of them lacks equipoise about the design of the trial, it would be wrong, and almost certainly counter-productive, to try to persuade them to participate against their better judgment.

8.6.2 Regular collaborators' meetings

The trial management group should organize regular, typically annual, meetings for all active and, when appropriate, potential collaborating centres. The purpose of these meetings is to discuss the progress of the intake and data collection. Reports presented include no information on trial outcomes by treatment group until the intake has been completed and analysed ready for publication (see Section 8.8). The reports are likely to include such items as are shown in Box 8.4.

Box 8.4   Items included in reports to collaborators' meetings

- Total accrual rate and accrual by centre
- Projected accrual, showing how soon the intake is likely to be completed
- Characteristics of patients at randomization, showing how balanced the intake is between the treatment groups, especially in relation to known prognostic factors
- Treatment received, showing whether the treatment regimens are being applied successfully
- Details of toxicity and of any treatment problems that are being encountered, provided interim results of a trial outcome measure by treatment group are not thereby disclosed
- Compliance by centres in providing data and quality of life questionnaires

Any areas of concern can be discussed and necessary action taken. It is important to allow plenty of time for collaborators to comment on the progress of the trial from their point of view and to discuss both what is going well and areas of difficulty.

8.7   Conferring with patient advocacy groups

The trial management group should already have established collaboration with suitable consumer representatives or patient advocacy groups in the design of the trial and the drafting of the protocol. During the conduct of the trial, there may well be topics, such as the following, on which their advice would be helpful and important.

- Recruitment may be slow because high proportions of potentially eligible patients are declining to take part. Patient advocacy groups may be aware of misunderstandings about the trial or of reasons why it might be unattractive to patients. They may be able to advise on the rewording of the patient information sheet, and may be able to allay patients' concerns through their publications or their direct contact with patients.

- They can publish articles in their newsletters or other publications, explaining why the trial is being done and why it is important.

- They can deal objectively with queries raised by patients over the telephone.

- They can inform patients about the trial, and advise them how to seek the chance to collaborate, if they wish to do so.

It is important to keep patient advocacy groups fully informed on the progress of the trial, to assure them of its continuing relevance and importance, and to answer any questions they raise.

8.8   Conducting analyses

Data analysis and interpretation are considered in detail in Chapters 9 and 10. The responsibility for ensuring that data relating to all the trial outcome measures are fully and correctly analysed, and that appropriate conclusions are drawn from the results, rests with the trial management group and more widely with the collaborators. This is consistent with the responsibility the trial management group bears for the successful conduct of the trial and for the preparation of reports.

Interim analyses for the data monitoring and ethics committee, undertaken while the trial intake is still in progress, contain confidential results on trial outcome measures presented by treatment group. They must therefore be prepared with great care. Interim results may suggest differences between treatment groups in either direction or no differences, and results may swing from one direction to another in the early stages of a trial. If they suggest differences, they might disturb clinicians' equipoise; if they suggest no differences, they might reduce interest in the trial. Either way, they could discourage further collaboration on wholly inadequate grounds, jeopardizing patient accrual and successful completion of the trial. The data monitoring and ethics committee should be totally independent of the trial coordinating team, are not involved in the care of patients in the trial, and can therefore make independent and objective recommendations (see Section 8.10.1). The analyses should be undertaken by the statistician, and the results must not be made available to anyone else involved in the trial, including the principal investigator, those with clinical responsibilities, expert advisers, independent assessors, or collaborating centres.

It is more debatable whether other members of the coordinating team (for example the clinical trials manager) should be aware of confidential interim results. The best principle to follow is that access to the unblinded data is restricted to the minimum number of people. Clinical trials managers might find it difficult in their day-to-day contacts with clinicians if they were aware of interim findings unknown to the clinicians.

In the final analyses, all the trial outcome measures stated in the protocol should be analysed. Careful thought needs to be given to the results, which may suggest additional analyses that need to be done to clarify some details. The interpretation of the analyses and their implications need to be fully discussed by all collaborators (see Chapter 10).

From time to time, for various reasons, trials fail to recruit and have to be terminated prematurely. The results of such trials should nevertheless be analysed and should always be reported in some format. It is almost always possible to learn something from them, even if only the reasons for their failure [3,4].

8.9   Preparing reports for presentation and publication

Preparing reports for presentation and publication is fully discussed in Chapter 10. Here we comment on important practical matters that need to be agreed between all those conducting and collaborating in a trial.

Publication policy, the authorship of main reports, the way acknowledgements are to be made and who is to be acknowledged, should be indicated in trial protocols. Collaborators in multi-centre trials should be encouraged to quote publications arising from the trials on their CVs and to cite them as their own publications, even when they are not named authors, making their role clear.

8.9.1   Style of authorship

Two styles of authorship are commonly used. It is important that collaborators agree on the style to be adopted. It will sometimes be necessary to explain to journal editors why the chosen style has been adopted, and that the choice was made with the agreement of those collaborating in the trial. It is better to do this at the time a paper is submitted than to correct editorial alterations made on a proof.

Group authorship

- The group responsible for the trial is named as the author and the members of the group are listed. For example, the authorship of a report is stated as: 'Medical Research Council Testis Tumour Working Party,' and the people who were members during the period of the trial are listed in a footnote.

- Those responsible for managing the trial and drafting the report, usually the trial management group, are named. This can be done in the form: 'Prepared on behalf of the working party and its collaborators by ...' immediately after the statement of group authorship.

This style of group authorship is almost always the appropriate style for reports of large international trials or meta-analyses involving other trials groups in addition to the group primarily responsible for conducting the study.

Named authorship

◆ Those responsible for coordinating and managing the trial, usually the trial management group, are named as authors. The working party or equivalent group can be named in the title or in parenthesis; for example, 'Name, Name, Name, on behalf of the Medical Research Council Testis Tumour Working Party'. Alternatively, 'a Medical Research Council Testis Tumour Working Party trial' can appear in the title.

◆ The named authors may include clinicians who have contributed at least an agreed minimum number of patients or an agreed proportion of the total intake, or who have made a uniquely important contribution to the success of the trial. It needs to be born in mind, however, that small centres may have randomized a far higher proportion of their eligible patients than large centres although the total numbers entered by large centres are higher.

◆ It needs to be appreciated that references in journals are often quoted in the form: *Name, Name, Name, et al.*; title; journal reference. The parenthesis: '*on behalf of the . . . Group*' may sometimes be omitted. This difficulty is avoided if the group provenance is included in the title.

In abstracts, it is usual to use named authorship; in this case, the person presenting the paper should be the first (or only) named author. If group authorship is used, the presenter's name can be given in the form: '*Group*, presented by *Name*.'

8.9.2 Acknowledgements

Full acknowledgement is important to help establish the scientific and independent status of the trial and the reliability of the results, and to nurture collaboration with colleagues, other trials groups, and sponsors.

◆ In every publication, care must be taken to ensure that acknowledgement is made to all consultants entering patients, to the sponsor, and to all providing any additional support. The way this is done will depend partly on the style of authorship.

◆ In naming clinicians who entered patients, it is usual to indicate the level of their involvement. This can be done in the form: 'The following consultants and their colleagues entered twenty, say, or more patients . . .; the remaining patients were entered by . . .'. Alternatively, only those consultants who entered at least a stated proportion (say 10 per cent) of the total intake are named, although it is preferable to acknowledge all collaborating consultants. Whichever style is used, the centres where the named consultants recruited patients should be stated.

◆ Acknowledge by name all the local coordinators.

◆ It is essential to name the sponsoring organization: for example, National Cancer Institute, Cancer Research UK, or Medical Research Council. This is usually done in either the title or the authorship.

◆ It is also essential to name other organizations, including pharmaceutical companies, contributing to the funding or providing others means of support.

◆ Any possible conflict of interest must be declared.

8.9.3 Drafting reports

Drafting a report on a trial is a collaborative effort and it is important to ensure that all members of the trial management group and collaborating clinicians have the opportunity to comment on drafts.

* The report should be drafted by the trial management group.
* In international trials involving other trials groups, one group usually takes the lead and will draft the report(s), but the other groups should be given the opportunity to comment and agree the final manuscript.
* The trial management group decides to which journal the report should be submitted, and drafts the report in the appropriate style. They should, however, inform all collaborators of their suggestion, and be prepared to alter their decision if good reasons for doing so emerge.
* Appropriate members of the trial management group should take the initiative in preparing reports for publication, submitting them, and ensuring that referees' comments are addressed, revising manuscripts as required, checking proofs, and ordering, paying for and distributing reprints.
* Reprints should be sent to all collaborators in the trial.

8.10 Independent data monitoring and supervision

All randomized trials, whether they are multi-centre or conducted within a single hospital or local group, require data monitoring and supervision by individuals who are independent in the sense that they have no conflict of interest with any aspect of the trial. The trial sponsor (see Section 7.4.1) is responsible for ensuring that independent data monitoring and supervision are provided. The data monitors, usually called the data monitoring and ethics committee or other similar title, assess the progress of the trial in the light of confidential interim analyses and make recommendations to the trial supervisors. The supervisors provide overall supervision of the trial and ensure that it is conducted in accordance with the agreed standards (see Section 7.3). The trial sponsor may delegate to the supervisors the responsibility of deciding whether a trial should be continued, modified, or stopped prematurely. Both data monitors and supervisors must give high priority to patient safety.

Independent data monitoring and supervision can be provided in a number of ways. They are often provided by a single committee, the data monitoring and ethics committee, but supervision may be provided separately by the sponsoring organization, by one or more members of the host institution, or by a trial steering committee, responsible for making decisions about the conduct of the trial in the light of recommendations from a purely advisory data monitoring and ethics committee. The point at issue is who is responsible for making recommendations about continuing, modifying or terminating the trial, and who is responsible for taking the final decision. This must be made clear.

We describe the membership and functions of the data monitoring and ethics committee and the trial steering committee separately below, recognizing that their functions will sometimes be undertaken together by a single committee.

8.10.1 Membership and functions of the data monitoring and ethics committee

The role of the data monitoring and ethics committee is to provide totally independent reviews and recommendations to the trial steering committee on the progress of a trial; see Box 8.5. Their principal concerns are patient safety and the ethics of either continuing or terminating the intake to a trial or of modifying its protocol.

Membership

The defining characteristic of the data monitoring and ethics committee is that they are totally independent of anyone involved in the trial, the sponsor, and any organizations providing support, and have no conflict of interest in its outcome. They have no other involvement in the trial except as members of the committee. They can therefore provide wholly objective advice and make correspondingly objective recommendations to the trial management group, trial steering committee and sponsor. The professional members must be experts in their field with experience in the conduct of clinical trials. Any lay member(s) should be fully aware of the issues involved in conducting trials.

The committee needs to ensure that it has available all information it is likely to need on the day-to-day conduct of the trial, and is able to provide independent review. In addition to an independent chairman and other independent members, it therefore needs to be able to call upon members of the trial management group. It may be helpful to include a member of a patient advocacy group for part of a meeting, but it is usually

---

Box 8.5 Membership and functions of the data monitoring and ethics committee

Membership

- Two or more clinicians with experience in the relevant fields, a medical statistician and, if considered appropriate, a lay person or persons

Functions

- Monitoring all aspects of the progress of the trial and reviewing its progress and the quality of the data regularly
- Reviewing confidential data from interim analyses, usually unblinded by treatment group, provided by the trial management group, after requesting any additional analyses or information they need to make their assessment
- Reporting to the trial steering committee and making recommendations on the continuation of the trial
- Considering any requests for the release of interim findings, making recommendations to the trial steering committee on the advisability of this
- Responding to specific requests from the trial steering committee, particularly about the need for additional support, and making recommendations to this committee and to the sponsor

preferable to seek advice from such groups on specific topics as and when required rather than during a data monitoring meeting.

Functions

Monitoring the progress of the trial   At their first meeting, relatively early in the course of the trial, it is useful for the committee to meet and agree with the trial management group the planned recruitment targets and the information they will need for assessing the progress of the trial. They should then usually meet at least annually, but if a trial is running well, without problems, discussion of its progress may be quite brief.

Meetings of the committee are usually organized by the trial management group, but the committee themselves can decide when and how often to meet. The trial management group provide the information and analyses on the progress of the trial. In reviewing its progress, the committee should pay particular attention to answering the following questions.

- Is the trial recruiting patients at a satisfactory rate? If not, are the likely reasons discernible? Can they be corrected?
- Is the protocol being adhered to? Are the patients eligible? Are they receiving their allocated treatment regimens? Is unexpected toxicity being encountered? Is the safety of patients being compromized? Are collaborating centres providing the data?
- Is the trial likely to be completed within the planned timescale and budget? If not, the likely reasons should be identified and the sponsor informed as soon as possible.
- Is the trial still relevant? Does information from other sources, or do the results of other related trials, make it desirable to consider whether or not to continue with the present trial?
- Are the current results of the trial sufficiently convincing to persuade the members of the committee that the intake should be stopped or the protocol changed?

An agreed person should draft minutes of all meetings and reports, and ensure that members of the committee agree them.

Reviewing confidential interim analyses   The analyses reviewed will usually be unblinded by treatment group and are therefore confidential, although, for the sake of security, the treatment groups may be identified merely as 'A', 'B', etc. in the written report and tables and the committee told verbally what the groups are. The results of the analyses must not be conveyed to any of the clinicians, expert advisers, or independent assessors involved in the trial. Indeed, unblinded analyses will often be undertaken by the trial statistician alone and even other members of the team will not be aware of the results. Confidentiality is essential to prevent hasty and inappropriate conclusions being drawn from analyses of immature data.

The committee must ensure that they have all the information they need for making recommendations about the progress of the trial. The trial statistician, or other appropriate member of the team, should be available to attend part of the meeting to present the analyses and in order that the committee can ask for clarification or further information if required. Other members of the trial management group may be asked to attend an open part of the meeting to discuss information apart from the unblinded

Box 8.6 Structure of a typical data monitoring and ethics committee meeting

- The committee meet in private to review the data they have, to discuss the progress of the trial, and to identify any questions they need to ask of the trial management group
- Members of the trial management group may be called upon to discuss matters relating to the conduct of the trial such as the rate of intake and the quality of the data, but not the confidential interim analyses
- The committee and the trial management group discuss the progress of other related trials being conducted by other groups
- The trial statistician is called in to present the analyses and respond to any questions the committee may have
- The committee discuss in private their collective view on the progress of the trial and their recommendations about whether the intake should be continued or terminated, or the protocol modified
- The committee convey their conclusions to the trial statistician and the principal investigator, with their reasons, and draft reports to the sponsor, the trial management group, and the trial steering committee

analyses. This could include information on the progress of similar trials conducted by other groups. Thus, the meeting typically has the structure shown in Box 8.6.

Reporting and making recommendations to the trial steering committee After each meeting, the committee should make a confidential report to the trial steering committee, taking care that this does not reveal confidential interim results. Their report should make recommendations on the continuation of the trial. If they recommend stopping the intake prematurely or making a major modification to the protocol, it must be made clear whom they should make such recommendations to, and the process by which a decision is reached. In the model we propose here, it is for the trial steering committee to decide whether to accept the data monitoring and ethics committee's recommendation.

Recommendations for major changes to the conduct of the trial should not be made lightly. If the reasons for undertaking the trial are still valid, it is important that the findings are as reliable as possible. The committee must appreciate the inherent unreliability of interim analyses based on immature data and avoid recommending too hasty termination of a trial (see Chapter 9). Nevertheless, they should not hesitate to recommend major changes if these are necessary for preserving the safety of patients or if the results of the primary outcome measures are already sufficiently convincing that it would be inappropriate and unethical to continue the intake.

Considering requests for release of interim findings Some trials groups present interim findings, even on primary outcome measures, at national or international conferences, sometimes even before the intake has been completed. This is an inappropriate and undesirable practice: it may jeopardize further recruitment or lead to unjustified changes in practice; and it throws into question the information available at the time the trial was planned and the statistical calculations on which the size of the trial was based. Interim findings based on immature data are inherently unreliable and conclusions based on them may well turn out to be incorrect. Moreover, groups planning or undertaking similar trials may find themselves subjected to considerable pressure to abandon their trials on the basis that the primary question has already been answered.

The data monitoring and ethics committee should therefore view with extreme caution any requests for the release of interim data. Nevertheless, it may be necessary to make collaborating clinicians aware of differences in toxicity, for example, if to do so could protect patients from avoidable risk. The committee should always make the reasons for their recommendations clear.

Responding to requests for additional support If the trial management group feels that it may need to apply for additional support to complete the trial satisfactorily, the data monitoring and ethics committee may be asked for their recommendations on the matter. This may be difficult because they know the interim results. In response to such a request, they should therefore confine their comments to reporting on the progress of the trial, the quality of the data, and the likelihood that, with additional support, the trial would be completed successfully and would provide results that are still likely to be scientifically important and clinically relevant in the revised timescale. In their report, they should provide evidence to support their recommendations but not reveal the results of interim analyses. They should include and comment on relevant information that may be available from similar trials conducted by other groups.

8.10.2 Membership and functions of the trial steering committee

The membership and functions of the trial steering committee are summarized in Box 8.7. Their role is to provide an element of independent supervision over the conduct of a trial and, in this sense, fulfill an executive role for the sponsor. They are thus responsible for ensuring that the trial management group is fulfilling all its roles satisfactorily, and that any problems are dealt with rapidly and appropriately.

Membership

The membership of the committee must enable it to have available all information it is likely to need on the day-to-day conduct of the trial, and yet to provide truly independent supervision. It should therefore include, in addition to the members of the trial management group, an independent chairman, at least one other independent member, and a representative of the sponsoring organization. Not all members of the committee will necessarily need to attend every meeting.

As for the data monitoring and ethics committee, the independent members must be truly independent of all those involved in the trial.

Functions

Supervising the progress of the trial It is helpful for the committee to meet soon after each meeting of the data monitoring and ethics committee, so that they can make decisions

Box 8.7 Membership and functions of the trial steering committee

Membership

♦ Members of the trial management group, an independent chairman, at least one other independent member, a representative of the sponsoring organization

Functions

♦ Supervising all aspects of the progress of the trial and reviewing its progress regularly

♦ Responding to reports and recommendations from the data monitoring and ethics committee and deciding whether the intake should be continued or the protocol modified

♦ Regularly reviewing relevant information from other sources and on other related trials

♦ Making recommendations to the sponsor and the trial management group on publicizing the trial in the media

♦ Reporting on all aspects of the above to the sponsor

about the progress of the trial based on the report and recommendations of the data monitoring and ethics committee.

An agreed person should draft minutes of all meetings and reports, and ensure that members of the committee agree them.

Responding to recommendations of the data monitoring and ethics committee   As indicated above, the recommendations of the data monitoring and ethics committee are based on confidential interim analyses, unblinded by treatment group, and on any relevant information from other sources. The data monitoring and ethics committee is particularly concerned with the ethics of continuing the trial and with patient safety. It is the responsibility of the trial steering committee to decide how to respond to these recommendations.

If they decide to comply fully with them, the reasons will have been made clear by the data monitoring and ethics committee. If they decide not to comply with their recommendations, or to comply with them only in part, they must fully justify their decision to the sponsor and make their reasons clear.

At each meeting, the committee should consider whether the intake to the trial should be continued or the protocol modified. If they decide to stop the intake prematurely or make a major modification to the protocol, it is essential that they make their reasons clear, particularly whether their recommendation is made for scientific reasons or because of organizational matters; they should specifically state whether the reasons for undertaking the trial are still valid.

Reviewing relevant information from other sources   It is the trial management group who should be best informed on the progress of similar, relevant trials being conducted by other groups and who first become aware of their results. This is because they keep in contact with the groups running these trials and usually attend conferences at which results are presented and discussed. It is the responsibility of the trial management group to ensure that the progress of, and findings from, these trials are discussed by the trial steering committee. In the light of such findings, the committee should consider what, if any, action to take: for example, changing the protocol, collecting additional data, or even terminating the intake.

Making recommendations on publicizing the trial in the media   We have discussed above the roles of the trial management group in promoting and publicizing trials within the scientific and medical community and patient advocacy groups (see Section 8.4). There are times, however, when it is appropriate to issue a press release, arrange a press conference or interview, or to inform the media in other ways about the progress or results of a trial. The trial steering committee should consider whether they should make recommendations about such action to the sponsor.

Reporting to the sponsor   In reporting to the sponsor after each meeting, the committee should give a full account of the progress of the trial. It should pay particular attention to the following principles.

- Justify any decisions taken, in particular those made in response to recommendations from the data monitoring and ethics committee.
- Report particularly on patient safety and on the ethics of any decisions made on continuing or modifying the trial.
- Indicate the steps that have been taken to obtain information on the progress or results of similar, relevant trials being conducted by other groups.
- Give a full account of any complaints or adverse comments that have been made, indicating their source.
- Express a clear opinion on whether the trial is likely to be completed within the planned timescale and budget. If this is considered unlikely, either because more patients than originally planned are needed or because the rate of intake has been slow, state whether additional funding over a longer period is likely to be sought, giving full justification if this is so. Indicate, if relevant, the steps that have been taken to keep the trial within the bounds of the originally agreed support.
- If additional support over a longer period is considered desirable, ask the trial management group to suggest revised plans.

In fulfilling its functions, the committee have a particular responsibility to patients, ensuring that their rights, safety and well-being are being protected above the interests of science and society.

8.11   Computing and information technology

8.11.1   Communication

Running trials requires excellent communication between the trial coordinators and collaborators. In addition to good telephone, voice-mail, facsimile (fax) and e-mail facilities, there should preferably be a telephone line dedicated to randomization. Randomizations should also be acceptable by fax and e-mail, and a number of groups can now accept 24-hour interactive randomizations through the Internet or on touch-tone telephone systems. This facility may be particularly useful for international trials, but security and confidentiality need to be assured. Some offices provide 24-hour manned telephone lines for randomization.

8.11.2   Randomization software

It is important that the randomization software is simple and can be used speedily. A good randomization program should have the following features.

+ Eligibility criteria automatically checked.
+ Stratification and minimization by many variables possible.
+ Interactive 24-hour secure randomization available over the Internet. (Other modes of randomization must be available for when access to the Internet is not available; randomization by telephone may be easier for many clinical centres.)
+ Patient entry directly confirmed by fax, e-mail or post.
+ Summary details of patients on trials available.
+ Downloading of randomization information onto a variety of databases, including data-management programs, statistical packages and ASCII files, possible.
+ Portable across many operating systems.

8.11.3   Clinical trials software

Clinical trials software is a fast developing field and it is therefore impossible to make detailed or specific recommendations. Nevertheless, the software needs to be capable of functioning well in the light of the following issues.

+ Trials often generate vast amounts of data, including demographics, disease characteristics, treatment given, and data on, for example, acute toxicity, long-term risks of adverse effects, tumour recurrence, metastatic spread, and quality of life.
+ A number of outcome measures may be of interest in addition to survival.
+ Follow-up is essential and can be prolonged or, indeed, indefinite.
+ Many types of case report form may be used, including a randomization checklist, an entry form, one or more types of treatment form, an end of treatment assessment form, more than one type of repeating follow-up form, and several special forms, such as forms for reporting serious adverse events, tumour staging, histology, and death.
+ Many trials include quality of life (or other) questionnaires completed by patients.

We recommend using a data management system that avoids the need for a new database to be programmed for each trial, a process that can take months to complete.

An appropriate clinical trials software package will possess many of the features shown in Box 8.8.

Box 8.8 Features of an appropriate clinical trials software package

- Simple to set up the database for a new trial rapidly in-house
- Flexible, allowing changes to be made to the structure with safeguards against inadvertent changes
- Includes automatic schedule checking and detection of missing data, and is capable of generating letters reminding clinicians when a form is due and giving details of problems
- Capable of handling the large amounts of data associated with multi-centre trials, particularly randomized phase III trials
- Accommodates longitudinal data involving several types of follow-up form
- Can handle large numbers of repeated variables as are involved, for example, in quality of life studies
- Allows the rapid interactive entry and correction of data, the merging of data, and the specification of repeated blocks of variables
- Includes detailed checks for the consistency and accuracy of data
- Maintains a list of data inconsistencies together with the status of any queries and the action taken
- Assists day-to-day trial administration
- Produces displays and printed listings required for interim analyses, data review and site visits
- Permits multi-user access. This is valuable for very large or complex trials in which different parts of the database may be monitored, updated or analysed by different users or centres
- Permits remote data entry
- Permits import and merging of data from external sources or databases
- Exports to common statistical packages
- Should allow a full audit trail that tracks all data entry and changes to be done

8.12 Data protection

The legal requirements for preserving the confidentiality of personal information about individual patients and other relevant persons and organizations (data subjects) vary from country to country. Nevertheless, the underlying principles are important and should be observed, whatever the legal requirements.

For example, the Data Protection Act 1998 for the UK implements the EU Data Protection Directive (95/46/EC). It contains data protection principles, a registration system, an independent supervisory authority to oversee data protection legislation, and the data subject's rights. It is supervised by the Information Commissioner. The Commissioner's introduction to the Act together with information and guidance is available on the Commissioner's homepage (http://www.dataprotection.gov.uk/). The Act itself can be found at http://www.legislation.hmso.gov.uk/acts/acts1998/19980029.htm. The Act applies to both paper records and those held on computers. Clinical researchers and trial coordinators should therefore observe the principles of data protection, whatever the form in which the data are stored, and comply with the law of their own country.

The eight principles of data protection as set out in the 1998 Act are based upon the provisions of the Council of Europe Convention on Data Protection. They are general in nature and form a suitable basis on which to formulate common-sense rules. They apply to all personal data. These are defined as data that relate to a living individual who can be identified from those data, or from those data and other information which is in the possession of, or is likely to come into the possession of, the data controller.

8.12.1 Principles of data protection

First principle

Personal data shall be processed fairly and lawfully. Patients must be informed how personal data are to be used and that confidentiality will be maintained. No unfair pressure must be applied in obtaining data. Patients must give their consent to data processing and/or processing must be 'necessary'. Processing for medical purposes, including medical research, is considered necessary.

Second principle

Personal data shall be obtained only for one or more specified and lawful purposes, and shall not be further processed in any manner incompatible with that purpose or those purposes. For patients in trials, the purpose is for research and statistical analysis. This principle is not breached by providing data to other collaborators involved in the clinical research programme (but see the eighth principle).

Third principle

Personal data shall be adequate, relevant and not excessive in relation to the purpose or purposes for which they are processed. This is a valuable principle to bear in mind when designing trial protocols and forms. Information should not be collected on the basis that it might possibly be useful in the future without a view of how it will be used.

Fourth principle

Personal data shall be accurate and, where necessary, kept up to date. This is a crucial principle of good data management. If and when inaccuracies are discovered, they should be corrected without delay.

Fifth principle

Personal data processed for any purpose or purposes shall not be kept for longer than is necessary for that purpose or those purposes. This principle is not breached by keeping data indefinitely, providing the purposes for doing so are clear.

Sixth principle

Personal data shall be processed in accordance with the rights of data subjects under this Act. This principle establishes the right of a person to have access to personal data and, where appropriate, to have such data corrected or deleted.

Seventh principle

Appropriate technical and organizational measures shall be taken against unauthorized or unlawful processing of personal data and against accidental loss or destruction of, or damage to, personal data. Efficient procedures must be instituted to ensure that this principle is observed. There should be documented security procedures and contingency plans for avoiding and/or dealing with emergencies such as theft, vandalism, fire and flooding, and all members of staff should be familiar with them. Backup procedures should permit rapid recovery of essential data and re-establishing office functions as soon as possible following an emergency.

Eighth principle

Personal data shall not be transferred to a country or territory outside the European Economic Area, unless that country or territory ensures an adequate level of protection for the rights and freedoms of data subjects in relation to the processing of personal data. The European Economic Area consists of the fifteen EU member states together with Iceland, Liechtenstein and Norway. This principle is complied with if data subjects give their consent to the transfer.

8.12.2   Common-sense rules for protecting data

The common-sense rules shown in Box 8.9 for protecting information on living individuals, based on the above general principles, should be adhered to. They apply to data not only on patients but also on staff processing data, collaborating clinicians and other relevant persons and organizations.

It is often possible and advisable to dissociate data from names by use of unique trial numbers; when this is done, ensure that lists of names and numbers are kept secure.

8.12.3   Encrypting data

There are many ways to encrypt data (see, for example, http://www.netsecurity.about.com/cs/encryptionrefs and http://www.rsasecurity.com/rsalabs/faq/sections.html). However, groups receiving data need to be able to de-encrypt them readily, and the aim should be to choose methods that are simple and secure.

8.12.4   Worldwide availability of data

While it is important that trial data be available to international collaborators as necessary for the successful conduct of a trial, it is equally important that they are revealed only to such people and to no others. Data should only be sent to offices with adequate data protection procedures in operation.

Patient information sheets should assure patients entering trials that the confidentiality of information about them will be preserved, and that such information will be made available only to those conducting the trial and for trial purposes.

Box 8.9   Common-sense rules on data protection

- Never reveal passwords to other people or write them down in any recognizable form
- Never send unencrypted confidential personal information over the Internet, in e-mails, on disks or by post in such a way that it can be identified
- When sending data, send it, if possible, without the patient's name or other such identifying information not essential for the recipient
- Never disclose confidential information to unknown persons over the telephone
- Always destroy, e.g. by shredder, unwanted paper documents giving personal information
- Always obtain authorization from the person concerned before divulging personal information to an external source
- Always use imaginary data or blank out names when preparing material for discussions of procedures, presentations, or case reports
- Always keep cabinets containing confidential data locked
- Ensure that only such data as are needed for the clinical research in hand are stored and for no longer than is necessary
- Ensure that confidential data are handled only by trained staff who appreciate data protection requirements and who are appropriately supervised
- Ensure the security of data storage and handling through access controls, both physical and logical, and audit trails that enable a comprehensive audit of accesses to the system, including failed access attempts

8.13   Research misconduct

Although misconduct does, unfortunately, occur in clinical trials, allegations of misconduct are uncommon [5]. The true scale of the problem is not, however, known, although an anonymous survey of its members conducted by the International Society for Clinical Biostatistics showed that the majority of participants were aware of a fraudulent project, but did not know whether the organization they worked for had a formal system for handling suspected fraud [6]. Allegations must be taken seriously because misconduct affects our responsibilities to, and our credibility with, patients, the scientific community and the public. It also brings the medical and scientific professions into disrepute. Several surveys have shown that a number of researchers know of cases of misconduct that have not been reported [7]. Allegations must be fully investigated and reports of confirmed misconduct made publicly available. The public must be protected and must have confidence in research results; they ought to be able to assume that researchers are honest and reliable. Correspondingly, researchers themselves must be protected from frivolous and malicious accusations. There is now international recognition of the need to tackle the problems honestly and realistically [8].

   The primary responsibility for establishing and maintaining standards and ensuring probity and integrity rests with the relevant professional bodies, senior investigators and employing institutions [9]. This requires guidelines, training in their use, and supervision.

8.13.1 Definition of misconduct

Scientific misconduct has been defined as fabrication, falsification, plagiarism, or deception in proposing, carrying out or reporting results of research and deliberate, dangerous, or negligent deviations from accepted practice in carrying out research. It includes failure to follow established protocols, if this results in unreasonable risk, and also the facilitating of misconduct by collusion in, or concealment of, such action by others. Misconduct does not include honest error or honest differences in the design, execution, interpretation, or judgement in evaluating research methods or results [5,10].

The types of misconduct most likely to be encountered in clinical trials are data fabrication and data falsification within a collaborating centre [6,11]. This is important, because such misconduct is usually intended to conceal inefficiency and missing data rather than to distort the results of a trial. We therefore restrict ourselves to commenting on misconduct within a collaborating centre.

8.13.2 Examples

Documented examples of misconduct in centres collaborating in trials include the following [7,11–14].

+ Forging patients' consent forms.
+ Adjusting eligibility criteria to make a patient appear eligible who does not meet these criteria.
+ Filling in results of repeated measurements that were not done, e.g. by repeating previous results.
+ Failing to report adverse events.
+ Filling in patient diaries retrospectively.
+ Destroying data to thwart the investigation of suspected misconduct.

8.13.3 Detecting possible misconduct and whistle-blowing

Each trial management group will need to decide how assiduously, if at all, it tests data for possible misconduct in a trial. In multi-centre trials, there are circumstances, such as the following, that should arouse suspicion; and statistical methods are available to detect the plausibility of data received from centres. These rely on the difficulty of fabricating plausible data: human beings are poor generators of random numbers. For a full description, see the report prepared by the International Society for Clinical Biostatistics Subcommittee on Fraud [11].

+ Data are unconvincingly tidy. Data from one centre can be compared with data from all centres with respect to the distribution of variables taken either in isolation (univariate) or jointly (multivariate). False data may lie 'too close' to the mean and lack variance and outliers. Multivariate observations may lack consistency and fail to correlate with other data in ways that would be expected.
+ False data may exhibit digit preference.

- Data may be normally distributed when in fact normal distribution is implausible.
- Compliance with the protocol may seem too good to be true.
- Changes over time and dates of attendances and records may be unlikely.

If a trial management group has possible evidence of suspect data, then it should first consider raising the matter with the person who provided the data. It needs to be recognized that assuming the role of whistle-blower is difficult. Most of us would be loath to make unjustified allegations, but willfully concealing misconduct is itself misconduct. Junior researchers, in particular, may fear reprisals, and there might even be the threat of libel. Both whistle-blowers and those they accuse must be treated justly; allegations can ruin the careers of both accused and accusers. Nevertheless, it is very important to report observed, suspected or apparent misconduct to the director of the group concerned. This should initially be done informally and confidentially. If it seems that misconduct may have occurred, the standard procedures for the group concerned should be set in motion.

Whistle-blowers are responsible for making allegations in good faith, maintaining confidentiality, and cooperating in any assessment or investigation that may be necessary.

8.13.4   Prevention

Research misconduct is best prevented by nurturing a culture of scientific integrity among all members of research institutions. Educating and training staff and collaborators and establishing ethical standards can help to prevent misconduct [9]. Within research establishments and collaborating centres, standard operating procedures can help to discourage misconduct. The following principles should help.

- Avoid requesting data that are unnecessary.
- Identify who is responsible in collaborating centres for supervising the collection and reporting of trial data and for sending them to the trials office.
- Conduct source data verification.
- Ensure that all information is clearly and legibly recorded and that laboratory reports are kept and filed logically and are available for verification, even after publication of the results of a trial.
- In the collaborating centre, keep copies of data forms sent to the trials office.

8.14   Conclusion

In this chapter, we have set out the principles of good clinical research in conducting trials and have recommended how these principles should be applied in practice. It is our experience that with good trial management and trial coordination, undertaken by well-trained and highly motivated staff, the majority of trials proceed to a successful conclusion without engendering major problems. Trials that are well conducted provide reliable conclusions and should influence clinicians of all relevant specialities and so benefit both patients and future research.

References

[1] McFadden, E. (1998) Chapter 5: Data Entry and Distributed Computing, in Management of Data in Clinical Trials, pp. 73–87. John Wiley, New York.

[2] Gibson, D., Harvey, A.J., Everett, V., and Parmar, M.K.B. on behalf of the CHART Steering Committee (1994). Is double data entry necessary? The CHART trials. *Controlled Clinical Trials*, 15, 482–8.

[3] Earlam, R. (1991) An MRC prospective randomized trial of radiotherapy versus surgery for operable squamous cell carcinoma of the oesophagus. *Annals of the Royal College of Surgeons of England*, 73, 8–12.

[4] Medical Research Council Lung Cancer Working Party (1999) Treatment of endotracheal and endobronchial obstruction by non-small cell lung cancer: lack of patients in an MRC randomized trial leaves key questions unanswered. *Clinical Oncology*, 11, 179–83.

[5] Medical Research Council (1997) *MRC Policy and Procedure for Inquiring into Allegations of Scientific Misconduct.* Medical Research Council, London.

[6] Ranstam, J., Buyse, M., George, S.L., Evans, S., Geller, N.L., Scherrer, B., Lesaffre, E., Murray, G., Edler, L., Hutton, J.L., Colton, T., and Lachenbruch P. for the ISCB Subcommittee on Fraud (2000) Fraud in medical research: an international survey of biostatisticians. *Controlled Clinical Trials*, 21, 415–27.

[7] Smith, R. (1996) Time to face up to research misconduct. *British Medical Journal*, 312, 789–90.

[8] Rennie, D., Evans, I., Farthing, M.J.G., Chantler, C., Chantler, S., Riis, P., Poloniecki, J., Irving, M., Berwick, D.M., Rubin, P., Treasure, T., and Klein, R. (1998) Dealing with research misconduct in the United Kingdom. *British Medical Journal*, 316, 1726–42.

[9] Evered, D., and Lazar, P. (1995) Misconduct in medical research. *Lancet*, 345, 1161–2.

[10] Evans, I. (1998) Dealing with research misconduct in the United Kingdom: conduct unbecoming – the MRC's approach. *British Medical Journal*, 316, 1728–9.

[11] Buyse, M., George, S.L., Evans, S., Geller, N.L., Ranstam, J., Scherrer, B., Lesaffre, E., Murray, G., Edler, L., Hutton, J., Colton, T., Lachenbruch, P., and Verma, B.L. for the ISCB Subcommittee on Fraud (1999) The role of biostatistics in the prevention, detection and treatment of fraud in clinical trials. *Statistics in Medicine*, 18, 3435–51.

[12] Martyn, C. (1996) Not quite as random as I pretended. *Lancet*, 347, 70.

[13] Atterstam, I. (1997) Karolinska Institute rocked by research misconduct. *Lancet*, 350, 643.

[14] White, C. (1998) Call for research misconduct agency. *British Medical Journal*, 316, 1695.

Chapter 9

Analysis

9.1 Introduction

In this chapter we present the principles of, and approaches to, analysis. A central component of this chapter are the practical issues for the analysis of a typical randomized trial, which should give the practitioner guidance on many aspects of analysis. Within this section there is, in particular, guidance on the analysis and presentation of quality of life data. There is also a statistical methods section which outlines the methods available for different types of data. This section is brief and can be omitted without loss of continuity. The aim is to emphasize principles and limit the number of formulae and equations. For a more detailed technical presentation of these methods the reader is referred to more specialized books, such as Altman [1].

Throughout this chapter, four examples will be used to illustrate some of the methods. The four examples are introduced below.

CR06 Colorectal Cancer Trial

The British Medical Research Council Colorectal Cancer Working Party conducted a randomized trial of three chemotherapy regimens for patients with advanced colorectal cancer. In this trial 905 patients were randomized between the de Gramont regimen, Lokich and raltitrexed chemotherapy regimens [2]. The de Gramont regimen was considered the 'control,' while there were two experimental arms, Lokich and raltitrexed.

BA06 Bladder Cancer Trial

An international collaboration of trialists randomized 976 patients with locally advanced bladder cancer between chemotherapy prior to local definitive treatment (radical surgery or radiotherapy) against local definitive treatment alone [3].

ICON2 Ovarian Cancer Trial

The ICON (International Collaborative Ovarian Neoplasm) collaborators randomized 1526 women with ovarian cancer between single agent carboplatin and the three-drug combination CAP (cyclophosphamide, doxorubicin and cisplatin) [4].

CHART Lung Cancer Trial

The CHART (continuous hyperfractionated accelerated radiotherapy) steering committee randomized 563 patients with non-small cell lung cancer to receive either CHART or conventional radiotherapy [5].

9.2 Significance testing and estimation

9.2.1 Significance testing

In a clinical trial comparing an experimental treatment against a control treatment, typically a primary question of interest is: is the experimental treatment better than the control? To address this question using the data from a clinical trial we actually answer a different but related question – we test the null hypothesis of 'no difference.' In a randomized clinical trial where we are aiming to show that the experimental treatment is better than the control treatment, the null hypothesis is that there is no difference between the experimental and control treatments in their effect on the main outcome measure. To test this null hypothesis, often denoted by H_0, we compare the results for the group of patients treated with the experimental with the group treated with the control. The goal of doing this is to reject the null hypothesis of 'no difference' in favour of an alternative hypothesis, that there is in fact a difference between experimental and control. A general approach to test this is to calculate the following 'Z' statistic for the main outcome measure

$$Z = \frac{\text{(observed difference between experimental and control)} - \text{(difference anticipated in the null hypothesis)}}{\text{standard error of the observed difference}}. \quad (9.1)$$

If the null hypothesis is true, then on average the observed difference should be zero (i.e. no difference), so that large values of Z represent more significant results, that is, smaller p-values. The standard error (SE) of the observed difference represents the variability inherent in estimating the observed difference. Generally, the larger the trial, the smaller the SE and therefore the larger Z will be.

The difference anticipated in the null hypothesis is usually zero. In this instance the Z-statistic simplifies to:

$$Z = \frac{\text{observed difference}}{\text{standard error of the observed difference}}. \quad (9.2)$$

Once the value of Z is calculated, its value is referred to standard tables to obtain a p-value. This resulting p-value answers the question: what is the probability that we would have observed this difference or a more extreme difference, if the null hypothesis is true? If the p-value is small, say less than 0.001, then we may conclude that the null hypothesis is unlikely to be true. On the other hand, if the p-value is large, say greater than 0.5, then we cannot conclude with any certainty that the null hypothesis is not true. Issues around interpreting and presenting p-values are presented in Chapter 10, and also discussed below.

9.2.2 Estimation

In contrast to testing the null hypothesis of no difference between treatments, we might ask the question 'how large is the difference between the experimental and control treatment?' The best estimate of this difference is given by the observed difference from the trial, and is called a point estimate. Alongside this, some indication of the precision of the estimate is required. This is provided by the confidence interval. It is conventional to quote the 95 per cent confidence interval, which gives a range of values around the estimate that we can be 95 per cent confident contains the true underlying value of the difference between treatments.

9.2.3 Differences and relationship between significance testing and estimation

The differences and relationship between significance testing and estimation are best shown using hypothetical examples.

The three rows in Table 9.1 shows the results of three hypothetical randomized trials, all estimating the same underlying true difference between treatments. The three trials differ only in terms of their size, with respectively 200, 2000 and 20,000 patients randomized. Although, because of the play of chance, in practice not all of these trials would produce exactly the same observed difference, we have assumed this for the purposes of this illustration. It can be seen that the first trial with 200 patients randomized has a corresponding p-value of 0.46. This trial may be reported to be a 'negative trial – showing no difference between the treatments.' This is of course wrong – the trial actually contains insufficient information, and is more correctly reported as an inconclusive trial. This can be seen by the width of the 95 per cent confidence interval, which shows that the difference between treatments could still be large in favour of either treatment, either 9 per cent in favour of the control treatment or 17 per cent in favour of the experimental treatment. The second trial with 2000 patients randomized has a p-value of 0.02, with a confidence interval ranging from 1 to 9 per cent. This p-value may be considered conventionally significant, in that it is less than 0.05. This is reflected in the 95 per cent confidence interval which excludes the value of no difference, i.e. zero. This displays the relationship between the significance level and confidence intervals – a p-value of exactly 0.05 will mean that the 95 per cent confidence interval just includes the value zero. Similarly a p-value of 0.01 will mean that the 99 per cent confidence interval will just include the value zero. In general a p-value of p will mean that the $100(1 - p)$ per cent confidence interval will just include zero. This 2000 patient trial provides us with more persuasive evidence in favour of the experimental treatment, the p-value is encouraging. However, the 95 per cent confidence interval is still wide ranging from 1 to 9 per cent in favour of the experimental treatment. Thus, this 2000 patient trial although encouraging still has some uncertainty about the size of the effect. The 20,000 patient trial has a p-value of less than 0.0001, and a 95 per cent confidence interval of (4%, 6%). This trial therefore provides extremely good evidence that there is a difference between the treatments, and the 95 per cent confidence interval is sufficiently narrow to suggest that the difference

Table 9.1 Three randomized trials of different size, each estimating the same difference of 5 per cent.

Number of patients	Estimated difference	95% Confidence Interval	p-value
200	5%	(−9%, 17%)	0.46
2000	5%	(1%, 9%)	0.02
20,000	5%	(4%, 6%)	<0.0001

has been estimated with reasonable accuracy. It is probably only this trial that allows a definitive statement to be made, in favour of the experimental treatment.

9.3 Statistical methods

9.3.1 Binary data

Outcome data from a cancer clinical trial will often be in the form of categories. For example, at a given time of assessment, in an individual patient we may observe a complete response, partial response, stable disease or progressive disease. In analysing these data the questions that are of central interest are, is there a difference between the experimental and control treatments, and what is the magnitude of any difference? These questions are first addressed for the special case when there are only two categories – called binary data. Suppose we have conducted a clinical trial in which patients have received either an experimental treatment or a control treatment and the response to each of the treatments has been reported in the form of a yes or no result for each patient. Data from such a trial could be reported as in Table 9.2.

In the table, of the $b + d$ patients receiving the experimental treatment b have responded, and of the $a + c$ patients receiving the control treatment a have responded. We would like to test the evidence against the null hypothesis that there is no difference between the experimental treatment and the control treatment. We can address this problem in one of two ways. Here we present the most easily accessible, which displays the link between hypothesis testing and estimation.

The proportion of responders on the experimental treatment is $p_{\text{experimental}} = b/(b + d)$, while the proportion of responders on the control treatment is $p_{\text{control}} = a/(a + c)$. The observed difference between experimental and control is therefore: observed difference $= p_{\text{experimental}} - p_{\text{control}}$ and this observed difference is the best estimate of the difference between the experimental and control treatments. If the numbers of patients in each group is not too small, then the standard error (SE) for this observed difference is given by:

$$SE(p_{\text{experimental}} - p_{\text{control}})$$

$$= \sqrt{\frac{p_{\text{experimental}}(1 - p_{\text{experimental}})}{b + d} + \frac{p_{\text{control}}(1 - p_{\text{control}})}{a + c}} \qquad (9.3)$$

Table 9.2 A table displaying whether patients have responded or not to the experimental and control treatments in a randomized trial

Response	Control treatment	Experimental treatment	Total
Yes	a	b	$a + b$
No	c	d	$c + d$
Total	$a + c$	$b + d$	$a + b + c + d$

and a 95 per cent confidence interval around this estimate is given by

$$p_{experimental} - p_{control} - 1.96 \times SE(p_{experimental} - p_{control}) \quad \text{to}$$

$$p_{experimental} - p_{control} + 1.96 \times SE(p_{experimental} - p_{control}). \tag{9.4}$$

The value 1.96 comes from considering the standard normal distribution with mean zero and variance 1 (see Section 5.4.1). Providing the trial is not too small, under the null hypothesis this is the relevant distribution for the statistics we calculate here. 2.5 per cent of this distribution lies above $+1.96$ and 2.5 per cent lies below -1.96; combining these probabilities gives a total of 5 per cent. Thus 95 per cent of the probability lies between -1.96 and $+1.96$, hence the 95 per cent confidence interval. To obtain a different width of confidence interval a different multiplier from 1.96 is used. For example to obtain a 99 per cent confidence interval we use 2.58 because 99 per cent of the standard normal distribution is contained within $(-2.58$ to $2.58)$, and to obtain a 90 per cent confidence interval we use the value 1.68.

In general, a $100(1 - \alpha)$ per cent confidence interval is given by:

$$p_{experimental} - p_{control} - Z_{1-\alpha/2} \times SE(p_{experimental} - p_{control}) \quad \text{to}$$

$$p_{experimental} - p_{control} + Z_{1-\alpha/2} \times SE(p_{experimental} - p_{control}). \tag{9.5}$$

To help understand this, if we are calculating the 95 per cent confidence interval, then $\alpha = 1 - 0.95 = 0.05$, and $(1 - \alpha/2) = 0.975$. Thus, looking at the normal distribution at www.anu.edu.au/nceph/surfstat/surfstat-home/tables.html gives $Z_{1-\alpha/2} = 1.96$.

To perform a test of the hypothesis that the underlying proportion of responders in the two groups is the same, we construct a similar framework, with interest focusing on $p_{experimental} - p_{control}$. However, we have an added consideration in this framework – the basic assumption is that in truth $p_{experimental}$ and $p_{control}$ should be the same, that is that the proportion of responders is the same on the experimental and the control treatments. The best single estimate of this proportion, p, is calculated by considering the two groups as one. In this instance

$$p = \frac{a + b}{a + b + c + d}, \tag{9.6}$$

$$SE(p) = \sqrt{\frac{p(1 - p)}{a + c} + \frac{p(1 - p)}{b + d}}. \tag{9.7}$$

It should be noted that this SE is not quite the same as the standard error used above to calculate the confidence intervals, because it is calculated on the basis that the null hypothesis, that these two proportions are the same is true. In contrast, the standard error when calculating confidence intervals is calculated on the basis of the observed differences in proportions.

The Z-statistic to test the null hypothesis is given by

$$Z = \frac{p_{experimental} - p_{control}}{SE(p)}. \tag{9.8}$$

To assess the significance of this result the equivalent p-value from this Z-value can be read from tables of the standard Normal distribution. As indicated above, such a table can be found at www.anu.edu.au/nceph/surfstat/surfstat-home/tables.html. This website allows the user to enter the observed Z-statistic and produces an exact p-value. An example of the analysis of this type of data is presented below.

Example. In the randomized trial, CR06 [2], comparing three chemotherapy regimens for patients with advanced colorectal cancer where clinical response of the disease was a secondary outcome measure, the following results were seen for two of the regimens twelve weeks from randomization (Table 9.3). It should be noted that although response was classified in four categories we have collapsed them into two for the purposes of this example. It should also be noted that a number of patients on each arm died before twelve weeks, these have been included as non-responders in Table 9.3.

Table 9.3 Response by treatment in the CR06 randomized trial

Response	Control treatment (de Gramont)	Experimental treatment (raltitrexed)	Total
Yes	59	46	105
No	193	204	397
Total	252	250	502

Following the methods outlined above,

$$p_{\text{experimental}} = p_{\text{raltitrexed}} = 46/(46 + 204) = 0.184,$$

$$p_{\text{control}} = p_{\text{de Gramont}} = 59/(59 + 193) = 0.234.$$

Thus,

$$p_{\text{experimental}} - p_{\text{control}} = 0.184 - 0.234 = -0.050.$$

To calculate confidence intervals we have to calculate

$$\text{SE}(p_{\text{experimental}} - p_{\text{control}}) = \sqrt{\frac{0.184(1 - 0.184)}{250} + \frac{0.234(1 - 0.234)}{252}} = 0.0362$$

A 95 per cent confidence interval for the estimate -0.05 is therefore given by $-0.05 - 1.96 \times 0.0362$ to $-0.05 + 1.96 \times 0.0362$, which gives -0.121 to 0.021.

To assess whether there is evidence of a statistically significant difference between these two treatments we need to calculate

$$p = \frac{59 + 46}{502} = 0.209,$$

$$\text{SE}(p) = \sqrt{\frac{0.209(1 - 0.209)}{250} + \frac{0.209(1 - 0.209)}{252}} = 0.0363.$$

It is interesting to note that this SE is only very slightly different from the SE calculated above for calculating confidence intervals. The Z-statistic is given by, $Z = -0.05/0.0363 = -1.377$. The corresponding p-value for this (which can be obtained from www.anu.edu.au/nceph/surfstat/surfstat-home/tables.html) is 0.169. Note that this is a 2-sided p-value (see below), in that we are considering differences in both directions. This result suggests that, from these binary data, there is no good evidence that the response rates are different in the de Gramont and raltitrexed groups. This conclusion is supported by the calculation of the 95 per cent confidence interval which includes the value zero.

Estimating and testing a single proportion

Together with estimating differences across groups we may be interested in estimating the proportion in just one group, say the experimental group. This can be done quite simply by setting c, d, and $p_{control}$ all as zero in the above formulations. In this way estimates and confidence intervals can be obtained. We can also assess whether the $p_{experimental}$ differs from a prespecified proportion of interest.

Example. In the CR06 colorectal cancer trial we may be interested in just the experimental arm (raltitrexed) and to assess whether there is good evidence that the response rate for this arm is more than 10 per cent. We note therefore that $p_{experimental} = 0.184$ and

$$SE(p_{experimental}) = \sqrt{\frac{p_{experimental}(1 - p_{experimental})}{250}}$$

$$= \sqrt{\frac{0.184(1 - 0.184)}{250}} = 0.0245.$$

Thus, the Z-statistic for testing whether the observed value is greater than 0.10 is given by:

$$Z = \frac{p_{experimental} - 0.10}{SE(p_{experimental})} = \frac{0.184 - 0.10}{0.0245} = 3.43.$$

Consulting the 1-sided normal distribution at www.anu.edu.au/nceph/surfstat/surfstat-home/tables.html, the corresponding p-value to this Z-statistic is 0.0003. (The reason why we are peforming a 1-sided test is because we are only interested in whether the estimate is greater than 10 per cent). This result shows that there is good evidence that the response rate in the raltitrexed arm is greater than 10 per cent. If we are also interested in the evidence that this response rate is greater than 15 per cent, we replace 0.10 by 0.15 in the above equation to give $Z = (0.184 - 0.15)/0.0245 = 1.39$. The corresponding p-value for this is 0.082, suggesting that we do not have good evidence that the response rate is greater than 15 per cent.

Continuity correction for the Z-statistic

When doing tests and calculating p-values, the methods described above use the fact that when the size of samples is reasonably large the Normal distribution is a good approximation of the Binomial distribution, which is the appropriate distribution when we have binary data. However, it should be noted that the number of responders can only take integer values whereas a normally distributed variable can take any value. For example, the number of responders on the experimental treatment can only take values 1,2,3, etc. To ensure a better correspondence between the Normal distribution and the Binomial distribution a value of 1/2 is subtracted from each observed frequency. Thus, we should, for example, take away 0.5 from the values a, b, c and d. It is advisable to use the continuity correction routinely when comparing two groups or when comparing a single proportion against a prespecified value (such as in Table 9.2). If it is not used, the Z-statistic tends to produce too large a value, and hence p-values are too small. The difference will not be large when the size of the study being analysed is reasonably large. However, it can have a considerable effect when the study size is small. In particular circumstances when one of the values of a, b, c or d is particularly small (less than five say) an alternative approach, called Fisher's exact test, is more appropriate (see below). It should be noted we do not consider adjustments for confidence intervals in the same way as for the test statistic, because we are not calculating probabilities from the tail area of a distribution.

Chi-square (χ^2) test

To test the null hypothesis of no difference between the true proportions responding to the experimental and new treatments, many analysts perform a chi-square test. This is done by comparing the observed value in each cell, a, b, c and d with its expected value $e_a, e_b, e_c,$ and e_d respectively under the null hypothesis and taking the sum of the squares between each respective pair. The calculation of the relevant statistic is:

$$X^2 = \frac{(a - e_a)^2}{e_a} + \frac{(b - e_b)^2}{e_b} + \frac{(c - e_c)^2}{e_c} + \frac{(d - e_d)^2}{e_d}, \tag{9.9}$$

where

$$e_a = \frac{a+b}{a+b+c+d} \times \frac{a+c}{a+b+c+d},$$
$$e_b = \frac{a+b}{a+b+c+d} \times \frac{b+d}{a+b+c+d},$$
$$e_c = \frac{a+c}{a+b+c+d} \times \frac{c+d}{a+b+c+d},$$
$$e_d = \frac{b+d}{a+b+c+d} \times \frac{c+d}{a+b+c+d}.$$

The expected values $e_a, e_b, e_c,$ and e_d are calculated on the basis that if the null hypothesis is true and there is really no relationship between response and treatment then the number in each cell of the table is just given by a simple multiplication of the row and column proportions in which that cell falls, the proportion of patients who are in that treatment group multiplied by the total number of responders in the trial as a whole. The X^2 statistic obtained through this calculation is compared against a chi-squared distribution with one degree of freedom. The reason there is one degree of freedom is because once all the row and column totals (that is $a + b, a + c, b + c, b + d$) have been specified we only have to specify one of the cells, such as a, to calculate all the remaining cells b, c and d. In general, for a table with r rows and c columns the chi square test has $(r - 1)(c - 1)$ degrees of freedom. In our case we have two rows and two columns and thus $(2 - 1)(2 - 1) = 1$ degree of freedom.

It can be shown that in most circumstances the X^2 statistic is equivalent to the square of the Z-statistic, presented above. Thus the two methods will give the same results.

However, the chi-square test provides just a test of the null hypothesis and unlike the methods presented above does not directly provide estimates and confidence intervals. Thus it is generally not the preferred approach for binary data. The chi-square test is not a good approximation in certain circumstances, and a rule of thumb is that none of the expected values should be less than five. If this is the case, then an alternative method of testing the null hypothesis, called Fisher's exact test, should be performed. Finally, as for the test of independent proportions, a continuity correction is needed for small sample sizes.

Fisher's exact test for two proportions

As mentioned above, the chi-square test for two proportions requires that all the 'expected' values are greater than five. Because of the direct correspondence between the chi-square test and the Z-test of two proportions, this condition holds for the detailed approach presented above as well. The reason for this is that when we are dealing with data as presented in Table 9.2, the data are essentially discrete and we are using continuous distributions to assess the Z and chi-square statistics. In these circumstances, Fisher's exact test is recommended. The reader is referred to specialist statistics texts [1] for a description of this test.

9.3.2 More than two categories

In many cancer clinical trials, the categories of interest will have a natural ordering. For example, the assessment of response may fall into one of the following four categories: complete response, partial response, stable disease and progressive disease. These four categories have a natural ordering with complete response the 'best' result and progressive disease the 'worst.' Two commonly used approaches for analysing such data are the chi-square test for trend and the Mann–Whitney test. We first illustrate the chi-square test for trend by an example.

Example showing the chi-square test for trend

In the CR06 colorectal cancer trial introduced above, patients were assessed for response at twelve weeks and there were actually five categories as shown in Table 9.4.

Table 9.4 All categories of response by randomized treatment for the CR06 colorectal cancer trial

Response	Control treatment (de Gramont)	Experimental treatment (raltitrexed)	Total
Complete response	4	3	7
Partial response	55	43	97
Stable disease	94	86	180
Progressive disease	60	68	128
Dead at 12 weeks	39	50	89
Total	252	250	502

There is clearly a set of four ordered categories of response here from complete response through to progressive disease. It is not clear how best to take into account those patients who have died by twelve weeks – the time of assessing response. We could include them as a separate category, or we could include them in the category of progressive disease, or we could exclude them from this analysis altogether. We discuss this problem further below in Section 9.5.2. For the purposes of the example only, we shall include these patients as a separate ordered category, 'worse than' progressive disease.

To analyse these data we first need to assign scores to each of the groups and a simple scoring may be one for 'complete response,' two for 'partial response,' three for 'stable disease,' four for 'progressive disease' and five for 'dead at twelve weeks.' This scoring, although arbitrary, shows the order of the categories; and the question we wish to address is: do patients receiving the experimental treatment generally have higher (or lower) scores than patients receiving the control treatment? A higher score would mean a generally poorer response, while a lower score would mean a generally better response. Unfortunately, the simplest way of calculating the chi-square test for trend does not show the derivation and nature of the method. To help the calculations we have to define some quantities. We focus on the raltitrexed group and define the five 'response' groups by their score 1–5; the number of patients in each of these response groups is r_i, thus r_1 is 3; the total across both the raltitrexed and deGramont groups will be referred to as n_i, thus n_1 is 7. Further, we let x_i be the score allocated to each group with, for example, for the complete response group, $x_1 = 1$. We then calculate the following quantities:

$$N = \sum_{i=1}^{5} n_i = n_1 + n_2 + n_3 + n_4 + n_5 \qquad R = \sum_{i=1}^{5} r_i,$$

$$p = R/N \quad \text{and} \quad \bar{x} = \sum_{i=1}^{5} n_i x_i / N.$$

The test statistic X^2_{trend} is given by the following equation:

$$X^2_{trend} = \frac{\left[\sum_{i=1}^{5} r_i x_i - R\bar{x}\right]^2}{p(1-p)\left[\sum_{i=1}^{5} n_i x_i^2 - N\bar{x}^2\right]}. \tag{9.10}$$

The statistic X^2_{trend} is then compared against the chi-square distribution with one degree of freedom. The reason for one degree of freedom is because in essence what we are doing is fitting a line to the responses in both experimental and treatment groups and then assessing whether the slope of this line is different across the two groups. Thus we are considering one variable. This example is worked through in more detail in Section 9.4.5.

The Mann-Whitney test

An alternative approach to analysing these data is to use the Mann–Whitney test. This is a more complicated test, which is based on ranks. The Mann–Whitney test is one of the 'non-parametric' tests, so called because it does not assume that the data come from any particular known distribution (such as the Normal distribution). In this test we first consider the two groups (raltitrexed and de Gramont) as one, that is a single sample. We then rank the patients in terms of response, assigning the value one to a complete response, two to a partial response, three to stable disease, etc . . . . Then the sum of the ranks for the raltitrexed group is compared to the sum of the ranks of the de Gramont group. If there are generally better responses in the raltitrexed group, then the sum of the ranks for the raltitrexed group should be lower than the sum of the ranks for the deGramont group. Statistics calculated from the sums of the ranks in the groups allows us to perform a significance test on the null hypothesis that there is no difference in response to these two treatments. For more details the reader is referred to Altman [1] (p. 194) or Bland [6] (p. 223). The Mann–Whitney test is also often referred to as the Wilcoxon two-sample test – although they have different derivations, they are in fact the same test. The Mann–Whitney test and the chi-square test for trend will generally produce similar results. As a rule of thumb, the chi-square test for trend is preferred if the number of categories is small (say five or fewer), while the Mann–Whitney test is preferred when there is a larger number of categories (six or more). When using the Mann–Whitney test some care must be taken if there are a large number of ties of ranks. This becomes more likely as the number of categories decreases. In this situation the basic Mann–Whitney test needs to be adapted. This is complicated but possible. It should, however, be emphasized that not all computer packages allow for this situation and thus may give incorrect results, the reader should therefore confirm that the package they are using allows for ties.

Estimation when there are more than two categories

There are no natural, easily accessible, estimates when there are more than two categories. Thus, in such situations it is common to use slightly different approaches for hypothesis testing (for example the chi-square test for trend) and estimation. To obtain estimates, it is common to collapse categories into a binary yes/no response; for example, the categories of complete and partial response may be collapsed into one single 'response' category, while stable disease and progressive disease may be collapsed into a 'no response' category. Then methods described above for estimating a single proportion for binary data to obtain estimates and confidence intervals, should be used. It is important to note that for the testing of the hypothesis, all the original categories should be retained as this maximizes the power of the test and retains maximum information in this analysis.

9.3.3 Continuous data

When comparing two groups of continuous observations the focus is usually the mean difference between groups. To perform a test of the hypothesis that there is no difference between groups we calculate the following statistic:

$$t = \frac{\bar{x}_e - \bar{x}_c}{\mathrm{SE}(\bar{x}_e - \bar{x}_c)}, \tag{9.11}$$

where $\bar{x}_e$ is the mean of the observations for the experimental group and $\bar{x}_c$ is the mean of the observations in the control group. The value $\mathrm{SE}(\bar{x}_e - \bar{x}_c)$ is the standard error of the difference between the means. The calculation of this standard error is straightforward, if a little cumbersome, and we have to define a number of terms first. Initially we need an estimate of a pooled variance, s^2,

$$s^2 = \frac{(n_e - 1)s_e^2 + (n_c - 1)s_c^2}{n_1 + n_2 - 2}, \tag{9.12}$$

where n_e is the number of observations in the experimental group, n_c, the number of observations in the control group, s_e, the standard deviation of the experimental group, s_c, the standard deviation of the control group.

The SE of the difference between means is then given by

$$SE(\bar{x}_e - \bar{x}_c) = s \times \sqrt{\frac{1}{n_e} + \frac{1}{n_c}}. \tag{9.13}$$

The statistic t which is obtained from this calculation is compared against a t-distribution (rather than Normal distribution used above) to obtain a p-value for this test. However, similar to the chi-square distribution, the t-distribution varies according to the degrees of freedom. In general, the degrees of freedom are given by the total number of observations (across both groups) minus the number of parameters estimated in the numerator of the statistic. Thus the degrees of freedom is given by: number of observations in the experimental group + number of observations in the control group − 2. The value two comes from the fact that we have estimated two means, one for each group. A 95 per cent confidence interval for the difference between means is

$$\bar{x}_e - \bar{x}_c - t_{0.975} \times SE(\bar{x}_e - \bar{x}_c) \quad \text{to} \quad \bar{x}_e - \bar{x}_c + t_{0.975} \times SE(\bar{x}_e - \bar{x}_c), \tag{9.14}$$

where $t_{0.975}$ is the 97.5 per cent percentile from the t-distribution with the degrees of freedom given as described above. To calculate a 90 per cent confidence interval $t_{0.975}$ is replaced by $t_{0.95}$, the 95 per cent percentile of t-distribution. The t-distribution is similar to the standard Normal distribution, in that it is symmetrical around zero. The major difference is for small sample sizes (small numbers of degrees of freedom) the t-distribution has fatter tails (at either end) than the Normal distribution. For larger sample sizes (large numbers of degrees of freedom) the t- and Normal distributions are very similar. Thus, when comparing groups with reasonable numbers of patients (for example more than twenty-five patients in each group), the t-statistic calculated above can be regarded as a Z-statistic, and compared as described above with a Normal distribution.

The methodology above assumes the data being analysed come from an approximately Normal distribution (see Chapter 5). Where there is doubt about this, alternative methods that do not assume any particular distribution for the data are generally applied. These are known as non-parametric tests, and the Mann–Whitney test described in the previous section is one such example. In fact the Mann–Whitney (or equivalently the Wilcoxon two-sample test) is again the appropriate test to use when one wishes to compare data from two groups where the Normality assumption is questionable. This is often the case with very small sample sizes. As for the categorical data example, the individual values from the two groups are combined and ranked and the sum of the ranks in the two groups compared. Though widely applicable, such tests are best used when there is clear evidence of lack of Normality, as they are less powerful than the t-test when the Normality assumption holds. The appropriate summary statistic for such data is the median; confidence intervals can be calculated but this is not straightforward, nor is it routinely offered by many statistical analysis packages.

More than two groups

Where more than two groups are being compared, the general approach is to carry out a 'global' test which examines whether there is any evidence of substantial differences between the groups (without indicating where this lies). Only if this test is positive are further, pairwise, comparisons carried out to isolate and explain the main differences. This is discussed further below with respect to time-to-event data. For Normally distributed data, the appropriate global test is an extension of the two-sample t-test, known as Analysis of Variance, often abbreviated to ANOVA. The non-parametric equivalent is the Kruskal–Wallis test. For details of both, we refer readers to a statistics text book such as Altman [1].

9.3.4 Time-to-event data

There are many examples in cancer where a time from one event to another is used. For example, the time a woman with ovarian cancer survives once the tumour has been removed by surgery, the time a man with testicular cancer treated with chemotherapy survives and remains free of disease. These times are triggered by an initial event: a surgical intervention, followed by a subsequent event, death, or recurrence of disease. The time between such events is known as the 'survival time.' The term survival is used because the first use of such techniques arose from the life insurance industry. The difference between 'survival' data and other types of numeric continuous data is that the time to the event occurring is not observed in all subjects. Thus in the above examples, in the lifetime of our study all the women with ovarian cancer may not die, or all the men with testicular cancer may not experience a recurrence of their disease. Such non-observed events are called 'censored.' Historically, much of the analysis of survival data has been developed and applied in relation to randomized cancer clinical trials in which the survival time is often measured from the date of randomization or commencement of therapy until death, and the early papers by Peto and colleagues [7,8] reflect this.

Estimation and summary statistics for time-to-event data

The Kaplan–Meier survival curve. The Kaplan–Meier estimate of the survival curve is often used as a means of summarizing 'survival' data. The survival rate estimate at time t, $S(t)$, will start from 1 (100 per cent of patients alive) since $S(0) = 1$, and progressively decline towards 0 (all patients have died) with time. It is plotted as a step function, since the estimated survival curve remains constant between successive patient death times. It drops instantaneously at each time of death to a new level. The graph will only reach 0 if the patient with the longest observed survival time has died. Patients who are still alive are included in the formation of the curve but are 'censored' from the time they were last known to be alive. In general the overall probability of survival at time t, $S(t)$, is given by:

$$S(t) = \left(1 - \frac{d_1}{n_1}\right)\left(1 - \frac{d_2}{n_2}\right)\left(1 - \frac{d_3}{n_3}\right)\cdots\left(1 - \frac{d_t}{n_t}\right), \tag{9.15}$$

where d_t represents a death at time t and n_t the number of patients still alive and being followed up (that is not censored) at time t. Thus the value of $S(t)$, changes only on times (days) on which there is at least one death. As a consequence the curve does not change during the times (days) when there are no deaths. The succesive overall probabilities of survival $S(1), S(2), \ldots, S(t)$ are known as the Kaplan–Meier (or product-limit) estimates of survival. If all the patients have experienced the event before the data are analysed the estimate is exactly the same as the proportion of survivors plotted against time.

The overall survival curve is much more reliable than the individually observed survival probabilities at each of the timepoints of which it is composed. Spurious (large) falls or (long) flat sections may sometimes appear. These are most likely to occur if the proportion of censored observations is large or when the number of patients still alive and being followed up may be relatively small. A guide to the reliability of different portions of the survival curve can be obtained by recording the number of patients 'at risk' at various stages beneath the time axis of the survival curve. The 'number at risk' is defined as the number of patients who are known to be alive at that timepoint and therefore have not yet died nor have been censored before the timepoint. These individuals are therefore 'at risk' of the event in the subsequent time interval. At time zero, which is the time of entry of patients into the study, all patients are at risk and hence the number 'at risk' recorded beneath $t = 0$ is the number of patients entered into the study. The patient numbers obviously diminish over time, because of both deaths and censoring. The deaths which happen at various times can be seen on the plot by the fact that the survival curve drops down; to help indicate the censored observations the survival curve is sometimes annotated with vertical ticks at each timepoint at which an individual patient is censored.

The reliability of the Kaplan–Meier estimate of $S(t)$ diminishes with increasing t. There is no precise moment when the right-hand side tail of the survival curve becomes unreliable. However, as a rule of thumb, the curve can be particularly unreliable when the number of patients remaining at risk is fewer than fifteen. The width of the confidence intervals (see below), calculated at these and other timepoints, will help to show the uncertainty in the estimate. Nevertheless, it is not uncommon to see the value of $S(t)$, corresponding to the final plateau, being quoted as the 'cure' rate, especially if the plateau appears to be long. This can be seriously misleading as the rate will almost certainly be reduced with further patient follow-up. Clearly, if there are no censored observations preceding the end of a plateau, then the plateau will not disappear with more patient follow-up. Even in such cases the plateau should be interpreted with considerable caution.

Median survival time

A commonly reported statistic in cancer studies is the median survival time. This statistic is particularly useful in studies of advanced disease, where prolongation of survival may be more relevant than cure. The median survival time is obtained by finding the time at which the proportion alive (and dead) is 0.5. This is done by reading across from the vertical axis at 0.5 and when the curve is hit, reading down to the timepoint at which this happens. As an example Fig. 9.1 shows the overall survival curves for the three groups (de Gramont, raltitrexed and Lokich) from the CR06 colorectal cancer trial discussed above. Reading across from 0.5, median survival for the de Gramont appears to be approximately nine months. More accurately, considering the data used to plot these curves, the estimated median survival is 294 days.

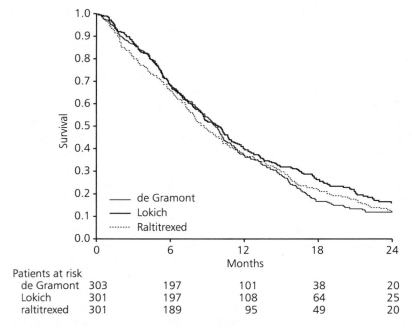

Fig. 9.1 Overall survival in the CR06 trial. Reprinted with permission from Elsevier Science (*The Lancet*, 2002, **359**, 1555–63).

Confidence intervals

Confidence intervals (CI) calculated at relevant points along the Kaplan–Meier survival curve will give an indication of the reliability of the curve at those points. There are several ways of calculating confidence intervals at given points. Popular approaches include those proposed by Greenwood, Peto and Rothman (see pp. 36–40 in Ref. [9]). We first present our preferred method – the transformation method. One of the reasons this a preferred method is because it constrains the confidence interval within zero and one, something not all methods will do.

We first transform $S(t)$ onto a scale which more closely follows a Normal distribution. It can be shown that $\log_e\{-\log_e[S(t)]\}$ has an approximately Normal distribution, with SE given by

$$\text{SE}_{\text{TR}}[S(t)] = \frac{\left[\sum_j d_j/[n_j(n_j - d_j)]\right]^{1/2}}{-\sum_j[(n_j - d_j)/n_j]}, \tag{9.16}$$

where d_j is the number of deaths on day j and n_j is the number of patients alive on follow-up at the beginning of day j.

To calculate the 95 per cent CI on this transformed scale we calculate the following two values:

$$\log_e\{-\log_e[S(t)]\} - 1.96\text{SE}_{\text{TR}}[S(t)] \quad \text{to} \quad \log_e\{-\log_e[S(t)]\} + 1.96\text{SE}_{\text{TR}}[S(t)].$$

We now return to the original scale by using $S(t)^{\exp(+1.96\text{SE}_{\text{TR}})}$ which is the upper 95 per cent confidence limit and $S(t)^{\exp(-1.96\text{SE}_{\text{TR}})}$, the lower 95 per cent confidence limit.

A simpler but less reliable way of obtaining a confidence interval is a method suggested by Peto. In this approach we first calculate a standard error as follows:

$$\text{SE}_{\text{TR}}[S(t)] = \left[\frac{S(t)\{1 - S(t)\}}{R_t} \right]^{1/2}, \tag{9.17}$$

where R_t is the number of patients recruited to the trial minus the number censored by the time under consideration. Thus $R_t = N - c_t$, where N is the number of patients in the trial and c_t is the number of patients censored before time t. R_t is sometimes termed the effective sample size. A 95 per cent confidence interval is then given by $S(t) - 1.96\text{SE}_{\text{TR}}[S(t)]$ to $S(t) + 1.96\text{SE}_{\text{TR}}[S(t)]$.

Comparison of two survival curves

Above, we described how the Kaplan–Meier estimate of a single survival curve is obtained. Within most clinical trials we shall want to compare two or more survival curves. For example, we may wish to compare the survival experiences of patients who receive different treatments. Before we describe the methods available to compare two survival curves, we note that it is inappropriate and usually very misleading to compare survival curves only at a particular point of the curve, for example, making comparisons of 1-year survival rates. The reason for this is that each individual point on the curve is not in itself a good estimate of the true underlying survival. Comparing two such estimates (one from each of the two curves) leads to an unreliable comparison of the survival experience of the two groups. Further, it makes very poor use of all the data available by concentrating on particular points of each curve and ignoring the remainder of the survival experience. The comparison of two (or more) survival curves is usually done by the logrank test, or some variant of it.

The Logrank test The Logrank test, like all hypothesis tests, is based on comparing the observed against the expected data under the null hypothesis of no difference between the experimental and control arms. To compare two survival curves, one for the experimental treatment and one for the control, we use the following test statistic:

$$X^2_{\text{Logrank}} = \frac{(O_e - E_e)^2}{E_e} + \frac{(O_c - E_c)^2}{E_c}, \tag{9.18}$$

where O_e is the observed number of deaths on the experimental arm, e, E_e, the expected number of deaths on the experimental arm, e, O_c, the observed number of deaths on the control arm, c, E_c, the expected number of deaths on the control arm, c.

This is a format which is similar to that for the standard chi-square test for a 2×2 table. The only difference is that the expected numbers of deaths in groups e and c are actually a summation of the expected numbers of deaths in each group calculated on each occasion that a death happens in either group. The expected number of deaths on the experimental and control arms is obtained by forming a 2×2 table at each timepoint at which there is an death in the trial. Under the null hypothesis of no difference between the groups the probabilty of an event in either group at a given time is proportional to the number of event free in each group at that time. Thus at each timepoint at which there is an event we can calculate the probability that the event should have been in either the experimental or control groups. Multiplication of this probability by the actual number of events (usually one) at that timepoint gives the expected number of deaths in the two groups at that timepoint. Summation of these expected values over all timepoints at which there is an event, gives the E_e and E_c in equation 9.18. The observed number of deaths O_e and O_c are simply the number of deaths seen in the trial on the experimental and control arms.

When there are two treatment groups the χ^2_{Logrank} statistic is compared against a chi-square distribution with one degree of freedom. In general, for G treatment groups the χ^2_{Logrank} statistic is compared with the chi-square distribution with $G - 1$ degrees of freedom. The logrank test is a hypothesis test, testing the (null) hypothesis that there is no difference in survival between the groups. We also need an estimate of the difference between the curves, and this is given by the hazard ratio.

The hazard ratio

The hazard ratio (HR) is defined as

$$\text{HR} = \frac{O_e/E_e}{O_c/E_c}. \tag{9.19}$$

The HR is the ratio of the relative hazards of the event in the two groups being compared. It compares the risk (hazard) of an event on the experimental arm (O_e/E_e) at any given time with the risk (hazard) of an event in the control arm at the same time. In this sense the HR can be considered to be a type of relative risk for time-to-event data. Thus, for example, a hazard ratio 0.75 represents a 25 per cent reduction of the risk of an event on the experimental arm compared to the control arm.

Confidence intervals for the hazard ratio can be calculated by considering the logarithm for the hazard ratio, because this is approximately Normally distributed. A $100(1 - \alpha)\%$ confidence interval for the logarithm of the hazard ratio is given by:

$$\log_e \text{HR} - [Z_{1-\alpha/2} \times \text{SE}(\log_e \text{HR})] \quad \text{to} \quad \log_e \text{HR} + [Z_{1-\alpha/2} \times \text{SE}(\log_e \text{HR})],$$

where $Z_{1-\alpha/2}$ is the upper $(1 - \alpha/2)$ point of the standard Normal distribution.
The $100(1 - \alpha)\%$ CI for the HR is then

$$\exp(\log_e \text{HR} - [Z_{1-\alpha/2} \times \text{SE}(\log_e \text{HR})]) \quad \text{to}$$
$$\exp(\log_e \text{HR} + [Z_{1-\alpha/2} \times \text{SE}(\log_e \text{HR})]).$$

In the expression above

$$\text{SE}(\log_e \text{HR}) = \sqrt{\frac{1}{E_e} + \frac{1}{E_c}}. \tag{9.20}$$

The Mantel–Haenszel estimate

The estimate of the SE($\log_e$ HR) given in equation 9.19 is not always reliable in situations when the total number of events in the study is small. A preferred estimate of the SE involves more extensive computation at each death time and requires the calculation of the variance, called the hypergeometric variance, V. This gives an alternative estimate of the hazard ratio and an alternative test called the Mantel–Haenszel test. The estimate of the hazard ratio is given by

$$HR = \exp\left(\frac{O_e - E_e}{V}\right). \qquad (9.21)$$

Describing follow-up maturity

In all studies with a survival-type endpoint there will usually be a mixture of subjects in which the critical event has been observed and those in which it has not. Mature data are those in which most of the events that have been targeted in the design of the trial have been observed. There are a number of ways in which to summarize the reliability and maturity of follow-up. The numbers at risk at various stages along the Kaplan–Meier survival curve and the indication of the censored data on these curves, together with SEs at specific time points, are useful measures. However, they do not give single concise measures. Simple summaries which have been suggested for this purpose include the median follow-up time of those individuals still alive, the minimum and maximum follow-up times of these individuals and the proportion of patients who have experienced the event.

In all trials the following statistics should always be calculated and reported (see Table 9.5): the numbers at risk at various appropriate timepoints on the survival curves: the targeted total number of events, and observed number of events. In trials in which a large proportion of the patients are expected to experience the event by the time of analysis, for example in trials of advanced disease, the most informative statistic to report is the proportion of patients with an event. In contrast, in trials in which less than say 60 per cent of patients have experienced the event by the time of analysis, the most informative statistic is the median follow-up of survivors.

For all trials, to check that there is no imbalance in follow-up between groups being compared it can be useful to calculate a Kaplan–Meier 'follow-up' curve. To do this, we label those patients who have 'died' as actually being 'censored' on their date of death, and those patients who are still alive as having an 'event' on the date they were censored. The estimated median follow-up can be read off the curves in the same way as median survival.

Table 9.5 Statistics to report follow-up from randomized trials

Statistic to report follow-up	Which type of trial?
Numbers at risk	All trials
Targeted total number of events	All trials
Observed number of events	All trials
Proportion of survivors followed to a timepoint of interest, e.g. two or five years	All trials
Proportion of patients with an event	Advanced disease trials

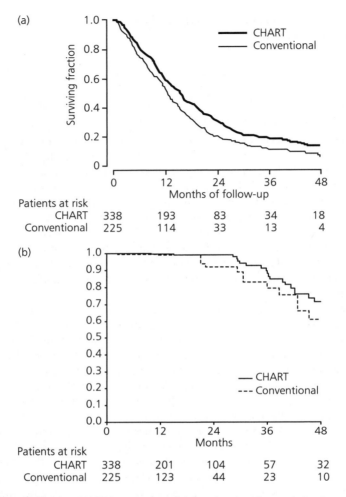

Fig. 9.2 (a) Survival in the CHART lung cancer trial. Reprinted with permission from Elsevier Science (*The Lancet*, 1997, **350**, 161–5) (b) Follow-up in the CHART lung cancer trial.

Example. Saunders and colleagues report a randomized trial of continuous hyper-fractionated accelerated radiotherapy (CHART) versus conventional radiotherapy in patients with locally advanced non-small cell lung cancer. Approximately 600 patients were planned to be entered into this trial, and a total number of deaths of approximately 475 was targeted to achieve the power and type I error for the targeted difference. A total of 563 patients were actually entered into the trial and a total of 444 deaths were observed, i.e. when the results of this trial were reported, events had been seen in the large majority, 79 per cent (444/563), of patients. The Kaplan–Meier survival curves for the two groups, are shown in Fig. 9.2a and the follow-up curve in Fig. 9.2b.

It can be seen that beyond two years the numbers at risk become relatively small, especially in the conventional radiotherapy group, with the numbers alive and at risk at three and four years of thirteen and four patients, respectively. Comparison of the

Kaplan–Meier curves gives a hazard ratio of 0.76 (95 per cent confidence interval 0.63 to 0.92; $p = 0.004$) indicating a 24 per cent reduction in the relative risk of death at any time with CHART.

The stratified Logrank test

In any study the outcome for patients will often be influenced by the characteristics of the patients themselves as well as by the treatments they receive. For example, for most cancers, patients with a more advanced stage of the disease generally have a shorter expectation of life than patients with less advanced disease. In making comparisons between two groups receiving, for example, different treatments, we need to ensure as much as possible that the differences observed between groups are due to the treatments and not due to the fact that the groups have inherently differing prognoses. In large trials randomization should ensure this, but we may wish to adjust for these prognostic variables when making comparisons between groups, especially in smaller trials. This ensures that 'like' is compared with 'like.' These individual comparisons are then combined to achieve an overall comparison of treatments. This is done by means of the stratified Logrank test.

The extension to equation 9.18 to obtain the stratified logrank statistic for comparing treatments is

$$\chi^2_{\text{stratified}} = \frac{\left(\sum O_e - \sum E_e\right)^2}{\sum E_e} + \frac{\left(\sum O_c - \sum E_c\right)^2}{\sum E_c}, \tag{9.22}$$

where $\sum$ denotes the sum over strata.

More than two groups

We have described how two groups may be compared using the logrank test. There are also situations where we may wish to compare more than two treatment groups in a clinical trial or compare outcomes for patients with differing characteristics. For example, we may wish to compare the survival times of patients with different stages of disease. Here we describe how the Logrank test can be extended to three or more group comparisons.

The general expression corresponding to equation 9.18 but for G groups is given by

$$\chi^2_{\text{Logrank}} = \sum_G \frac{(O_G - E_G)^2}{E_G} \tag{9.23}$$

with G groups the degrees of freedom is $G - 1$.

This test is a general test and does not identify where any differences occur. This information may be sought in an informal way from the Kaplan–Meier plots, or by making further, usually pairwise, statistical tests in subgroups of the G groups. However, we need to take some care, when comparing more than two groups, because as pointed out below in Section 9.5 as the number of tests performed increases, the probability of finding a spurious 'positive' result increases. One practical solution to this is to use what is called a 'closed' analysis, which helps protect against this. In this 'closed' analysis, a single logrank analysis is performed across all the groups to assess whether there is overall evidence of differences between groups. Only if this analysis is significant at a pre-specified level (for example, if the observed p-value is less than 0.05), are further pairwise comparisons performed between groups. If the initial overall p-value is not significant at this level then the conclusion is reached that there is no good evidence of a difference anywhere between the groups and no further analyses are done.

Cox's proportional hazards model

Cox's proportional hazards model is used extensively in the analysis of survival data. The use of the model includes comparing treatment effects in trials and adjusting these comparisons for baseline characteristics. A further use of these models is to assess variables for prognostic significance. The basic assumption for this model is that the ratio of hazards of an event at a given time in the groups being considered is proportional over time. It is beyond the scope of this book to consider how one might test this assumption, and the reader is referred to more specific books on survival analysis for these (such as Ref. [9]). Despite this apparently rather limiting assumption, the proportional hazards model has been extensively used, partly because experience suggests that it works well in practice in many situations, but also because it is available in nearly all major statistical packages.

In studying a group of patients we might wish to relate the duration of their survival to various clinical characteristics that they have at diagnosis, for example age, stage of disease, grade of disease, performance status, etc. In survival analysis terms we model the probability of dying at a given time, t, given the patient has survived to that time. This is called the instantaneous death rate or the hazard rate and denoted as $\lambda(t)$. The proportional hazards model relates this to an overall average hazard for the whole group $\lambda_0(t)$, using the following expression:

$$\lambda(t) = \lambda_0(t) \exp(\beta x), \qquad (9.24)$$

where x is the group of variables representing the characteristics of the patient, for example their age, stage of disease, grade of disease, etc., and β are a set of parameters which need to be estimated from the data. For example if we are trying to evaluate the risk of dying at a particular time, given survival to that time, and given the patient's age, stage of disease and grade of disease:

risk of dying at time t = average risk of dying at time t

$$\times \exp(\beta_1 \times \text{age} + \beta_2 \times \text{stage} + \beta_3 \times \text{grade}). \qquad (9.25)$$

The parameters $\beta_1, \beta_2, \ldots$ (together with their standard errors) give an indication of the relative importance of each of the variables. In most situations when comparing two treatments in a randomized trial, the Cox model with the treatment group as the only variable in the model will give very similar results to the logrank test described above, and the hazard ratio will be given by $\exp(\beta)$.

It is clear from the above that the logrank test and the Cox model can both be used for the same purposes, usually with little difference between the results. We discuss the pros and cons of both approaches in Box 9.1.

It can be seen from Box 9.1 that, except for the simplest analyses, the Cox model although more complicated, provides a more general framework for the analysis of time-to-event data.

Box 9.1   Comparison of the logrank test and the Cox model

	Logrank test	Cox model
Provides estimates and standard errors	yes	yes
Assume proportional hazards	no	yes
Stratified analyses with binary or categorical data	yes, but number of strata limited	yes
Stratified analyses with continuous data	no	yes
Factorial trials, with interaction term	yes, with some manipulation	yes

9.3.5   Longitudinal data (repeated measures)

For each patient, data from a clinical trial are sometimes in the form of repeated assessments over time. In such a trial observations are taken on more than one occasion for each patient over the period of the trial. An example of such data is given in the randomized clinical trial LU19 conducted by the Medical Research Council Lung Cancer Working Party [10]. In this trial the control arm of six cycles of ACE chemotherapy given 3-weekly was compared to the experimental arm of 6 cycles of ACE + G-CSF given 2-weekly. For each patient, clinicians were asked to complete a symptom assessment form before starting treatment and then after each cycle of chemotherapy, 3-weekly for the ACE arm and 2-weekly for the ACE + G-CSF group. In both groups after the completion of chemotherapy (eighteen weeks for the ACE arm, twelve weeks for the ACE + G-CSF arm) reports were to be completed each month up to six months.

Longitudinal data pose many problems for analysis which can include data missing at particular timepoints, repeated (and therefore correlated) data on each patient and the difficulty that we shall probably be performing multiple comparisons and thus we shall be increasing our chance of finding a 'positive' result by chance alone (see subgroup analysis and interim analysis sections below). Whatever the form of longitudinal data (binary, categorical or continuous) there are two principal methods for analysing them, using summary measures or model-based approaches. In cancer clinical trials longitudinal data most often occur in the form of 'quality of life data' and the presentation and analysis of such data is best done through practical example. Thus the reader is referred to Section 9.4.9 for a presentation and discussion of analysis of these data.

9.4   Practical guidance in analyzing the data from a randomized trial

9.4.1   Intention-to-treat analysis

A major source of bias in a randomized trial can be the exclusion of patients from the analysis. Patients may be excluded for a variety of reasons including:

- further tests carried out after randomization show the patient is ineligible,

- the patient does not receive any of their allocated treatment,
- the patient receives some, but not all their allocated treatment,
- the patient is not assessed for the outcome of interest, such as response,
- an independent review reports the patient as ineligible.

Although all these may appear to be legitimate and sensible reasons to exclude patients from analysis, it actually transpires that most are likely to introduce bias into the analysis. The reasons for this are discussed below.

Further tests carried out after randomization shows the patient is ineligible

Most trial protocols will list investigations that must be performed before randomization to determine whether a patient is eligible. However, often because of the nature of one of the treatments, further investigations may be performed on one arm (typically the experimental arm) after randomization, the findings of which may mean the patient is 'ineligible.' As an example, in a trial of interstitial versus conventional radiotherapy for patients with brain tumours, it may be tempting to exclude those patients with multifocal tumours who have a poor prognosis and are unlikely to benefit from either type of radiotherapy. However, such tumours are only readily detectable in those patients having interstitial radiotherapy. To exclude these patients from the analysis would have been inappropriate, because there are probably a similar number of patients with undetected multi-focal tumours in the conventional radiotherapy arm. Exclusion of such patients would therefore introduce systematic differences between the two arms and lead to a biased analysis. This displays the general point that excluding patients on the basis of an investigation performed after randomization is likely to introduce bias, particularly when one treatment group is more likely to undergo the investigation, and such patients should generally be included in the analysis.

Patients who do not receive any of their allocated treatment

In most randomized trials a (usually small) proportion of patients will never receive the allocated treatment. The reasons for this may include: the patient changes their mind, or the patient's condition deteriorates (or improves) rapidly, or an administrative error means the patient receives the wrong treatment. In this circumstance they may receive the alternative treatment in the trial, another treatment altogether or no treatment at all. It may be tempting to exclude such patients from the analysis. However, in general patients who do not receive any of their allocated treatment are likely to be those with a poorer prognosis. This is perhaps most obvious in trials comparing an active treatment against a 'no-treatment' control group – in this situation the active treatment group may have patients receiving none of their allocated treatment. It may be tempting to exclude these patients from the analysis. However, it is almost impossible to identify and exclude a similar group of patients from the control arm, because we cannot predict who would have failed to receive the treatment if they had been allocated it. Thus exclusion of such patients on the experimental arm from the analysis means that we are introducing systematic differences between the arms and are likely to introduce bias in favour of the more aggressive, usually new, treatment. It should be noted that including these patients in the analysis according to their allocated treatment group, does itself introduce a form of bias, because the difference between the experimental and control arms will be underestimated (as patients who receive none of the allocated treatment cannot benefit from it). Nevertheless, such an approach is inherently conservative and is to be preferred to overestimating the difference (by an unknown amount) in favour of the experimental therapy.

Patients who receive some, but not all their allocated treatment

For many cancers, treatment is given over a period of many weeks, months or sometimes years. As a consequence, it is almost inevitable that some patients will not complete all their allocated treatment. This may happen because the patient dies during treatment, or the patient's disease progresses (or improves) rapidly making further treatment inappropriate, or the patient experiences unacceptable toxicity and refuses further treatment, or the doctor considers it not in the patient's best interests to continue with it. Generally, patients who do not complete the allocated treatment are likely to have an inherently poorer prognosis than those who do complete it, and this poor prognosis is not a consequence of their non-completion of the course of treatment. Further, in cancer, the experimental treatment is likely to be more toxic than the control treatment and thus lead to more patients stopping treatment early. Hence, exclusion of such patients from the analysis will again introduce systematic differences between the two groups being compared, and this bias will be introduced into the analysis and results. An extreme example of this is if we are comparing six courses of adjuvant cytotoxic therapy versus no adjuvant cytotoxic therapy. In many trials it is common to find that only approximately 80 per cent of all patients actually receive all six courses of adjuvant therapy, with those perhaps least well stopping therapy early. If we exclude these patients then we are comparing the 80 per cent most 'well' patients in the adjuvant therapy group with 100 per cent of patients in the no adjuvant therapy group, leading to a clearly biased estimate of the difference between the two.

Patients who are not assessed for the primary outcome

In most trials, outcome measures are measured many months and sometimes years after randomization. It is therefore possible that some of these patients will be 'lost to follow-up' before the outcome measure has been observed. For example, if the analysis is focusing on the response at twelve weeks, then some patients may have died, others may not be assessed because they are too ill and do not turn-up, while, perhaps more rarely, others do not turn up because they are well. If these missing data are more common in one group than another then bias in the comparison can creep in; even if the numbers of patients with missing data are similar in the two groups the reasons for the missing data may be different in the two groups. This situation is perhaps more difficult than those above, because the data on these patients are just not available for inclusion in the analysis. Options in these circumstances include regarding patients with missing data as 'failures' on therapy, making the general assumption that this is the prime reason data are missing. This may not be appropriate for all outcome measures, such as quality of life, where imputation of missing values is possible, but potentially dangerous. We discuss how these issues may be addressed for different outcome measures of response (Section 9.4.5) and quality of life (Section 9.4.9). This difficulty emphasizes the importance of concentrating on an outcome measure that can be assessed in all randomized patients such as, for example, duration of survival (see Section 5.2)

Independent review says the patient is ineligible

Many trials will incorporate central review of eligibility, for example pathology or radiology, where a small group of experts will review all the patients in a trial and confirm, or not, their eligibility according to the protocol. Whether or not this has the potential to introduce bias depends on whether the reviewers have information on the patients' treatment or outcome which could conceivably influence their diagnosis. Of course anyone intent on bias could, in the knowledge of treatment allocation, declare ineligible all those patients in one treatment group with the features indicating poor prognosis. A more subtle bias may creep in if the reviewer has knowledge of the patients' outcomes. For example, a neuropathologist reviewing slides for brain tumour patients entered into a trial of high-grade glioma may, on the basis of the limited material available to him, be unsure whether some patients have a grade 2 (low grade) or grade 3 (high grade) tumour. If the review was being done retrospectively, and he was aware of the patients' survival times, he may be steered towards a diagnosis of grade 2 (ineligible) for those with longer survival and grade 3 (eligible) for those with shorter survival, since this would be in keeping with the usual prognosis of these patients. If in fact the reason for the longer survival for some patients was that they had been allocated a particularly effective treatment, their exclusion would bias the results against this treatment. These issues are avoided if central reviews are conducted 'blind' to treatment allocation and outcome, the latter being helped by conducting the review prospectively. Where review is blind, the question is whether it is appropriate to exclude a patient on the basis of an expert opinion, when that opinion would not routinely be available to patients outside the trial. This issue is discussed further in Section 4.2.3.

The difficulty with all but the last of the situations outlined above is that the reason for exclusion is very likely to be related to the treatment that the patient has been allocated, leading to the potential for systematic differences between the experimental and control groups being analysed. Unless we can be absolutely sure that the reasons for exclusion are completely independent of the allocated treatment, then the best, least biased and most conservative approach is to include all patients in the analysis. This is called the 'intention-to-treat' or 'ITT' analysis (see Box 9.2) defined as including all randomized patients and analyzing them according to the treatment to which they were allocated irrespective of the treatment that they actually received. In contrast, examples of when exclusion of patients might be justified are when an independent review has been done of pathology, blind of the treatment allocated and also in 'equivalence' trials, and this is discussed in Section 9.4.2.

9.4.2 Intention-to-treat analysis and equivalence trials

One situation when an intention-to-treat analysis may not be the only primary analysis is in equivalence or non-inferiority trials (see Section 4.2.2 for a full definition for this type of trial). In such trials it is typically anticipated that for the main outcome measure (such as duration of survival) the new treatment will be no worse than the control treatment, while the new treatment may have a better toxicity profile. As

Box 9.2 Intention-to-treat (ITT) analyses:

- include all patients randomized in the analysis according to their allocated treatment, whether or not they actually received it
- are the preferred form of analysis of trials which are planned to show a difference between two treatments
- minimize bias
- are likely to produce 'conservative' estimates of the difference between treatments
- may be supplemented (but not replaced) by analyses excluding certain groups of patients; if this is done, then the exclusion of patients should be justified, and the likely bias that these exclusions bring to the analysis should be fully discussed.

intention-to-treat analyses tend to dilute an effect between treatments, an ITT analysis in an equivalence trial may make the treatments appear to be more similar than they actually are. Thus, for equivalence trials a 'per protocol analysis' (PPA) could be regarded as 'conservative' and therefore is often given as much emphasis as an ITT. A PPA is defined as the analysis of the set of data generated by the subset of patients who have complied with the protocol sufficiently that they are likely to show the effects of the treatment. Thus, for example, in an equivalence trial comparing two chemotherapy regimens PPA analysis may concentrate on those patients who received at least two courses of treatment.

9.4.3 Patient characteristics

When analysing a randomized trial, generally the first table to be presented is a table of pre-treatment or patient characteristics. This is presented for two reasons, first, to show the population of patients that have entered into the trial and second to 'display' how effective the randomization has been in achieving balance on these known patient characteristics. For the BA06 bladder cancer trial [3] a subset of the table of patient characteristics are shown in Table 9.6.

It is important that in such a table, for each characteristic each randomized patient is accounted for, even if they have missing data. For example, ten patients have missing data for size of tumour (four in the chemotherapy arm, six in the no chemotherapy arm). This table shows that all these characteristics are well balanced between the two groups. It is of interest to note that the median age of the patients in this trial is sixty four, which is perhaps lower than the population of patients with this disease. This is probably because the nature of the new treatment (chemotherapy) dictates that patients have to be relatively fit, indicated by their generally good performance status, and as a consequence this group of patients are somewhat younger than the population as a whole.

Sometimes it is common to see a hypothesis test being performed to assess whether there is a 'statistically significant' imbalance in patient characteristics between the randomized arms. Further, it is sometimes suggested that any observed 'imbalances' should

Table 9.6 Subset of patient characteristics for the BA06 bladder cancer trial. Reprinted with permission from Elsevier Science (*The Lancet*, 1999, **354**, 533–40)

Patient characteristic	Chemotherapy (*n* = 491)	No chemotherapy (*n* = 485)
T-category		
T2	169 (34%)	165 (34%)
T3	285 (58%)	282 (58%)
T4a	37 (8%)	38 (8%)
Age		
Median	64	64
Sex		
Male	433 (88%)	430 (89%)
Female	58 (12%)	55 (11%)
Histological grade		
G1	6 (1%)	2 (0.4%)
G2	52 (11%)	61 (13%)
G3	433 (88%)	421 (87%)
Not known	0	1
Tumour size (cm)		
≤2.5	82 (17%)	93 (19%)
2.6–5.0	306 (62%)	315 (65%)
5.1–6.9	88 (18%)	63 (13%)
≥7.0	11 (2%)	8 (2%)
Missing	4	6
Median	4	4

be allowed for in a stratified analysis. For example, in Table 9.6 interest may focus on whether there is an imbalance in the size of the tumour across the two arms of the trial. As Senn [11] and others have pointed out, it is inappropriate to perform a significance test for the number of reasons. Firstly, in doing this standard advice for hypotheses tests is ignored. In particular, null and alternative hypotheses are not clearly stated, a lack of significant difference between arms is treated as a 'proof' of equivalence and no adjustment is made for multiple testing. Further, if randomization was carried out 'appropriately,' then it is almost impossible to address these issues in any sensible way, and it transpires that all that is tested is that the process of randomization was concealed in the way planned, rather than whether randomization achieved the desired effect of 'balance.' Thus it is inappropriate to perform such tests of significance. Rather, the best use of these characteristics is set out in Box 9.3.

9.4.4 Treatment and compliance

For most trials it is useful to report how much of the allocated treatment has been received by the patients in the trial. One useful way of doing this particularly for chemotherapy is graphically. This is best displayed by an example. In the ICON2 ovarian cancer trial [4],

Box 9.3 How to use patient characteristics in the analysis of a randomized trial

- When designing the trial, from previous trials identify characteristics of prognostic value. From these, identify a small number (perhaps no more than five) of the most important characteristics which can be included as 'stratification' characteristics in the randomization process (see Chapter 4).

- For all the characteristics identified – and only these characteristics – at the beginning of the trial, include them in a stratified/adjusted analysis (either using simple stratified analyses or an appropriate model – such as the Cox model).

- State whether the adjusted analysis or the unadjusted analysis is the primary one; for large trials an unadjusted analysis is probably appropriate, while for small trials a (prespecified) adjusted analysis may preferable.

interest focused on two components of the treatments given, the total dose and the dose intensity of CAP and carboplatin treatments achieved across patients.

For total dose, for each patient and each drug we calculate the actual total dose given and divide it by the planned protocol total dose that should have been given if the treatment had been given in full. Figure 9.3 shows how these data might be presented. The two panels on the left represent the total dose achieved of the two treatments and they are to be interpreted as follows. Fifty eight per cent of patients allocated single agent carboplatin actually received 100 per cent or more of their planned total dose, while 90 per cent of patients received 60 per cent or more of their planned total dose. This graph of total dose tells us about reductions of the dose of drugs, but does not give any information on delays in giving the drugs. This is done in the right hand panels of Fig. 9.3 and points are calculated as follows. For each patient and each drug we consider the total dose given and note the total time taken to give this dose, td. This is then divided by the total dose which should (theoretically) have been given over the this total time, td.

If a considerable proportion of patients did not receive their allocated therapy then the reasons for this should be given. For example in the BA06 bladder cancer trial of the 491 patients assigned chemotherapy, one patient received four cycles, 392 received three cycles, thirty-seven received two cycles, thirty-three received one cycle and twenty-eight received no cycles. Thus ninety-nine patients did not receive all three cycles of chemotherapy and the reasons for this are set out in Table 9.7.

9.4.5 Response

In the CR06 colorectal cancer trial, clinicians assessed the response of the disease twelve weeks from the start of treatment. The results are shown in Table 9.8.

These data can be analysed in a number of ways. For example, we may be interested in the proportion of responders in each treatment group, or we may be interested in the proportion of patients with progressive disease in each treatment group. In both these situations we are considering the data as binary – forming two groups from the large

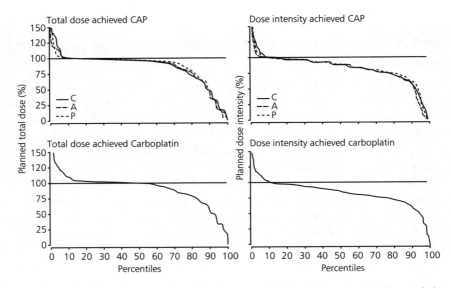

Fig. 9.3 Total dose and dose intensity curves from the ICON2 trial. Reprinted with permission from Elsevier Science (*The Lancet*, 1998, **352**, 1571–6)

Table 9.7 Reasons for not receiving three cycles of chemotherapy in the BA06 bladder cancer trial. Reprinted with permission from Elsevier Science (*The Lancet*, 1999, **354**, 533–40)

Reasons	Number of patients
Renal toxicity/reduced renal function	23
Other toxic effects of chemotherapy	18
Disease progression/death	14
Protocol errors/unspecified	23
Patient refusal	21
Total	99

Table 9.8 Response to the three chemotherapy regimens used in the CR06 colorectal cancer trial. Reprinted with permission from Elsevier Science (*The Lancet*, 2002, **359**, 1555–63)

	de Gramont (control)	Lokich	raltitrexed
Complete response	4	1	3
Partial response	55	57	43
Stable disease	94	80	86
Progressive disease	60	66	68
Dead at twelve weeks	39	32	50
Total	252	236	250

number of groups available for analysis. To analyse the data in this way we could use methods introduced for binary data in Section 9.3.1. Alternatively we could consider the full data as presented and consider the ordered categories from complete response being the 'best' category to progressive disease being the 'worst' category. Whichever approach is adopted, an important decision to be made is whether the patients who have died by twelve weeks and therefore could not be assessed for response should be included in the analysis. A number of these patients will have died from the toxicity of the treatments, others will have died from progressive disease which has not been catalogued; a very small number may have died from other causes. One can think of many, if not all, these patients as having failed therapy, and thus they could be naturally added to the 'progressive disease' category. This is recommended for analyses of such data. If these data are ignored, then it is entirely possible that inappropriate (biased) conclusions can be reached.

Considering the data as binary

If interest focuses on the proportion of responders (complete response + partial response) in the three groups the results in Table 9.9 are seen.

Table 9.9 Response rates in the three groups in the CR06 colorectal cancer trial

	de Gramont (control) (%)	Lokich (%)	raltitrexed (%)
Response rate (excluding deaths)	28	28	23
Response rate (including deaths)	23	25	18

It can be seen that excluding the patients who die, increases the response rate for all three treatments, particularly for the raltitrexed therapy which had the largest number of deaths. Using the nomenclature introduced in Section 9.3.1, we have

$$p_{\text{experimental}}(\text{excluding deaths}) = p_{\text{raltitrexed}}(\text{excluding deaths}) = 46/(250 - 50) = 0.23,$$
$$p_{\text{experimental}}(\text{including deaths}) = p_{\text{raltitrexed}}(\text{including deaths}) = 46/250 = 0.18,$$

$$p_{\text{control}}(\text{excluding deaths}) = p_{\text{de Gramont}}(\text{excluding deaths}) = 59/(252 - 39) = 0.28,$$
$$p_{\text{control}}(\text{including deaths}) = p_{\text{de Gramont}}(\text{including deaths}) = 59/252 = 0.23,$$

Thus,

$$p_{\text{raltitrexed}}(\text{including deaths}) - p_{\text{de Gramont}}(\text{including deaths}) = 0.18 - 0.23$$
$$= -0.05,$$

$$\text{SE}(p_{\text{raltitrexed}} - p_{\text{de Gramont}}) = \sqrt{\frac{0.18 \times (1 - 0.18)}{250} + \frac{0.23 \times (1 - 0.23)}{252}} = 0.036.$$

Thus a 95 per cent confidence interval for the estimated difference of -0.05 is given by $-0.05 - 1.96 \times 0.03644$ to $-0.05 + 1.96 \times 0.036$. When this is evaluated this gives -0.121 to 0.021, i.e. -12 per cent to $+2$ per cent. To perform a test of the hypothesis that the proportion of responders in the two groups is similar, we calculate the following:

$$p = \frac{46 + 59}{250 + 252} = 0.209,$$

$$SE(p) = \sqrt{\frac{p(1-p)}{250} + \frac{p(1-p)}{252}}$$

$$= \sqrt{\frac{0.209 \times (1 - 0.209)}{250} + \frac{0.209 \times (1 - 0.209)}{252}} = 0.0363.$$

The Z-statistic to test the null hypothesis of no difference in the response rate between the two treatments is given by:

$$Z = \frac{(p_{\text{raltitrexed}} - p_{\text{de Gramont}})}{SE(p)} = -0.05/0.0363 = -1.377.$$

If we look up this Z-statistic in the tables at www.anu.edu.au/nceph/surfstat/surfstat-home/tables.html then the p-value of 0.084 is obtained. This indicates that although the estimate of the response rate is higher in the de Gramont treatment when compared with the raltitrexed treatment, from these data there is no clear evidence that it is significantly better. We need to ensure that this result is not a consequence of how the data have been analysed – we have collapsed the five ordered categories into two (binary) categories. This is addressed below.

Considering the data as five ordered categories

In the publication of this trial these data were analysed using the Mann–Whitney test (see Section 9.3.2), considering all five categories in the order presented in Table 9.8. The comparison of de Gramont against raltitrexed gives a p-value of 0.20, again suggesting no evidence of a difference in response rates between these two groups. Thus in this situation we reach the same conclusions as for when we considered the data as binary. This may not be true for all datasets.

9.4.6 Toxicity

Toxicity data will be collected and presented in nearly all trials. For example, in the ICON2 ovarian cancer trial [4], data on the toxic effects of treatment were collected on 875 of the patients randomized. A subset of these data is presented in Table 9.10.

Issues raised in the analysis of toxicity data are the same as those for quality of life data and the reader is referred to Section 9.4.9 for a full discussion of the analysis of such data. Some more general issues are covered here.

There is a strong temptation to perform significance tests for each toxicity. However, it is usually inappropriate to do this because standard advice for significance tests is not usually followed. In particular, as described with reference to Table 9.6, null and alternative hypotheses are not clearly stated, a lack of significant difference between arms is treated as a 'proof' of equivalence and adjustment is not always made for multiple testing. Further, it should be noted that the trial alone is unlikely to be the only source of toxicity data for the treatments being compared. For example, in the above ICON2 trial it would not be informative to perform a significance test of whether the rate of alopecia

Table 9.10 Number of patients with grade 3 or 4 toxic effects reported (using World Health Organization criteria) during treatment in the ICON2 ovarian cancer trial. Reprinted with permission from Elsevier Science (*The Lancet*, 1998, **352**, 1571–6)

Toxic effects	CAP (*n*=430)	Carboplatin (*n*=455)
Alopecia	300 (70%)	20 (4%)
Leucopenia	153 (36%)	44 (10%)
Nausea and vomiting	84 (20%)	39 (9%)
Thrombocytopenia	26 (6%)	73 (16%)
Anaemia	12 (3%)	5 (1%)

is different in the two treatments, before other issues are addressed. Issues are: how important is the side effect of alopecia to patients and what sort of differences between alopecia are important? Thus, if the relative toxicity of the treatments are likely to be critical in deciding between treatments, then this needs to be stated at the beginning of the trial, and hypotheses should be specified and power calculations should be performed for the most important toxicities. For the remaining toxicities, the information should be presented as in Table 9.10, perhaps allied to confidence intervals for the difference between percentages.

9.4.7 Time-to-event

Time-to-event data occur frequently in cancer clinical trials. Relevant outcome measures which are analysed using time-to-event methods include duration of survival, time to disease progression and time to local recurrence. In this section we cover some practical issues in the analysis of such data.

Relative and absolute measures of effect

The hazard ratio introduced in Section 9.3.4 is a relative measure of effect. Thus, when comparing two treatments, an experimental and control, a hazard ratio of 0.75 represents a 25 per cent reduction in the relative risk of an event on the experimental group compared to the control group at any given time. This is a useful scale on which to conduct and report analyses. In reporting results it is useful to report an absolute difference as well as this relative difference. It is not good practice, though, to read survival figures off the two Kaplan–Meier curves, as individual points on the curve are unreliable, even though the whole curve is a good summary of the overall experience of the two groups. One means of calculating an absolute difference at a particular timepoint is as follows:

$$\text{Absolute difference at time } t = \exp\{\text{hazard ratio} \times \log_e[\text{control survival at time } t]\}$$
$$- \text{ control survival at time } t. \tag{9.26}$$

This approach implicitly assumes that the hazards are proportional in the two groups, that is the relative risk of an event in the two groups is constant over time. Although this a slightly limiting assumption, it is generally preferable to reading off differences between the Kaplan–Meier curves at individual timepoints.

Example. In the BA06 bladder cancer trial [3] comparison of the duration of survival of the chemotherapy and no chemotherapy groups gave a hazard ratio of 0.85 with a 95 per cent confidence interval of 0.71–1.02. This estimate represents a 15 per cent reduction in the risk of death with chemotherapy. Reading from the Kaplan–Meier curves the 3-year survival in the no chemotherapy group is approximately 50 per cent (i.e. control survival is 0.5). Applying equation 9.25 gives an absolute difference of 5.5 per cent. Thus, we estimate that 3-year survival is improved to 55.5 per cent in the chemotherapy group. To obtain a 95 per cent confidence interval for this absolute difference, we can use equation 9.25 again, and this time use the upper and lower end of the confidence of the hazard ratio, i.e, $\exp\{0.71 \times \log_e[0.50]\} - 0.50 = 11.0$, and $\exp\{1.02 \times \log_e[0.50]\} - 0.50 = -0.7$. Thus the 95 per cent confidence interval for the absolute difference of 5.5 per cent is given by (-0.7 per cent to 11.0 per cent).

To translate relative differences to differences in median survival we can use the following equation:

$$\text{Median survival in experimental group} = \text{Median survival in control group/hazard ratio.} \tag{9.27}$$

This approach assumes that the two Kaplan–Meier curves both follow approximately exponential distributions, which is a more limiting assumption than proportional hazards for the absolute difference calculations, but again is preferred to reading values off the survival curves. To continue the BA06 bladder cancer trial, median survival in the no chemotherapy group is approximately thirty-six months, thus the estimated median survival in the experimental group is given by $36/0.85 = 42.4$ months, a difference of 6.4 months. Confidence intervals for this can be obtained by again inserting the confidence intervals of the hazard ratio into equation 9.25, giving an approximate confidence interval of the absolute difference in medians of approximately -0.7 months to 15 months.

It is important to note that the relative difference is always larger in magnitude terms than the absolute difference, thus it is important to report both. Further, the absolute difference varies as the underlying control group varies with a maximum absolute difference at 50 per cent reducing as we move away from 50 per cent in both directions. Thus, the same relative difference may have different interpretations depending on the underlying control group rate. This is discussed also in Section 11.5.7.

Assessing maturity and reliability of data

The Kaplan–Meier survival curves for the BA06 bladder cancer trial [3] are shown in Fig. 9.4. The report gives the median follow-up of patients still alive at four years. We can see from this figure that the curves, and therefore their comparison, are still reliable at five years (an important timepoint in this disease), since the total numbers at risk in the chemotherapy and no chemotherapy groups at five years are ninety-three and eighty, respectively. In the design, the plan was to reliably detect (approximately 90 per cent power, 5 per cent significance level) a difference at two years from 50 per cent survival in the no chemotherapy group to 60 per cent survival in the chemotherapy group, and to recruit 915 patients, and observing 460 deaths. The trial was actually reported when 485 deaths have been observed. Finally, 53 per cent (485/915) of patients have died. All these observations taken together show that this trial was reported as planned and is appropriately mature.

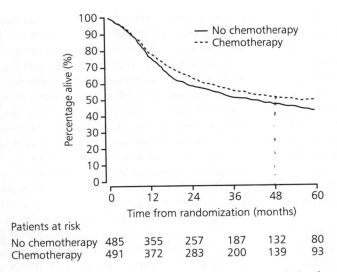

Fig. 9.4 Overall survival, BA06 bladder cancer trial. Reprinted with permission from Elsevier Science (*The Lancet*, 1999, **354**, 533–40).

Event-free survival, event-free interval and cancer-specific survival

It is common to compare, analyse and report the time to an event which is not death. When doing this it is not always clear what to do with patients who have died before the event. For ease of discussion and without loss of generality we shall consider the event of disease progression to make it easier to understand and discuss the issues.

It is possible to include patients who have died before documented progressive disease by defining an event as progression of disease or death, using the phrase progression-free survival time to describe this outcome measure. Alternatively, it is possible to define an event as progression of disease only, censoring those patients who have died before their disease has progressed, using the phrase progression-free interval to describe this outcome. Which of these is most appropriate depends on the situation. In cancers where only a relatively small proportion of deaths are due to causes other than the cancer (less than 20 per cent, say), then it is safest (and conservative) to focus on the outcome measure progression-free survival. The reason for this is that a proportion of patients who have apparently died before documented progressive disease have probably died from their disease, but their disease has progressed too quickly to allow a formal assessment to be made. Further, a small proportion of patients may have died from toxicity of the treatment, and censoring of these patients could bias the analysis in favour of the more toxic treatment. Therefore, the noise introduced in the analysis by inclusion of patients who have died without documented evidence of progressive disease is likely to be relatively small. For example, in trials of women with advanced ovarian cancer, progression-free survival is widely used as an outcome measure, because the large majority of women with this disease will die from their disease (or its treatment), and only a small proportion will die from other causes.

In contrast, in cancers where a large proportion of deaths are due to causes other than the cancer (more than 50 per cent, say) then there may be a stronger argument to focus on the outcome measure progression-free interval. The reason for this is that including deaths, a large proportion of which may be from causes other than the cancer under study, may plausibly dilute and hence obscure any difference between treatments and in some situations, through the play of chance, may enhance the difference. For example, in trials of men with early prostate cancer, progression-free interval is widely used as an outcome measure because many of the men with this disease will die from causes other than prostate cancer. As a safeguard against too much misclassification for this outcome measure, the information on cause of death is often examined so that patients who are reported as dying from this disease are included as 'event' even though they may previously have had no reported evidence of progressive disease. Although this may be helpful, it is widely known that in nearly all countries cause of death is poorly classified.

There are similar difficulties when we consider the choice between the outcome measures overall survival and cancer-specific survival. The reasons for using cancer-specific survival rather than overall survival are the same as those given above for using progression-free interval, in that if there are a reasonable proportion of deaths from non-cancer causes, then this may obscure (or sometimes enhance) any difference between treatments. The principal difficulty with this outcome measure is that it is based on a reliable classification of the cause of death, which often cannot be guaranteed. This is a particular difficulty if unexpected toxicities occur. This problem was observed in the a meta-analysis of randomized trials [12] which compared surgery plus radiotherapy against surgery alone for women with early breast cancer. In this meta-analysis there was clear evidence of an effect of radiotherapy in improving cancer-specific survival. However, in contrast there was no evidence of a difference in overall survival. This was because although the radiotherapy had an impact on the disease and thus prevented some deaths, it was also the cause of some deaths from long-term toxicity from radiotherapy on the cardiovascular system, some of which is irradiated when the breast is being irradiated.

It is important that the approach to analysis is pre-specified in an analysis protocol and the reasons for the choice of outcome measure should be made clear. If possible disease and cause-specific measures should generally be avoided as the primary outcome measure. If they are chosen as the primary outcome measure, then it should be made clear how issues of possible bias and subjectivity are going to be addressed. As a rule, analysis of overall survival should always be performed, whatever the primary outcome measure. In rare circumstances where there is little information at the start of the trial and it is not clear which approach should be adopted it is probably best to perform both analyses. If they broadly agree, then for trials aiming to show a difference between treatments the least extreme result should be emphasized, and for trials aiming to show 'equivalence' between treatments the most extreme result should be emphasized. If the results of these two analyses disagree, then the reasons for the disagreement should be reported and explored. In these situations neither result should probably be emphasized above the other.

9.4.8 Subgroup analysis

Nearly all randomized trials will recruit patients with a variety of characteristics, and therefore there is often interest in investigating whether we can identify subgroups of patients in whom the relative effects of treatment are different. For example, in a trial showing an experimental treatment is better than a control treatment, we may ask whether the experimental treatment is more effective in younger patients than older patients. There are many difficulties in undertaking such analyses and considerable care needs to be taken in performing and interpreting these analyses.

The first and main problem is that usually such analyses will (quite properly) be exploratory in nature and therefore there is a danger that the data will be analysed in a number of different ways in the hope of finding some significant result. The problems with doing this are similar to those for interim analysis below, in particular the chance of finding a significant result increases as the number of tests we perform increases. An example of the dangers of searching through multiple subgroups has been shown by Collins and colleagues [13], who showed that in a trial for patients with suspected acute myocardial infarction the benefit of treatment was restricted to patients born under Scorpio and four times as great as compared to the effect of treatment for patients born under all the other birth signs considered together. This is of course quite implausible. A further reason for being wary of subgroup analyses claiming positive results is because the trial is usually powered for detecting a difference in all patients. As a consequence when examining subgroups of patients there is usually very limited power to detect different sizes of effect in these subgroups.

Some guidance to the analysis of data in subgroups is given in Box 9.4.

Box 9.4   Guidance for the analysis of subgroups

- Treat all subgroup analyses with a degree of scepticism. In the protocol pre-specify a few important subgroups which are to be analysed, providing a rationale for why the effect of the experimental treatment is likely to be different in the different groups. Regard all other subgroup analyses as exploratory.

- Report all subgroup analyses (whether pre-specified or not), even if this is only in summary form (see examples below of how this might be done).

- Subgroup analyses *should not be* performed by comparing the experimental group against the control group and reporting a *p*-value separately for each subgroup, for example performing and emphasizing separate analyses for older and younger patients.

- Subgroup analyses *should be* performed by performing an analysis looking at the difference between the results in subgroups by performing a test for interaction (see below).

- Different results in different subgroups are probably *more plausible* when the overall result comparing experimental treatment against the control treatment is itself positive and statistically significant. This is because then we are looking for quantitative differences between subgroups, for example is the effect in younger patients larger than the effect in older patients?

- Different results in different subgroups are less plausible when there is no evidence of a difference between the experimental treatment against the control treatment. This is because then we are looking for qualitative differences between subgroups, for example, is the effect in younger patients in favour of the control treatment, while the effect in older patients in favour of the experimental treatment? Such qualitative differences are usually inherently biologically less plausible.

Box 9.4 *(continued)*

- If there is evidence of a different size of effect in different subgroups in the main outcome measure, such as survival, consider other internal evidence from the trial by examining secondary outcome measures, such as recurrence.

- If there is an indication of a different size of effect in different subgroups, then consider whether there is evidence external to the trial, for example from other similar trials, that support (or contradict) this result. A systematic review (see Chapter 11) may help in doing this.

Test for interaction

As mentioned above the appropriate test to perform when considering subgroups is a (single) test for interaction assessing the consistency of the overall effect across the groups, rather than a separate test for significance for each subgroup. Although the basic principles are the same, the exact details of the test vary with the type of data. The basic principles are that the estimate in each subgroup is compared with the overall estimate from the whole trial. The squared difference of this comparison is then weighted by the relative amount of information in the subgroup. The test statistic for the test of interaction is given by the sum across subgroups of these weighted squared differences. Under the null hypothesis that there is no interaction, i.e. that the effect is consistent across subgroups, this test statistic follows a chi-square distribution with one degree of freedom. Altman [1] gives more details for different types of data.

Example. The Sarcoma Meta-Analysis Collaboration [14] performed a systematic review and meta-analysis of fourteen randomized trials which compared surgery plus chemotherapy against chemotherapy alone for patients with soft-tissue sarcoma. As part of this meta-analysis nine factors were examined to assess whether the effect of chemotherapy was similar across the subgroups defined by these nine factors. The results of these analyses are presented in Fig. 9.5. The figure shows the nine factors considered ranging from age to use of radiotherapy. For each factor the results for each subgroup are displayed. To understand this plot consider the factor sex and its two obvious subgroups, female and male. The numbers alongside the subgroup give the number of deaths and the number of patients randomized to the chemotherapy and control groups. The horizontal line alongside each subgroup gives the estimate of the hazard ratio (centre of black square) and 95 per cent (inner ticks) and 99 per cent (outer ticks) confidence intervals around the estimate. The size of the square is proportional to the amount of information in that subgroup, so the larger the square the more events have happened in that subgroup. There are similar total numbers of deaths in the female and male subgroups, so the squares are similar in size. The vertical line running through the plot is the unity line, representing a hazard ratio of 1. From the plot it can be seen that the estimates of the hazard ratio for the female and male groups are approximately 1 and 0.7, respectively. Further, it can be seen that the 99 per cent confidence interval for the male group just touches the HR = 1 line, suggesting the *p*-value for the chemotherapy effect in this group is approximately 0.01, while quite clearly the result for the female group suggests no evidence for the effect of chemotherapy. Does this mean that chemotherapy

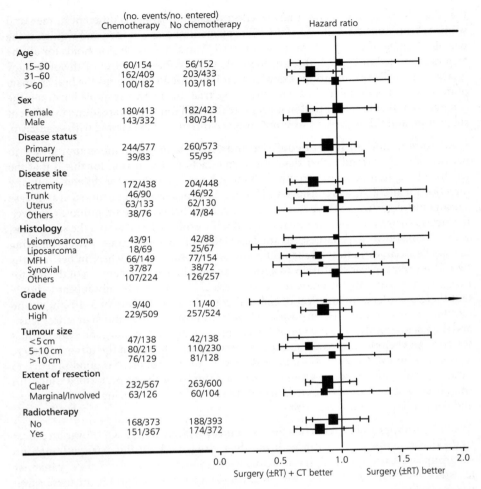

	(no. events/no. entered)		Hazard ratio
	Chemotherapy	No chemotherapy	
Age			
15–30	60/154	56/152	
31–60	162/409	203/433	
>60	100/182	103/181	
Sex			
Female	180/413	182/423	
Male	143/332	180/341	
Disease status			
Primary	244/577	260/573	
Recurrent	39/83	55/95	
Disease site			
Extremity	172/438	204/448	
Trunk	46/90	46/92	
Uterus	63/133	62/130	
Others	38/76	47/84	
Histology			
Leiomyosarcoma	43/91	42/88	
Liposarcoma	18/69	25/67	
MFH	66/149	77/154	
Synovial	37/87	38/72	
Others	107/224	126/257	
Grade			
Low	9/40	11/40	
High	229/509	257/524	
Tumour size			
<5 cm	47/138	42/138	
5–10 cm	80/215	110/230	
>10 cm	76/129	81/128	
Extent of resection			
Clear	232/567	263/600	
Marginal/Involved	63/126	60/104	
Radiotherapy			
No	168/373	188/393	
Yes	151/367	174/372	

0.0   0.5   1.0   1.5   2.0

Surgery (±RT) + CT better   Surgery (±RT) better

Fig. 9.5 Subgroup analyses in the soft tissue sarcoma meta-analysis. Reprinted with permission from Elsevier Science (*The Lancet*, 1997, **350**, 1647–54).

is effective in males and not in females? This would be an incorrect conclusion. The reason is that we are not posing the question correctly. The question that needs to be posed is, is there evidence that the effect of chemotherapy is different in the males and females? We can assess this visually by considering whether the confidence intervals for the effects in the two subgroups overlap markedly, and on inspection, they do. More formally we can test this, by performing a test for interaction, which simply compares the estimate in each subgroup with the overall estimate (appropriately weighted) and produces a chi-square statistic on one degree of freedom. If there is no interaction the results in the subgroups would differ only randomly from the overall result. For the factor sex, we obtain a chi-square statistic of 3.86 to give an associated *p*-value of 0.049. For such exploratory analyses, where we have performed a number of tests, this could be considered to be far from levels considered significant, and thus we would conclude that there is no good evidence that the effect of chemotherapy is different in men and women. Thus our best estimate of the effect of chemotherapy in men and women is the overall estimate of effect seen in the whole trial. The same conclusion holds for all the factors examined in Fig. 9.5, there is no good evidence that the effect of chemotherapy is larger or smaller in subgroups examined, and thus for all subgroups the best estimate of the effect is the overall estimate for the whole trial. In fact this example illustrates the general point that in cancer trials it is very rare that different effects are found in different subgroups, and this is perhaps why any observed differences are viewed with scepticism.

For some factors such as tumour size and age, it is probably more appropriate to perform a test for trend rather than test for interaction. The reason for this is that the test for interaction poses no structure on the subgroups, looking for differences in any direction for all subgroups considered. This may be appropriate for factors such as disease site and histology, where there is no natural structure between the subgroups. However, for factors such as tumour size we may reasonably expect a trend across the subgroups, with <5 cm showing the largest (or smallest) effect of chemotherapy, >10 cm showing the smallest (largest) effect of chemotherapy, with 5–10 cm somewhere in between the two. This ordering leads naturally to a test for trend which is an extension of the test for interaction. Examining the figure for tumour size this may superficially appear to imply that there is evidence of an effect of chemotherapy in the subgroup of 5–10 cm, but no effect in the <5 cm and >10 cm groups. This clearly does not make much practical sense, and the test for trend gives a p-value of 0.96, suggesting that we have no good evidence that the effect of chemotherapy varies (linearly) according to the size of the tumour. If there is a process of categorizing continuous data to form subgroups, it is good practice to generally have more than two groups so that a test for trend can be performed, since this will generally give more power to detect differences than categorizing into two groups and performing a test for interaction.

Example. An approach of reporting these succinctly is given in the ICON2 ovarian cancer trial [4] comparing carboplatin with the three drugs CAP. In this trial, although no subgroups were pre-specified, seven factors were investigated in an exploratory manner to assess whether the observed effect was consistent within subgroups of these seven factors (Table 9.11).

It should be noted that the test for interaction (and to lesser extent trend) is generally not a very powerful test, not least because we usually do not anticipate large differences between subgroups. Nevertheless, chance positive results can still occur, especially as many subgroups are often examined. In these circumstances, scepticism is important and the reader should ensure they follow the guidelines in Box 9.4, before the urge to report a 'new and exciting' result takes hold.

9.4.9 Quality of life (including longitudinal) data

It is clearly important that patients and clinicians are able to use and interpret the results of the analysis of quality of life (QL) data, in addition to more traditional outcome measures, to make informed decisions. However, there are considerable problems with the analysis and presentation of QL data including (i) the data are multi-dimensional (data on many symptoms and functions are collected) (ii) there are often many missing data due to patient attrition and non-compliance, and (iii) the data are longitudinal

Table 9.11 Results of chi-square tests to assess whether CAP or carboplatin was more or less effective in different subgroups of seven factors on the endpoint of overall survival (chi-square on one degree of freedom, except for histology which is a chi-square on five degrees freedom; tests for interaction were performed on the factors coordination centre and histology, while tests for trend were performed on the remaining five factors). Reprinted with permission from Elsevier Science (*The Lancet*, 1999, **352**, 1571–6).

Factor (subgroups)	Chi-square statistic	*p*-value
Coordination centre (Italy, UK)	0.98	0.32
Age in years (<55, 55–65, >65)	2.16	0.14
FIGO stage (I, II, III, IV)	0.36	0.55
Residual bulk (none, <2 cm, >2 cm)	0.76	0.39
Differentiation (poor, intermediate, good)	0.03	0.87
Histology (serous, mucinous, endometrioid, clear cell, undifferentiated, other)	4.73	0.45
Number of patients entered by each hospital (<5, 5–10, >10)	0.80	0.52

Box 9.5 Key elements of plan to analyse quality of life data from a trial

- Descriptive tables including a distribution of baseline and follow-up data and a report on compliance
- Analysis of the stated hypotheses as outlined in the protocol
- Expanded and sensitivity analyses to explore the key results
- Exploratory analyses to generate new hypotheses

(data are collected over several timepoints). All of these aspects are difficult enough to deal with individually, but combined they represent formidable problems.

As for more traditional outcome measures it is useful to have a general plan for the analysis which should include the components set out in Box 9.5.

Features of QL data

Multi-dimensionality. All widely used questionnaires consist of multiple items, but for simplicity and robustness rather than analyse individual items, the common approach is to combine items into subscales. Scoring manuals to form these subscales are available for all major questionnaires, see, for example, Refs [15,16]. There is a psychometric reason for asking more than one question about one aspect of QL as discussed in Chapter 6, but there is also a statistical reason, in that error terms for individual questions tend to be large and summation across questions reduces the variability and therefore improves reliability.

Compliance and missing data   It is important to present information on patient compliance and to assess whether the compliance is approximately of the same level and follows a similar pattern in each treatment group. It is also important to show how representative the population from whom QL data have been collected is of the whole trial population. Hopwood and colleagues [17] have defined compliance as the number of forms completed as a proportion of those expected, where the anticipated number of forms is the total number that should have been completed by each patient according to the protocol schedule but taking account of the date of death.

Not only is it important to indicate what forms have been received, but whether they were completed at the scheduled times. Let us assume, for example, that the scheduled QL assessment day is day forty-two. If the corresponding QL form is not completed until say, day seventy-two, the responses recorded may not reflect the patient's QL at the timepoint of interest. However, it is necessary to recognize the variation in individual patients' treatment and follow-up, and so a reasonable time frame (or window) should be allowed around each scheduled protocol assessment timepoint, as introduced in Chapter 6. Clearly such time windows may be different for different timepoints. For example for the pre-treatment quality of life form the window may be narrow, such as seven days, and asymmetrical, i.e. before the start of treatment. Alternatively, for a three-monthly form a symmetrical window of one month may be used, with possibly wider windows for later timepoints which are more widely spaced.

One of the major problems with quality of life data is missing data. There are two aspects of missing data: missing forms and missing items. In cancer trials, some missing forms are unavoidable. When such forms are termed to be 'missing completely at random' (MCAR), then the missing data do not depend on any characteristics of the patient or the condition of the patient, and the missing data can be relatively simply imputed. If the forms are 'missing at random' (MAR), that is not related to the condition of the patient but related to other observed factors e.g. performance status, it is possible to model what would have happened if those data had been collected, based on what is known about the patient and what is known about other patients. However, in the assessment of QL the proportion of missing forms increases as patients' health deteriorates and particularly as they approach death. Thus the majority of forms are 'not missing at random' (NMAR), which means the reasons for the missing data are related to the unobserved factors, for example the condition of the patient. The standard methods for imputing missing data, extrapolating in some way from within (or outwith) the data set, cannot be used. It would be illogical to impute data for patients who are ill and unable to complete forms from patients who are fit and well and have completed forms. There are some methods of multivariate analysis that allow missing values to be ignored, and some statistical methods of imputing NMAR data, but in QL analyses all such methods must be used with extreme caution.

As opposed to missing forms, very few papers report the extent of missing items on forms or how these were handled in the analysis. Trials groups such as the Medical Research Council and the European Organization for the Research and Treatment of Cancer regularly report between 0.5 per cent and 1 per cent missing items, which seems trivial. However, as most questionnaires include 30–40 items, this can mean that at each assessment between 15 and 40 per cent of forms have missing items, and if patients are expected to complete 4–6 questionnaires, there is the potential for there to be no patients at all with complete data at all timepoints.

Most standard questionnaire manuals suggest methods of dealing with missing items so that missing individual items do not necessarily mean the loss of data. For instance, if the patient has answered three of four items relating to, say, anxiety, in a positive way, it is reasonable to presume they would have answered the 4th in the same manner. The recommendation is to estimate summary scale scores using the mean of the other observed scale items. However, caution should be exercised in doing even this. Most of the questionnaire manuals [15,16] include an algorithm for allowing imputation. They usually state that as long as data are available for at least 50 per cent of the items the scale can be formed and standardized to 0–100 accordingly. Nevertheless, this has dangers, and Fayers *et al.* [18] summarized a number of checks that should be made (Box 9.6) before applying such imputation (Box 9.7).

Box 9.6   Checks that should be performed before imputation of missing values (adapted from Ref. [18])

- Are patients with missing items different from other patients?
- Do items comprising the scale all have similar mean values?
- Is the scale ordered or hierarchical?
- Do items comprising the scale have high correlations with each other?
- Do items comprising the scale have similar standard deviations?
- Is the item correlated with external factors or baseline variables?

Box 9.7   Options for imputation of missing values (adapted from Ref. [18])

- If any one item is missing, call the scale missing, although this results in a much-reduced sample.
- Estimate scale score from the mean of those items that are available. This assumes missing items would have had a score equal to the average of the non-missing items. This is usually restricted to cases where the respondent has completed at least half of the items in the scale. One disadvantage is that imputing may result in numbers between the expected discrete numbers. This might affect summarizing data using presentations such as histograms, although an alternative is to estimate the score to the nearest 'real' score.
- Use general model-based imputation methods. The object here is to replace missing data by estimated values which preserve the relationship between items and which reflect as far as possible the most likely true value.

It is unlikely that patients who complete all QL forms will be truly representative of the whole group of patients, for example they will have to be survivors. This need not effect the comparison between treatments, as in many trials the reasons for non-completion of QL forms will be the same across treatment arms. Any differences between arms in compliance should be investigated and, if possible, explained.

If properly carried out, imputation can reduce the bias that results from ignoring non-response, can restore balance to the data and permit simpler analysis. Hence imputation is an attractive procedure, provided one can be sure that the conditions are appropriate and that unintended bias is not being introduced. Although there are increasingly complex methods of imputation, in QL analysis the aim should always be to reduce the need for imputation and, when it is necessary, to explain exactly what has been done and why. It is important to remember that any inferences in the presence of incomplete data are not as convincing as inferences based on a complete data set. It should be emphasized that if there is a bias in the amount of missing data in the arms being compared, imputation of data can magnify this bias.

Approaches to analysis

Widely accepted standard methods of analysing QL data are not available, therefore only general guidelines can be given (see Box 9.8).

Box 9.8 General guidelines for the analysis and reporting of QL data

- A small number of hypotheses should be pre-specified to allow definitive analysis to be performed on them (see Chapter 6). All other analyses should be regarded as exploratory and hypothesis generating.

- The statistical methods of analysis must be described in sufficient detail so that other researchers could repeat the analysis.

- In all analyses all patients must be accounted for.

- It is often useful to analyse the data in more than one way to confirm any differences observed are not model dependent.

- It is important to specify how patients who died before reaching the endpoint were dealt with in the analysis.

- Graphical presentations can be helpful. In such presentations, where possible, it is important to specify the number of patients at risk (or contributing to each section of the plot) by treatment group beneath the time axis in the plot, similar to that for a Kaplan–Meier plot introduced in Section 9.3.4.

- Non-parametric tests, such as the Wilcoxon or the Mann–Whitney test may be more appropriate for QL data as the data are often skewed with ceiling or floor effects (for example, patients with no symptoms cannot get better, while patients with the worst category for a symptom cannot get worse).

Box 9.9　Alternative approaches to analysis of QL data

- Graphical summaries
- Scores at a common specific assessment point (landmark analysis)
- Summary measures such as mean or worst score
- Time to, or duration of, an event
- Complex models

A number of alternative methods for analysing the difference between treatment are available, and the general approaches are summarized in Box 9.9. We then go on to discuss each of these analyses in more detail.

In the absence of a clear rationale to use one analytical approach ahead of another, it is useful to conduct a number of types of analyses to ensure that any conclusions are not just a function of the (arbitrary) analytical approach adopted. In a detailed analysis of longitudinal data from a randomized clinical trial in lung cancer Qian and colleagues [19] employ a variety of summary scores and a complex model-based approach to assess the sensitivity of any conclusions to the analytical approach. They show, that for this dataset at least, the different approaches generally produce the same broad conclusions. They also emphasize that by examining the reasons for inconsistent results using different approaches allowed them to reject some conclusions, which they otherwise might have inappropriately emphasized.

Whichever approach is used a major problem that is always present is how to include individuals with missing data and in particular how we should allow for those individuals who have died during the course of collecting QL data. Approaches to missing data were discussed above. Hollen *et al.* [20] strongly encourage adjusting for death (scoring death as the worst possible score) and give an example where without such adjustment, QL erroneously appears to improve with time. However, while it is logical to put patients who have died in the worst category if you are assessing, say, response, it may not be logical for other symptoms such as cough.

Graphical summaries

Summary statistics, however calculated, are unlikely to encapsulate all the subtleties of QL data. Therefore it is important to first examine the data graphically before performing detailed analysis. This will also help readers interpret the data. For example, plotting the scores against the time from randomization will give a better feel for the range of data and the variability of completion over time.

Figure 9.6 shows a scatter plot of data of HADS depression scores [21], calculated as the sum of seven individual item responses for each patient providing data during the first year from an MRC Lung Cancer Working Party trial, plotted against the actual assessment date. The scheduled assessment times are indicated for the first year as vertical hatched lines. The horizontal lines represent agreed definitions of 'clinically normal' with a score of ≤ 7, those with 'clinical depression' with a score of ≥ 11 who would probably need

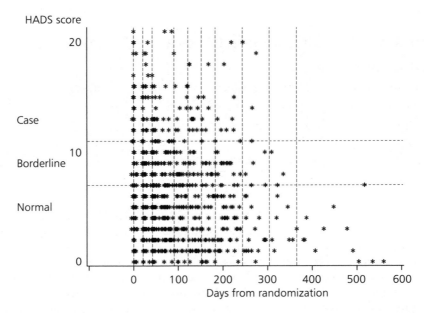

Fig. 9.6 Scatter plot of HADS depression score against actual assessment by the patient for the ten scheduled assessments in the first year (Reprinted with permission from John Wiley & Sons Ltd from reference [21]).

medical assistance whereas the 'borderline' patients with HADS of 8, 9 or 10 may require further assessment. This plot illustrates the increasing amount of missing data over time (after the baseline assessment) and the departure of assessments from the planned times.

It can also be useful to plot individual patient profiles as this will indicate the patterns of change and the number of patients with incomplete data.

Figure 9.7 shows the data for the symptom 'lack of appetite' for twelve patients in the CHART lung cancer trial [22], six from the conventional radiotherapy group and six from the CHART group. These data shows the variability both within and across patients in the profile of 'lack of appetite' over time and also show that missing data are common. This is useful to remember, because summary data averaged over patients is unlikely to show such variability. The figures in the right-hand corner of the boxes are explained below.

It is possible to plot the percentage of patients falling into a particular category (or categories) – i.e. a dichotomy of the scale, to show the proportion of patients experiencing a particular symptom over time. Alternatively we could use another statistic, such as the mean score. However, such plots, which are often found in the literature, can be very misleading as the number of patients completing forms at each timepoint will differ and usually decrease over time, and it is important to indicate the number of patients returning forms at each time on the plot. The obvious way around this is to restrict the dataset to only those patients who have returned complete data up to a certain timepoint. However, the sample size may become greatly reduced, and as these data will have come from patients who survive and complete forms, and thus may have better physical and psychological status, the result may not be generalizable to the whole trial population.

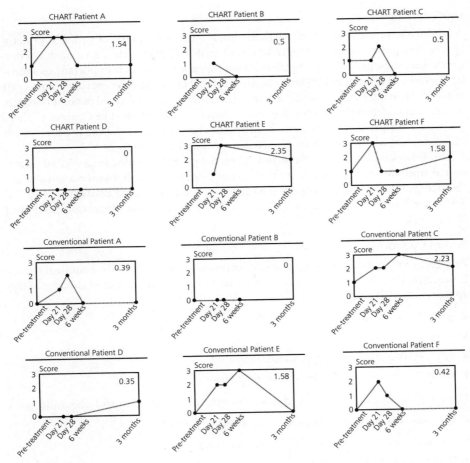

Fig. 9.7 *Lack of appetite* profiles for a sample of six patients from each treatment group (for the CHART trial) – A point represents an observed score and the lines between points are interpolations of the score between times.

Bias will occur if more patients drop out of one arm. Nevertheless, such plots (even if just produced for internal consideration) can provide valuable insight into the data.

Graphical summaries do not provide statistical tests of hypotheses, nor do they provide summary estimates. Nevertheless, because exploratory and descriptive analyses are often less concerned with significance testing, graphical methods may be especially suitable for presenting QL results. These have a number of advantages over purely numerical techniques. In particular, judicious use of graphics can succinctly summarize complex data that would otherwise require extensive tabulations and can clarify and display the complex interrelationships of QL data. At the same time graphics can be used to emphasise the high degree of variability in QL data. This contrasts with numerical methods, which may often lead to results being presented in a format which leads readers to assume there is greater precision than the measurements warrant.

Landmark analyses

A landmark, or cross-sectional, analysis simply gives a snapshot of patients' QL at a specific timepoint. One advantage of landmark analyses is that all the data available at that timepoint can be used. Choosing the most appropriate timepoint is important, as shown by Curran and colleagues [23] who compared global QL at six different timepoints in an analysis of two regimens for locally advanced breast cancer, and showed major differences in treatments depending on the timepoint. Indeed, as mentioned in Chapter 6, there is always a danger that the landmark timepoint chosen may not be the point at which differences are occurring or may give an unrepresentative picture.

Simple landmark analyses give no indication of how patients have improved or deteriorated since the start of the trial or the start of treatment. An alternative is to calculate the change in score i.e. the score at the timepoint minus the score at baseline. The disadvantage is that it limits the analysis to only those patients with data available at both timepoints.

Summary scores

An effective way of dealing with multiple scores over time is to derive a summary score for each patient, such as the mean, median, best or worst score. The advantages of this approach are that

+ analyses are focused,
+ statistics are valid,
+ missing data can be accommodated,
+ the methods are computationally straightforward.

There are a number of options to choose. For example, for each patient one could use:

+ the worst score (the usual method of assessing toxicity),
+ the best score (for example, the assessment of response),
+ the mean or median score,
+ the area under the curve (AUC),
+ the last available score.

It should be emphasized that the conclusions may depend on the summary score chosen, thus some thought should be given to its choice. One might choose the worst score in a trial evaluating a new and potentially less toxic regimen, and the best score in a trial of palliative treatments where the aim is to reduce baseline symptoms. The mean or median might highlight the frequency of episodes or the duration of symptoms. However, the mean or median can often mask a proportion of patients with severe symptoms, and worst score takes no account of duration. The choice of summary measure may be determined by the pattern of severity over time. Thus a relevant summary measure for an increasing or decreasing line might be the regression coefficient, final value, or time to reach a particular value, while for a peaked curve, the mean, maximum or time to maximum would be more appropriate [24]. Constructing individual patient plots may clarify the summary measure to use and/or whether the data need to be transformed to give an approximate normal distribution (for example the log or cube root may be taken) before the summary score is calculated. The choice of summary measure will also depend on the patient population (e.g. lung or testicular cancer), the treatment (adjuvant or palliative) and the trial design (equivalence or difference). Hollen *et al.* [20] suggest using slope analysis as a summary. Thus, if there are three data points the slopes between points 1 and 2, 1 and 3, and 2 and 3, are calculated and the median taken.

The choice of summary measure requires a good understanding of the patterns of change likely to be observed. This of course emphasizes the point made in Chapter 6 about forming a clear hypothesis at the start of the trial and if necessary conducting a pilot study. For instance, two treatments might both cause nausea and vomiting, but the duration of this side effect may be much longer in one than in the other. Summarizing by comparing the most severe effect experienced by the two groups may show no difference, comparing the duration of side effect may detect a clear difference.

The summary score AUC is a popular summary measure and an example of it is shown for each patient in the right-hand corner of each box in Fig. 9.7. It can be seen that to calculate this value we have to allow for missing intermediate response by connecting two datapoints with a straight line (e.g. CHART patient A). For some symptoms the AUC can be used to take account of both the length and quality of survival by plotting the patient's score over time and calculating the AUC [25]. This is an interesting method of summarizing data, and the advantage of using AUC with variables such as the performance status is that, if required, death can be scored as the worst category (5).

All summary measures suffer from the problems: (a) they assume that the precision of the summary measure is the same across patients, which is obviously not strictly true, and (b) there is no way of explicitly assessing the correlation between repeated measures. The summary measures 'worst score minus pre-treatment score' and AUC may also be influenced by the defined numerical value for each category of a symptom. A further problem specific to the AUC is that it can be influenced by long time periods between assessments.

Time to, or duration of, an event

Time-to-event analyses are frequently used in cancer trials, usually of course time to death, but this can equally be used to assess the time to worst, or best, QL. This is probably a valid comparison when the two therapies have similar survival, but if there are differences, censoring at death can give a biased result. This is because, with the Kaplan–Meier analyses, censored patients are assumed to follow the same pattern of response or side-effects as those with full information. This is perfectly reasonable if a patient is censored because they have not been in the trial very long, or have been lost to follow-up, but is often not so logical if they are censored because of death.

More complex analyses

Most of the more complex analyses involve fitting a mathematical model to the data. The two most common approaches are a multivariate analysis of variance (MANOVA) or mixed effect (multilevel) models. Model-based analyses are theoretically more efficient than all the analyses presented above, because they explicitly allow for correlation of repeated measures by including a covariance structure. Adjustment for other possible variables can be made, and time or time-dependent variables can also be included in the model so that time-changing patterns can be considered. However, model-based analyses make a number of assumptions and pose a large number of restrictions. For instance, MANOVA models only use complete cases in the analyses (and thus some form of imputation is required), while mixed models assumed data are missing at random, which is not always an easy assumption to justify. The reader is referred to more specialist texts for a detailed presentation of these models [26].

Clinically meaningful changes in QL scores

Although most methods of analysis can provide us with a *p*-value and 95 per cent confidence intervals to indicate the statistical significance of a comparison between two treatments, this inevitably needs to be translated into clinical significance to be useful. For example, given a large enough sample of patients even a 1 per cent difference will be statistically significant, but such a difference would rarely influence practice.

Given that most of the standard questionnaires require individual items to be summed into subscales and their score converted to a 0–100 scale, this poses problems in interpretation, as this is a scale without clinical meaning. For instance what does a score of thirty on emotional functioning mean, and would a patient notice the difference between thirty on one treatment and thirty-five on another treatment? Osoba *et al.* [27] asked patients to complete not only the EORTC QLQ-C30 on repeated occasions but also to rate their perception of change since the previous assessment. Associating the replies, they found that when the functional scale scores changed by 5–10 points patients described their change as a little better (or worse). A change of 10–20 points was associated with a moderate change, and 20+ points with very much better (or worse). How widely such general definitions can be applied is debatable, as King [28] collating data from fourteen studies, concluded that definitions of large changes differed for different scales. As a corollary, it should be noted that such definitions of change can have major impact on the sample size calculations, as relatively small numbers of patients are required if large differences are expected.

Integration of survival and QL

The concept of combining QL and survival into a single statistic is very appealing, as it overcomes the subjective balancing of quality and quantity of life. An argument against simple survival analysis is that there are only two 'states,' alive and dead [29]. Amongst those alive a patient who is bedridden with severe symptoms is considered equivalent to one who is active and asymptomatic. Quality Adjusted Life Years (QALYs) are calculated on the basis that a value between zero and one can be assigned to various health states, and that the time spent in each state can be multiplied by this value to express survival in terms of QALYs.

The QALYs require firstly the definition of a number of health states, and secondly weights to be assigned to each. How to achieve this is not obvious, although some have attempted to do this [30]. Clinicians and trialists have in the main not embraced QALYs. There is a feeling perhaps that this is oversimplification, and there is still a desire to consider the various domains and items of QL separately and make individual treatment decisions, although this puts a particular onus on clarity of presentation of the results.

An alternative method of combining QL and survival is TWIST (time without symptoms or toxicity) which is a summation of survival time during which patients had no symptoms or toxicity [31,32]. It is calculated by subtracting from the overall survival time, periods of time when symptoms, or other clinical events, were present. This requires defining what events (or what severity of events) are relevant and what the time penalty for each should be. It is important that all patients are beyond the period of toxicity before calculations are performed, as different patterns of toxicity (i.e. early or late) may be different in the different groups. A variant of TWIST is Q-TWIST (quality adjusted time without symptoms or toxicity) [33]. Here again health states that are clinically relevant to the disease and/or treatment are chosen (such as toxicity, asymptomatic, relapse), and scores between zero and one are assigned to each. The particular score assigned is called a utility, in effect the weight of importance placed on each health state, and these can be generated from patients, clinicians or previous work.

Summary

Standard statistical methods exist for the analysis of longitudinal data of which QL data are of one type. However, there are further specific problems outlined here, including missing data, multiple symptoms and clinical relevance that are important in QL data. This makes simple application of these standard methods hazardous. It is clear that the analysis of QL data is an evolving field but one where simplicity and clarity of presentation should be the aim.

9.5   Interim analyses

Nearly all randomized clinical trials in cancer will accrue patients over a period of many months and often years. During this period of accrual, events on the planned outcome measures will also be observed. During the period of accrual there is both an ethical and practical obligation to monitor the accumulating data from the trial to ensure that there is no large difference in the primary outcome measure between the arms. The ethical obligation is the need to minimize the number of patients receiving a clearly inferior treatment, while the practical obligation is to conclude the trial as soon as possible. Thus monitoring of the primary outcome measures is done in most trials and specific statistical analysis procedures have been developed to aid in such monitoring.

Example. In a randomized trial comparing CHART radiotherapy with conventional radiotherapy for patients with non-small cell lung cancer, patients were accrued from 1991 to 1995. During this time, information on toxicity, relapses and deaths was becoming available [34]. In particular, the number of patients entered and number of deaths at approximately annual intervals was as shown in Table 9.12. The data were analysed approximately annually in order to assess whether it was appropriate to continue the trial.

The fundamental problem with regularly and continually analysing the emerging data from a trial is that we are performing more than one statistical test. For example, if we perform two statistical tests on two independent outcome measures, that in truth are no different in the groups being compared, the probability that one of these tests is incorrectly significant at the 0.05 level is:

$$p = 1 - (1 - 0.05)^2 = 0.0975.$$

Thus the probability that one of these two tests is positive is 9.75 per cent, rather than 5 per cent if we were performing just one test. This problem increases as we increase the number of tests we do as seen in Table 9.13.

It can be seen from the table that the probability of incorrectly claiming significance, when in truth there is no difference, increases quickly as the number of tests increase.

Table 9.12 Data from the CHART lung-cancer trial showing the accumulation of deaths over the period of accrual of patients to the trial [34]

Year	Number of patients	Number of deaths
1991	119	12
1992	256	78
1993	380	192
1994	460	275
1995	563	379

Table 9.13 Relationship between the number of independent tests performed and the probability of incorrectly claiming at least one significant result at the 0.05 level

Number of independent tests performed	Probability of one incorrect significant result
1	0.05
2	0.0975
3	0.143
5	0.226
10	0.401
100	0.994

This situation is analogous to the one of performing a number of interim analyses, for example in the CHART lung cancer trial a total four analyses were done over the years 1992–1995 on the primary outcome measure of length of survival. The situation is slightly more complicated for monitoring the accumulating results of a randomized trial as the tests being formed are correlated, because, for example, the data used in the second analysis include the data used in the first analysis and similarly the data used in the third analysis include the data used in the first and second analyses. As they assume independence this means that the probabilities shown in Table 9.13 are conservative estimates of the probability of incorrectly claiming significance at the 5 per cent level, given in truth there is no difference.

Numerous different solutions have been proposed for this problem [35–38]. However, although many of these approaches are technically complicated, the general approach can be summarized quite easily in the following way. Assume that when the trial has been designed, the type I error (significance level) is set at 5 per cent (see Chapter 4). If we plan to do just one analysis and actually perform just one analysis, then the p-value from this analysis is tested in the usual way against 0.05. Thus, if the observed p-value is less than 0.05, then we can claim a conventionally significant result. If the plan is to perform two analyses one during the course of the trial and the other at the planned end of the trial, then each of the p-values from these analyses need to be tested against significance (α) levels less than 0.05 to ensure the overall significance level over the two analyses is 0.05. One way of doing this is to aportion out the 0.05 significance (α) level, between the two analyses, perhaps with 0.001 at the first analysis and 0.049 at the second. This approach has the benefit that for the second, final and primary analysis, the α level used of 0.049 and is very close to 0.05, and we have also catered for an interim analysis. This approach also has the benefit that at the first (and interim) analysis the observed p-value has to be lower than 0.001 to claim a significant result and consider stopping the trial. It should be noted that if the trials were stopped in such a situation, because of the analysis plan and even though the observed p-value is less than 0.001, we should report only a conventionally significant result, i.e. that we have a result significant at the 0.05 level. It is easy to see that this approach can be extended to any number of interim analyses with the α level being spread over all the analyses – this is called the α-spending approach [38]. It should be emphasized that the more the α is used at the interim analyses, the less is available for use at the final analysis.

Examples of approaches to interim analyses

During the course of a trial suppose the plan is to perform four analyses, three interim analyses and one final analysis. Suppose also that these analyses will be performed at approximately equal intervals, then three ways of spending this 0.05 level over the four analyses are presented in Table 9.14.

In Table 9.14, it can be seen that the more of the α that is spent in analyses one, two and three the less remains for the final (and primary) analysis. It is for this reason the most widely used approaches are O'Brien and Fleming and the Peto-Haybittle procedures, as they retain the large portion of α for the final analysis. Despite these proposed solutions for spending the α it should be stressed that there are many difficulties and assumptions associated in monitoring the accumulating results of a trial and, in particular, in stopping a trial as a consequence of the results at an interim analysis. Some of these issues are discussed below.

Estimating the size of the treatment effect

As emphasized at the beginning of this chapter, an important statistic that should always be calculated when a clinical trial is analysed is the estimate of the difference between

Table 9.14 Three approaches to spending a 0.05 significance level over the four analyses to be performed in a trial, made up of three interim analyses and one final analysis

Analysis number	Pocock	O'Brien and Fleming	Peto-Haybittle
1	0.018	0.001	0.001
2	0.018	0.004	0.001
3	0.018	0.019	0.001
4	0.018	0.043	0.0049

the treatments being compared. Although this is a relatively simple idea and is straightforward at the planned end of the trial, the calculation of an estimate becomes very complicated during interim analyses. We discuss below the reason.

Table 9.15 shows the CHART randomized clinical trial discussed above, and the results of the trial at each annual analysis. The rows show how the estimate has changed over the life of the trial, including the time at which reports were finally published. It can be seen that the estimate reached a peak at 20 per cent in 1992 more than twice its final value of 9 per cent reported in 1997. This trial was not monitored using any of the methods presented in Table 9.13, but using Bayesian methods and as a consequence was not stopped before its planned end.

Table 9.16 shows when the trial would have been stopped using the various approaches in Table 9.14. It can be seen that depending on the α-spending approach used, this trial may have been stopped in either 1992 or 1993 and reporting an estimated 2-year survival improvement of 20 per cent or 15 per cent, respectively. Both these estimates are much larger than the final 9 per cent that was reported. This shows that a trial which is stopped early for a positive result will typically have stopped on a 'random high' with the estimate of the difference between treatments being 'overestimated.' Proposals to adjust the estimate to allow for this overestimation have been made [39], but none provide a completely satisfactory solution and thus most trials which have stopped early present the simple unadjusted estimate. If this had been done with the CHART trial in 1992, then it would have reported an estimate of treatment effect more than two times larger than the final reported (and more reliable) estimate. Readers should bear this in mind reviewing the results of such trials. The attendant difficulties involved in assessing the accumulating

Table 9.15 Results of the CHART lung cancer trial at approximately annual intervals during the accrual of patients to the trial from 1992 to 1995, and at the time of reporting of the results of the trial in 1997. Reprinted with permission from Elsevier Science (*The Lancet*, 2001, **358**, 375–81)

Year	Hazard ratio	Estimated 2-year survival improvement (%)	p-value
1992	0.55	20	0.007
1993	0.63	15	0.001
1994	0.70	12	0.004
1995	0.75	9	0.006
1997	0.76	9	0.004

Table 9.16 Estimates of when the CHART lung cancer trial would have stopped using three different approaches to monitoring together with the estimated improvement in 2-year survival

α-spending function	Date trial would have been stopped	Estimated 2-year survival improvement (%)
Pocock	1992	20
O'Brien and Fleming	1993	15
Peto-Haybittle	1993	15

efficacy and safety results of a trial, and reaching incorrect premature conclusions has led to the formation of independent data monitoring committees. This committee, which is made up of individuals completely independent of the trial, will typically review the results of such trials in a confidential manner, and recommend continuation and early termination as appropriate. The structure and format of these committees are discussed further in Section 8.10.

Summary of disadvantages of stopping trials early

The advantages of stopping a trial early are reasonably obvious and have been discussed above. The disadvantages of stopping a trial early are set out in Box 9.10.

With all such considerations, it should be emphasized that the decision to stop a trial at an interim analysis before its pre-planned time should not be guided only by statistical considerations, but also a variety of practical and clinical considerations. For this reason, any statistical 'rules' for early termination are usually termed guidelines.

Example. Dillman and colleagues performed a trial of chemotherapy and radiotherapy against radiotherapy alone in patients with non-small cell lung cancer [40]. The authors do not give a hazard ratio, but reading from the Kaplan–Meier survival curves report that two and three year survival was 'doubled' by the use of chemotherapy. In a letter criticizing the stopping of this trial early Souhami and colleagues [41] make the following points: the reported estimate is likely to be an overestimate; no confidence intervals are presented and thus the reader is left with no idea of the likely size of the difference; finally, only 155 of the 180 patients have been analysed. Souhami and colleagues conclude: 'In

Box 9.10   Disadvantages of stopping a trial, as a consequence of an interim analysis, before the planned final analysis

- The risk of a false positive is increased. This problem and possible solutions have been discussed above.
- The trial is likely to have an overestimate of the difference between the treatments being compared. Although a number of solutions have been proposed for this problem, none provide a completely coherent and satisfactory solution.
- The trial will be relatively small and the estimated difference will generally be large. In most diseases, large differences between new and old treatments are relatively rare and therefore any such claimed difference will lack credibility, and often be insufficient to influence practice.
- The trial will tend to be relatively small and thus the confidence intervals around the estimated difference are likely to be very wide, giving considerable uncertainty as to its true value.
- For a time-to-event outcome measure the results at interim analyses will usually represent results in the early part of the Kaplan–Meier curve, longer term results may be quite different.

Table 9.17 Results of the EORTC randomized trial looking at the role of hormone therapy and chemotherapy in addition to surgery in the treatment of women with breast cancer when the trial was stopped (May 1985) and when the trial was published (March 1988). Reprinted with permission from John Wiley & Sons Ltd from reference [42]

Date	Patients	Deaths	Results						
			Hormone therapy			Chemotherapy			
			p-value	HR	95%CI	*p*-value	HR	95% CI	
May 1985	399	86	0.16	0.75	0.49–1.13	0.004	0.53	0.35–0.82	
March 1988	410	202	0.06	0.77	0.58–1.02	0.23	0.84	0.64–1.12	

our view, no firm conclusions can be drawn from such a small study presented in this way'. To support this view, further trials of adding chemotherapy to radiotherapy were initiated after this report.

Example. The European Organization for the Research and Treatment for Cancer (EORTC) conducted a factorial randomized trial looking at the role of hormone therapy and chemotherapy in the treatment of women with locally advanced breast cancer [42]. The data monitoring committee was not independent. Instead, the accumulating data from the trial were inspected by the trial statistician on a 6-monthly basis, and if they were 'statistically significant' they were discussed with the study coordinator and possibly with the main clinicians participating in the trial. The trial started in December 1979 and was closed soon after May 1985, because of 'slow accrual.' The slow accrual was probably a consequence of the results at the time being shown to the participating clinicians. The results were published in March 1988, as shown in Table 9.17.

It can be seen in Table 9.17 that the results when published appear to be quite different from those when the trial was effectively closed in May 1985. In May 1985, the effect of chemotherapy was encouraging with a large observed effect and an extreme *p*-value. In contrast at that time the results for hormone therapy looked less encouraging. When the trial was published the results for hormone therapy were actually more encouraging than those for chemotherapy – a complete reversal of the results seen at the interim analysis which led to the trial being stopped.

Interim analyses and stopping for futility

Increasingly, there are methods appearing which consider the trend of 'no difference' between the treatments being compared. These methods are beyond the scope of this book and the reader is referred to specialist articles on this issue [43,44]. Nevertheless, many of the principles attached to the issue stopping for a positive result equally apply to the problem of stopping for 'no difference.'

9.6 Conclusion

The analysis of the data from a randomized trial should be approached with considerable care. In this chapter, we have provided approaches to minimize the bias and address many of the difficulties which arise. We have paid particular attention to practical issues and purposely limited mathematical presentations. It is important that an experienced statistician, preferably with a knowledge of the disease, is involved in the analysis of such data. Nevertheless, it is important that readers as well as practitioners are aware of the possible pitfalls and possible solutions. The advice presented in this chapter together with the advice presented in Chapter 10 on reporting results, should provide all with a basic grounding on the major issues in the analysis of data from a randomized trial.

References

[1] Altman, D.G. (1991) *Practical Statistics for Medical Research*. Chapman and Hall, London.

[2] Maughan, T.S., James, R.D., Kerr, D.J., Ledermann, J.A., McArdle, C., Seymour M.T., Cohen, D., Hopwood, P., Johnston, C., and Stephens, R.J. for the British MRC Colorectal Cancer Working Party. (2002) Comparison of survival, palliation, and quality of life with three chemotherapy regimens in metastatic colorectal cancer: a multicentre randomised trial. *Lancet*, 359, 1555–63.

[3] International collaboration of trialists. (1999) Adjuvant cisplatin, methotrexate, and vinblastine chemotherapy for muscle-invasive bladder cancer: a randomised controlled trial. *Lancet*, 354, 533–40.

[4] The ICON2 Collaborators. (1998) Randomised trial of single-agent carboplatin against three-drug combination of CAP (cyclophosphamide, doxorubicin, and cisplatin) in women with ovarian cancer. *Lancet*, 352, 1571–6.

[5] Saunders, M., Dische, S., Barrett, A., Harvey, A., Gibson, D., and Parmar, M. (1997) Continuous hyperfractionated accelerated radiotherapy (CHART) versus conventional radiotherapy in non-small-cell lung cancer: A randomized multicentre trial. *Lancet*, 350, 161–5.

[6] Bland, M. (1987) *An Introduction to Medical Statistics*. Oxford University Press, Oxford.

[7] Peto, R., Pike, M.C., Armitage, P., Breslow, N.E., Cox, D.R., and Howard, S.V. (1976) Design and analysis of randomised controlled trials requiring prolonged observation of each patient. I. Introduction and design. *British Journal of Cancer*, 34, 585–612.

[8] Peto, R., Pike, M.C., Armitage, P., Breslow, N.E., Cox, D.R., and Howard, S.V. (1976) Design and analysis of randomised controlled trials requiring prolonged observation of each patient. II. Analysis and examples. *British Journal of Cancer*, 35, 1–39.

[9] Parmar, M.K.B., and Machin, D. (1995) *Survival Analysis: A Practical Approach*. John Wiley, New York.

[10] Thatcher, N., Girling, D.J., Hopwood, P., Sambrook, R.J., Qian, W.D., and Stephens, R.J. (2000) Improving survival without reducing quality of life in small-cell lung cancer patients by increasing the dose-intensity of chemotherapy with granulocyte colony-stimulating factor support: results of a British Medical Research Council multicenter randomized trial. *Journal of Clinical Oncology*, 18, 395–404.

[11] Senn, S.J. (1989) Covariate imbalance and random allocation in clinical trials. *Statistics in Medicine*, 8, 467–75.

[12] Early Breast Cancer Trialists Collaborative Group. (2000) Favourable and unfavourable effects on long-term survival of radiotherapy for early breast cancer: an overview of the randomised trials. *Lancet*, 355, 1757–70.

[13] Collins, R., Gray, R., Godwin, J., and Peto, R. (1987) Avoidance of large biases and large random errors in the assessment of moderate treatment effects: the need for systematic overviews. *Statistics in Medicine*, 6, 245–50.

[14] Tierney, J.F., Stewart, L.A., Parmar, M.K.B., Fletcher, C.D.M., Jones, G., Mosseri, V., Patel, M., de Elvira, M.C.R., Souhami, R.L., Sylvester, R., Tursz, T., Alvegard, T.A., Sigurdsson, H., Antman, K., Bacchi, M., Baker, L.H., Benjamin, R.S., Brady, M.F., Bramwell, V., Bui, B.N., Edmonson, J.H., Leyvraz, S., Omura, G.A., Rouesse, J., Ryan, L., van Oosterom, A.T., and Yang, J.C. (1997) Adjuvant chemotherapy for localised resectable soft-tissue sarcoma of adults: meta-analysis of individual data. *Lancet*, **350**, 1647–54.

[15] Cella, D. (1997) FACIT manual.

[16] Fayers, P.M.F. Scoring manual for the EORTC QLQ-C30.

[17] Hopwood, P., Harvey, A., Davies, J., Stephens, R.J., Girling, D.J., Gibson, D., and Parmar, M.K.B. (1998) Survey of the administration of quality of life (QL) questionnaires in three multicentre randomised trials in cancer. *European Journal of Cancer*, **34**, 49–57.

[18] Fayers, P.M., Curran, D., and Machin, D. (1998) Incomplete quality of life data in randomized trials: missing items. *Statistics in Medicine*, **17**, 679–96.

[19] Qian, W., Parmar, M.K.B., Sambrook, R.J., Fayers, P.M., Girling, D.J., and Stephens, R.J. (2000) Analysis of messy longitudinal data from a randomized clinical trial. *Statistics in Medicine*, **19**, 2657–74.

[20] Hollen, P.J., Gralla, R.J., Cox, C., Eberly, S.W., and Kris, M.G. (1997) A dilemma in analysis: issues in the serial measurement of quality of life in pateints with advanced lung cancer. *Lung Cancer*, **18**, 119–36.

[21] Machin, D., and Weeden, S. (1998) Suggestions for the presentation of quality of life data from clinical trials. *Statistics in Medicine*, **17**, 711–24.

[22] Bailey, A.J., Parmar, M.K.B., Stephens, R.J. on behalf of the CHART Steering Committee. (1998) Patient-reported short-term and long-term physical and psychologic symptoms: results of the continuous hyperfractionated acclerated radiotherapy (CHART) randomized trial in non-small-cell lung cancer. *Journal of Clinical Oncology*, **16**, 3082–93.

[23] Curran, D., Aaronson, N., Standaert, B., Molenberghs, G., Therasse, P., Ramirez, A., Koopman-schap, M., Erder, H., and Piccart, M. (2000) Summary measures and statistics in the analysis of quality of life data: an example from an EORTC-NCIC-SAKK locally advanced breast cancer study. *European Journal of Cancer*, **36**, 834–44.

[24] Matthews, J.N.S., Altman, D.G., Campbell, M.J., and Royston, P. (1990) Analysis of serial measurements in medical research. *British Medical Journal*, **300**, 230–5.

[25] Little, J.M. (1987) A method of calculating the value of palliative care of cancer patients. *Australian, New Zealand Journal of Surgery*, **57**, 393–7.

[26] Lindsey, J.K. (1999) *Models for Repeated Measurements* (2nd ed.). Oxford University Press, New York.

[27] Osoba, D., Rodrigues, G., Myles, J., Zee, B., and Pater, J. (1998) Intrepreting the significance of changes in health related quality of life scores. *Journal of Clinical Oncology*, **16**, 139–44.

[28] King, M.T. (1996) The interpretation of scores from the EORTC quality of life questionnaire QLQ-C30. *Quality of Life Research*, **5**, 555–67.

[29] Kaplan, R.M. (1993) Quality of life assessment for cost/utility studies in cancer. *Cancer Treatment Reviews*, **19** (supp A) 85–96.

[30] Olschewski, M., and Schumacher, M. (1990) Statistical analysis of quality of life data in cancer clinical trials. *Statistics in Medicine*, **9**, 749–63.

[31] Gelber, R.D., and Goldhirsch, A. (1986) A new endpoint for the assessment of adjuvant therapy in post-menopausal women with operable breast cancer. *Journal of Clinical Oncology*, **4**, 1772–9.

[32] Feldstein, M.L. (1991) Quality of life adjusted survival for comparing cancer treatments; a commentary on TWIST and Q-TWIST. *Cancer*, **67**, 851–4.

[33] Goldhirsch, A., Gelber, R.D., Simes, R., Goldhirsch, A., Gelber, R.D., Simes, R., Glasziou, P., and Coates, A.S. (1989) Cost and benefits of adjuvant therapy in breast cancer: a quality adjusted survival analysis. *Journal of Clinical Oncology*, 36–44.

[34] Parmer, M.K.B., Griffiths, G.O., Spiegelhalter, D.J., Altman, D., and Souhami, R.L. On behalf of the CHART Steering Committee. Monitoring of large randomised clinical trials: a new apprroach with Bayesian methods. (2001) *Lancet*, **358**, 375–81.

[35] Pocock, S.J. (1982) Interim analysis for randomized clinical trials: the group sequential approach. *Biometrics*, **38**, 153–62.

[36] McPherson, K. (1982) On choosing the number of interim analyses in clinical trials. *Statistics in Medicine*, **1**, 25–36.

[37] O'Brien, P.C., and Fleming, T.R. (1979) A multiple testing procedure for clinical trials. *Biometrics*, **35**, 549–56.

[38] De Mets, D.I., and Lan, K.K.G. (1994) Interim analysis: the alpha spending function approach. *Statistics in Medicine*, **13**, 1341–52.

[39] Todd, S., and Whitehead, J. (1996) Point and interval estimation following a sequential clinical trial. *Biometrika*, **83**, 453–61.

[40] Dillman, R.O., Seagren, S.L., Propert, K.J., Guerra, J., Eaton, W.L., Perry, M.C., Carey, R.W., Frei, E.F., and Green, M.R. (1990) A randomized trial of induction chemotherapy plus high-dose radiation versus radiation alone in stage-iii non-small-cell lung cancer. *New England Journal of Medicine*, **323**, 940–45.

[41] Souhami, R.L., Spiro, S.G., and Cullen, M. (1991) Chemotherapy and radiation-therapy as compared with radiation-therapy in stage III non-small-cell cancer. *New England Journal of Medicine*, **324**, 1136.

[42] Sylvester, R., Bartelink, H., and Rubens, R. (1994) A reversal of fortune: practical problems in the monitoring and interpretation of an EORTC breast cancer trial. *Statistics in Medicine*, **13**, 1329–35.

[43] Berntsen, R.F., Rasmussen, K., and Bjornstad, J.F. (1991) Monitoring a randomized clinical-trial for futility – the North-Norwegian Lidocaine Intervention Trial. *Statistics In Medicine*, **10**, 405–12.

[44] De Mets, D.L., Pocock, S.J., and Julian, D.G. (1991) The agonising negative trend in monitoring of clinical trials. *Lancet*, **354**, 1983–88.

Chapter 10

Reporting and interpreting results

10.1 Introduction

The ultimate aim of most trials is to influence clinical practice and/or clinical research, and this will generally only be achieved once the trial results have been presented, subjected to peer review and published in an appropriate journal. In this chapter, we discuss not just the typical format of trial publications and presentations, and what should be reported, but also why, when, how and by whom.

10.2 General principles

When reporting the results of a randomized trial, one should keep two goals in mind. Firstly, the onus is on the authors to show that the trial has been designed, conducted and analysed to appropriate standards – or if it has not, to explain why and discuss the possible impact of any limitations on the interpretation of the results. As other chapters demonstrate, the fact that a trial is referred to as randomized is not sufficient to confirm true randomization with adequate concealment; further, the use of proper randomization does not imply that all other aspects of the trial design will render it free from bias; and even the conduct of a well designed, properly randomized trial does not preclude the possibility of bias being introduced in the analysis. The first goal should therefore be to report the results in a structured way, which includes all the information necessary for a reader to judge whether these standards have been reached. For randomized trials, many aspects of structure have been formalized in the 'CONSORT' statement, which is discussed in detail later.

The second goal is to present all the data necessary to make a decision on the overall merits of one treatment compared with another. It is important to recognize that such a decision may often involve a complex weighing up of several advantages and disadvantages, and that decision makers – for example, patients or clinicians – will weight the individual components differently. A trial report should therefore not attempt to dictate – though of course as the people closest to the trial, the authors' opinions will be of interest – but to inform. Key to this, as discussed in Chapter 9, is the need to provide estimates of treatment effect on all relevant outcome measures and not simply the p-value resulting from a hypothesis test.

10.3 Structure and content of a trial report – CONSORT

The importance with which randomized controlled trials (RCTs) are held has meant that many of the leading medical journals not only undertake routine statistical review, but also apply specific checklists for the reporting of clinical trials. This was formalized, in 1996 [1] (updated in 2001 [2]), by the publication of the 'Consolidated standards of reporting trials' (CONSORT) statement (see also http://www.consort-statement.org). This statement includes a checklist of twenty-one items, mainly related to the description of the methods and results, and the discussion section of a randomized trial, which the CONSORT group has deemed essential in order to evaluate the 'internal and external validity' of a trial report. Table 10.1 shows the key items included in the CONSORT checklist together with a brief descriptor. Some journals ask for a table such as this to be submitted with a trial report, with the descriptor column replaced by one indicating the page of the report on which each item appears. CONSORT further recommends the inclusion of a flow diagram which follows the group of patients considered for, and randomized and analysed, in the trial, detailing the reasons for patients failing to be included at any stage (see Fig. 10.1).

10.3.1 The CONSORT guidelines – justification

Below we explain the importance of each item on the CONSORT checklist and then describe some additional items, which can usefully be added for completeness. All these points are discussed in detail on the CONSORT website (http://www.consort-statement.org) based on a paper by Altman *et al.* [3]. The numbers of the paragraphs below refer to the CONSORT checklist.

Title and abstract

1. It is important to identify a trial as randomized, not just to capture the casual reader, but also to ensure the report is classified as a randomized trial when indexed for databases such as MEDLINE. This in turn helps to ensure it can be identified as a randomized trial by those conducting systematic reviews. The word randomized should therefore be included in the title. As a rule, it is best to avoid 'declaratory' titles along the lines of 'x significantly improves survival in y cancer'; the title should describe the trial and not its results.

Abstract: Most journals now state their preferred abstract format covering background, methods, results and conclusions, often with a word limit. Abstracts deserve a great deal of thought and time being spent on them, as many readers will read no further, yet still draw conclusions from what you say in only 2–300 words. The provision of abstracts, but not full text, on many literature search engines increases the chance that a high proportion of those who see the abstract will never see the full paper. It is therefore better to state specific aspects of the results (e.g. the main outcome measure) in some detail, and others sufficiently vaguely that the reader will clearly have to look further to gain the full picture. Avoid statements such as 'there was no difference $p = 0.3$' in an abstract just as you would in a full report – it is better to give estimates and confidence intervals as well as p-values, or say nothing.

Introduction

2. *Background* This section describes the rationale: why you did the trial when you did it, why you designed it as you did, summarizing briefly the state of knowledge at the time the trial was designed. It is appropriate to indicate here any changes to the trial design or hypotheses during its conduct, and the reasons for them. It is important to be clear

Table 10.1 CONSORT checklist for reporting a randomized trial

Heading	Item number	Descriptor
Title and abstract	1	Identify the study as a randomized trial
Introduction		
Background	2	Scientific background and rationale
Methods		
Participants	3	Eligibility criteria for participants and the settings and locations where the data were collected
Interventions	4	Precise details of the interventions intended for each group and how and when they were actually administered
Objectives	5	Specify objectives and hypotheses
Outcomes	6	Clearly defined primary and secondary outcome measure(s) and, when applicable, any methods used to enhance the quality of measurements (e.g. multiple observations, training of assessors)
Sample size	7	How sample size was determined and, when applicable, explanation of any interim analyses and stopping rules
Randomization		
Sequence generation	8	Method used to generate the allocation sequence, including details of any restriction (e.g. blocking, stratification)
Allocation concealment	9	Method used to implement the random allocation sequence (e.g. numbered containers, central telephone) clarifying whether the sequence was concealed until interventions were assigned.
Implementation	10	Who generated the allocation sequence, who enrolled participants, and who assigned participants to their groups?
Blinding (masking)	11	Whether or not participants, those administering the interventions and those assessing the outcomes were aware of group assignment. If not, how the success of masking was assessed.
Statistical methods	12	Statistical methods used to compare groups for primary outcome(s); methods for additional analyses, such as subgroup analyses and adjusted analyses.
Results		
Participant flow	13	Flow of participants through each stage (a diagram is strongly recommended). Specifically for each group report the numbers of participants randomly assigned, receiving intended treatment, completing the study protocol, and analysed for the primary outcome. Describe protocol deviations from study as planned together with reasons.
Recruitment	14	Dates defining the periods of recruitment and follow-up.
Baseline data	15	Baseline demographic and clinical characteristics of each group
Numbers analysed	16	Number of participants (denominator) in each group included in each analysis and whether the analysis was by 'intention to treat.' State results in absolute numbers when feasible (e.g. 10/20 not 50 per cent).
Outcomes and estimation	17	For each primary and secondary outcome, a summary of results for each group, and the estimated effect size and its precision (e.g. 95 per cent CI)
Ancillary analyses	18	Address multiplicity by reporting any other analyses performed, including subgroup analyses and adjusted analyses indicating those prespecified and those exploratory.
Adverse events	19	All important adverse events or side effects in each intervention group
Discussion		
Interpretation	20	Interpretation of the results, taking into account study hypotheses, sources of potential bias or imprecision and the dangers associated with multiplicity of analyses and outcomes
Generalizability	21	Generalizability (external validity) of the trial findings
Overall evidence	22	General interpretation of the results in the context of current evidence

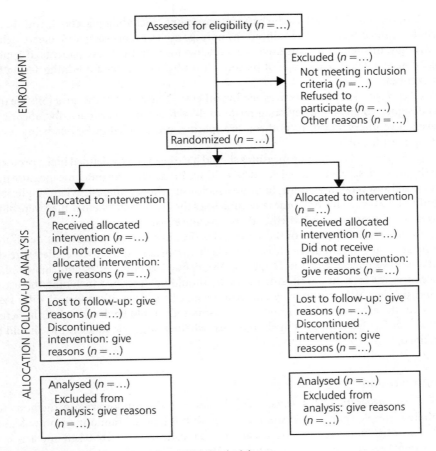

Fig. 10.1 General flow diagram of a randomized trial.

and honest about which additional analyses were pre-planned, which were suggested by events or information emerging independently of the trial and which were data-driven, since the confidence which can be attached to the results of the analyses decline in this order.

Methods

3. Participants Specification of eligibility criteria allows readers to assess the extent to which the trial population may represent the population they are interested in. You should describe the rationale for any inclusions/exclusions, which might be considered unusual and in particular justify any limits imposed on continuous criteria such as age. The method of recruitment – for example by referral or self-selection – may also be relevant.

Settings and locations; this will define whether or not it is a multi-centre study, whether it was carried out in specialist centres, generally give further information necessary to help a reader determine whether the results are relevant to their own setting.

4. Interventions   As well as the basic interventions (including placebos), you should include planned treatment modifications in response to events such as toxicity; rightly or wrongly, this report may be used as a guideline for treating future patients. If applicable, describe who (or the type of person who) was responsible for administering the interventions.

5. Objectives   Specific objectives and hypotheses. Objectives are the questions the trial was designed to answer. They often relate to the efficacy of a particular therapeutic or preventative intervention. Hypotheses are specific, prespecified questions being tested to help meet the objectives.

6. Outcomes   The outcome measures should have been clearly defined in the protocol, but should be described in equal detail here. In addition, where an outcome measure may be assessed at several timepoints, indicate which is of primary interest. Where applicable, specify who assessed the outcome, any guidelines they followed, whether they were blind to treatment allocation and whether there was more than one assessor.

7. Sample size   The basis of the sample size should be given in sufficient detail that the reader could reproduce it. It is particularly important to justify the effect size the trial was powered to detect (see Chapter 5). Pre-defined stopping rules/guidelines and/or procedures for interim monitoring of results should be described including the use of an independent data monitoring and ethics committee. Even if no formal rules were followed, the extent to which results were monitored should be described. If the actual trial size differs from that planned originally, whether larger or smaller, this should be explained.

Randomization

8. Sequence generation This section should describe the randomization method; for example if simple (pure) randomization was used, if blocked randomization was used and, if so, what block size was chosen, and if prognostic factors were taken into account, for example by stratification or minimization (see Chapter 4). It is not sufficient to state that 'computerized' randomization was used – the underlying method must be stated – but you should state if randomization lists were prepared in advance, or whether a computer program was used to produce allocations interactively. Also state here the randomization ratio.

9. Allocation concealment   Concealment of the allocation is essential to ensure that those responsible for entering a patient into a trial will not know in advance what the patient will be allocated, and therefore be in a position to decide whether or not to enter them on that basis. Where randomization is effected by calling a central randomization service or other independent group, or where 'dynamic' randomization is used, it may be clear that concealment is in place; where pre-prepared lists are used it would be necessary to state how they were prepared and stored until needed.

10. Implementation   This point clarifies further, if necessary, who was responsible for preparing the randomization schedule, who was responsible for inviting patients to join the trial and discussing it with them and who ascertained the treatment allocation (i.e. made the telephone call or opened the envelope). It is important to distinguish preparation and performance. For example, for sealed envelope randomization, an independent individual should prepare the randomization list and the accompanying sealed envelopes which, in due course, a participating clinician will open. If the preparation or performance of randomization was carried out by someone involved in delivering the intervention this may be questionable.

11. Blinding (masking)   Describe whether or not interventions or assessments were blinded to patients, clinicians, assessors or analysts. Also, describe steps taken to ensure any blinding was maintained, and any problems which you were aware of.

12. Statistical methods   Describe the methods of analysis used in general for specific outcome measures, or specific types of data, but remember that you may also need to indicate the methods used when describing the results (for example whether parametric or non-parametric methods were used for a given outcome). Explain here how you dealt with complications such as missing data. When discussing additional analyses, mention the use (or not) of adjusted *p*-values for multiplicity of comparisons if appropriate.

Results

13. Participant flow   It can be useful to describe these features in a flow diagram of the type illustrated in Fig. 10.1. It should though be pointed out that, for many multi-centre trials, the first two boxes may be difficult to complete. For such data to be useful or appropriate, it would be necessary to log, prospectively, every patient with the relevant diagnosis and to record in detail the reasons for not entering the trial. To do this comprehensively is no small task for an individual centre, and extremely difficult for a multi-centre trial coordinator to audit. While the intention is to give an indication of the 'representativeness' of the population actually randomized, it fails to do this because there will always be patients who, through lack of time, organizational problems or even investigator bias are never approached about the trial. Often therefore it will be appropriate for the diagram to begin with the 'randomization' box, and certainly all the remaining box items are important to document, if not in a diagram, then in the text. Deviations from the allocated treatment should be described by group, as should any other deviations from the protocol, for example in the way patients were assessed or followed-up. It is important to quantify the degree of compliance with protocol interventions and the reasons for non-compliance; if good results are achieved despite non-compliance it may indicate potential areas for simplification. Conversely, if 'negative' results are associated with poor compliance, could anything be done in the future to improve compliance? If not, then inability to comply is an important conclusion of the trial, if yes, further trials may be needed to determine whether improved compliance is associated with better results.

14. Recruitment   It is always important to know the time period over which patients were accrued, partly to place it in its historical context, partly to see how long it took to accrue patients. It may be that some aspects of patient care or assessment have changed over the course of a trial.

15. Baseline data   A table of patient characteristics by allocated treatment is one of the first things that should be reported. It serves to demonstrate the characteristics of the actual population entered into the trial (which may be a small subset of those potentially eligible, which the eligibility criteria themselves describe). It also demonstrates the success, or otherwise, of randomization in achieving approximate balance between the treatment groups with respect to important prognostic variables. As discussed more fully in Chapter 9, it is not necessary to demonstrate balance by carrying out a formal test for the comparability of the groups with respect to each factor, as is sometimes done. If treatment allocation was truly random, differences can only be due to chance.

In addition, prognostic variables are often correlated, and so chance imbalance in one may well be reflected in a similar imbalance in others, without this providing increased evidence of flawed or inadequate randomization. As described in Section 9.4.3, tests for baseline balance are also unhelpful in determining whether, and how, analysis of the main outcome measure should be adjusted for prognostic factors.

16. Numbers analysed   The number of patients contributing to various statistics or outcome measures in a trial report may well vary; stating results in absolute numbers makes it clear when patients have been excluded or data are missing.

17. Outcomes and estimation   As described in Chapter 9, it is not sufficient to give trial results simply in terms of *p*-values from hypothesis tests, which are dependent not just on the size of difference observed between groups, but also the sample size. Providing a relevant estimate, and appropriate confidence interval, both for the individual groups and for the measure of difference between them will indicate if statistically non-significant results actually provide some indication of what may potentially be a clinically worthwhile effect. Equally, in a large trial, provision of these details will help ensure that the clinical relevance of statistically significant results can be evaluated. Always give exact *p*-values for all analyses (and argue the case with journals that impose their own constraints) and never use NS (non-significant), and always report the results of all relevant analyses on the primary and secondary outcome measures, not just those which produced 'significant' results.

18. Ancillary analyses   Indicate which analyses were pre-specified and justify any that were not. If adjusted analyses of the main endpoint were used, both unadjusted and adjusted results should be presented. The choice of variables for adjustment should be justified (these should have been prespecified see Section 9.4.3).

19. Adverse events   Provide estimates of the frequency of the main serious adverse events in each treatment group, and specify any grading system used (e.g. common toxicity criteria).

Discussion

20. Interpretation   A useful structure has been proposed comprising the following elements: a brief synopsis of the key findings; possible explanations and mechanisms; comparison with other relevant results; limitations of the present study and any attempts made to address these; and a summary of the clinical and/or research implications of the results. The trial discussion should include a critical review not just of its strengths but also of its limitations, particularly those that may be apparent only to those who conducted the trial.

21. Generalizability   Indicate, but only if there is good justification, if the trial results can be extrapolated to groups not involved in the trial, for example different ages or genders, or to different classes of the intervention studied.

22. Overall evidence   This aspect requires comparison or integration with other relevant results, some of which may support the results and some of which may not. It may be impractical to conduct a full systematic review, but an attempt should be made to identify relevant sources of information so that the trial results can be placed in the context of other relevant results; does it confirm or contradict them? What are the possible reasons for contradiction, and do they cast any shadow on the trial? How does it add to the totality of evidence – what proportion of the total information does your trial represent? It is not necessarily essential to conduct a formal systematic review and meta-analysis to quantify the contribution and impact of the trial, but it is worth considering if this is feasible or at least highlighting what such an approach may bring to the debate.

10.3.2   Other points to include

The CONSORT statement is seen as something to be revised and updated when required; the website will indicate the current recommended version. Some items not present in the 2001 version, but which are useful to include, are the following:

Title
- Wherever possible, include the International Standard Randomized Controlled Trial Number (ISRCTN, see Chapter 11) in the title; failing this it should appear in the abstract.

Protocol
- What type of ethics review was done?
- How was the study managed – was there a steering group? Did it have independent members? (see Section 8.10).
- Was there an independent data monitoring and ethics committee? (see Section 8.10).

Methods
- How were data collected and checked; was any source data verification carried out?

Results
- Give the date of analysis/freezing of database for analysis.
- How many centres randomized patients?
- Quantify the maturity of time-to-event data by stating both the number of events and the minimum, maximum and median follow-up time in each group (see Section 9.3.4).

Appendices or footnotes
- State the trial sponsors, funders and any conflicts of interest.
- List all participants and describe their roles.

10.4   Presenting results – relative or absolute measures?

We have emphasized the importance of providing estimates of treatment effect to aid the clinical interpretation of data (see also Chapter 9). However, in many situations, there will be more than one way to present estimates of treatment effect. One distinction, introduced in Chapter 5, is between absolute and relative measures. In general, absolute measures use differences while relative measures employ ratios. Many outcome measures can be expressed in both absolute and relative terms. With respect to survival data, the difference in the proportions surviving to a given time point in two treatment arms gives an estimate of the absolute difference in survival. For example, if the 5-year survival rate for one treatment is 40 per cent and for the other is 50 per cent, the absolute difference in survival is 10 per cent. The hazard ratio on the other hand is a measure of the relative treatment effect; a survival hazard ratio of 0.76 implies that the relative risk of death at any given time is 24 per cent less in one treatment group than the other. This may sound like a more impressive difference than an absolute difference of 10 per cent. In fact, under the assumption of proportional hazards, an absolute increase from 40 per cent to 50 per cent is equivalent to a hazard ratio of 0.76. In general, relative measures will sound 'bigger' than absolute measures. A small absolute increase in a very rare event (for example the risk of a second, treatment-related cancer) may generate dramatically large relative risks, which can cause an unnecessary degree of alarm. It is therefore important to provide actual event rates in addition when using relative measures. It has been argued that absolute measures of treatment effect are most relevant at an individual patient level, and relative measures of more relevance at the population level.

A further measure which has gained popularity in the setting of a binary treatment outcome is the 'number needed to treat (NNT) [4]'. This is intended to describe the number of patients who must be treated with a new intervention for one patient to benefit, or for one adverse outcome to be avoided. For binary data, this is obtained as the reciprocal of the absolute difference in the proportion of patients with the outcome of interest. For example, if 40 per cent of patients respond on standard therapy and 50 per cent respond on a new therapy, the absolute difference is 10 per cent and the NNT is $1/0.1 = 10$, i.e. ten patients need to be treated for one patient to benefit. The NNT can provide a useful measure which can be compared in many different settings, particularly useful perhaps for those comparing the cost of introducing different treatments. Confidence intervals can (and should) be calculated for the NNT [5]; it is a measure which is all too easily taken simply at face value forgetting the uncertainty in the data from which it was generated. Furthemore, caution must be applied to the use of NNT for time-to-event data, for which there is debate about its role. Essentially, there is no single NNT for such data, since it will depend on the time point chosen and the number of patients at risk at that time [6]. In general the NNT will fall as the time from start of treatment increases. Furthermore, when a relative measure of treatment effect is the appropriate summary statistic, the absolute difference and hence the NNT is dependent on the baseline risk of the population to which it is applied [7] (see also Chapter 11). The NNT remains a controversial statistic, as a paper by Hutton and subsequent discussion illustrates [8].

10.5 Practical issues in reporting

This section discusses some of the more practical issues to consider when contemplating submitting a trial report. Authorship style is always an important issue, but one best dealt with in advance by specifying the rules to be followed in the protocol; therefore this is discussed in Section 8.9.

10.5.1 Always publish

Whatever the results, always aim to publish the trial in some format, irrespective of whether or not it was completed as planned, and whether or not there were problems with its conduct that may make the results difficult to interpret. Even when all trials are registered (see Section 11.5.4), publication of results will still be the best way to ensure that the totality of evidence concerning a particular treatment is readily available to those for whom the results are relevant – including 'consumers' of evidence (both clinicians and patients) and those planning new research. This principle is increasingly recognized not just by those conducting trials, but also by many of the medical journals. Sadly, however, there is still evidence of publication bias, with some journals far more likely to publish trials with 'positive' results (see Chapter 11). This makes the aim of publishing all trials difficult to achieve, but nonetheless it should be pursued. If the trial is not accepted as a full article (and not just by your first choice of journal), then there is still the possibility of putting the basic results in a letter and/or publishing electronically. There is often much to be learnt from trials which 'fail'; reporting your attempts to conduct a trial, the problems you encountered, the solutions you attempted whether or not they were successful, all provides valuable information for those working in the area – it is often the most interesting trials which are the most difficult to carry out successfully. Finally, there is an ethical imperative to publish in order to acknowledge the contribution which patients who took part in the trial have made.

10.5.2   When should the first results be published?

For time-to-event data, the number of events (and associated number of patients) required to provide the desired power should have been specified up front, and when this is the case it provides a simple guide as to the 'right time' to publish. This will depend both on the event rate and the accrual rate; the slower the rate of accrual, the longer the median follow-up at the closure of the trial and the shorter the time required after closure for the required number of events to accrue. It is necessary to bear in mind that those running trials have an obligation to the patients who agree to enter trials that they should contribute to the final results. Therefore presentation of results should not generally take place until all patients have at least completed their treatment. Exceptions to this may occur, firstly when the trial treatment is very long-term – for example ten years of hormone therapy for prostate cancer – and secondly when a trial stops early because of unequivocal evidence of superiority of one treatment over another. In this latter situation it is important to publish the results, *as they were when the decision was made to close the trial*, as soon as possible. In this situation, careful thought must be given as to how these results are communicated to patients, particularly those who may be still receiving treatment and those treated with the inferior therapy. If the results change with further follow-up, then subsequent publication may be appropriate, subject to the guidance given in the next section.

10.5.3   How often should trial results be updated for publication?

For all trials with time-to-event outcomes there remains the possibility of additional events being reported after the main study publication. When is it appropriate to update the results? Ideally one should pre-specify a frequency with which data will be examined post-publication and some guidelines as to what would warrant publication. These should generally be based on either the accumulation of specific durations of follow-up (e.g. there may be interest in examining the results, when all surviving patients have a minimum of five or ten years follow-up) or accumulation of a given number of additional events. There should be no need for frequent reviews – the dangers of too-frequent analyses may be just as great after the closure of a trial as they are during its accrual phase, and similarly the timing of any analysis should be decided independently of the results. For example, one may be prompted to update results by the publication of other, relevant, papers, or may receive a request to provide updated data for an individual patient data meta-analysis. In the absence of other 'prompts,' the accumulation of perhaps 15–20 per cent more events, or 5-year intervals of follow-up, may be a rule of thumb to trigger an updated analysis. Bear in mind though, that with long-term follow-up, particularly in trials with reasonably high overall survival rates, an increasing proportion of late events will not be disease-related. Generally this is simply a consequence of the age of the trial population. However, it may also represent late effects of treatment. For example, with respect to radiotherapy for early breast cancer, treatment-related mortality did not become apparent until 20–25 years after treatment, and meant that analysis of mature data found no overall benefit to radiotherapy with respect to all-cause mortality [9].

10.5.4 Choosing an appropriate journal

The appropriate journal may not always be the most 'high profile.' There is no harm in aiming high, and many of those conducting trials will need to satisfy the demands of research assessors who often judge output in terms of journal impact factors. But to avoid delaying the dissemination of the results of your work too much through repeated submission and rejection, give careful thought to whether the higher profile journals – which are often general rather than disease-specific – are really appropriate. Does the trial have relevance on an international scale? Across clinical disciplines? Does it address points of principle which are relevant across many disease areas? If the answer to all of these is really yes – and not just from your own, inevitably biased viewpoint – then high impact general medical journals are worth considering. If not, then in choosing your journal bear in mind that your target readership will have paper-based and electronic access to many journals, but that it is impossible to read them all in detail – Chapter 11 highlights this problem. Suppose, for example, that a trial compared two different radiotherapy schedules, widely used in a particular country but not elsewhere. However striking the results, they might most appropriately be targeted at clinical oncologists in that country. The best way to do that *and to provide the highest chance that they will be read in full,* may be to publish in a journal which all clinical oncologists in that country should receive, principally the journals of professional bodies and associations such as the Royal College of Radiologists in the UK (Clinical Oncology), European Society for Therapeutic Radiology and Oncology in Europe generally (Radiotherapy and Oncology) or the American Society for Therapeutic Radiology and Oncology in the USA (International Journal of Radiation, Oncology, Biology and Physics). If it is of particular importance, for whatever reason, to publish results quickly, one could argue that it is best to submit immediately to the journal which would most clearly recognize the importance of the trial in that disease area. Alternatively, some journals now provide a fast-track procedure for such studies, and these too might be considered.

10.5.5 The covering letter

Wherever you submit, *do not underestimate the importance of the covering letter to the editor,* justifying your choice of journal and explaining why the editors should be interested in publishing the report. Submitting a trial report with a covering letter stating simply 'please find enclosed a report on trial X, which we would like you to consider for publication' misses an opportunity to make it stand out from the crowd. Take advantage of the fact that busy editors can quickly read a short but informative covering letter, and decide whether it is of potential interest. When submitting to a high profile, general journal, attention to the covering letter is of particular importance.

10.5.6 Publishing data from sub-studies

An increasing number of trials collect not just the clinical data necessary to evaluate a treatment, but also additional data or information in all or a subset of patients. Examples include quality of life or health economics data as well as data arising from sub-studies such as tissue collection for evaluation of prognostic and predictive markers. The question then arises as to how much of these data should be included in the main study report without making it unwieldy. The key question to ask is, could these additional data potentially influence the overall assessment of the relative merits of the treatments? If the answer is yes, then at least the key results should be included in the main study report. For example, if some specific quality of life (QL) hypotheses were specified in advance, data pertaining to these should be included alongside the clinical data. As QL can generate a vast amount of data, it may well be appropriate to publish a more detailed analysis separately. In such a report, data on all the QL items and subscales can be presented, and exploratory analyses conducted, with appropriate cautionary notes relating to multiplicity of outcome measures and absence of pre-defined hypotheses (see Chapter 9). One such example is the MRC/EORTC factorial trial of three versus four cycles of BEP chemotherapy over three versus five days for good prognosis metastatic germ cell tumours. This was an equivalence trial and as such the QL results could potentially have had a major influence on the interpretation of the results. Therefore, the main study report [10] focused on the clinical data but included a summary of the findings of the QL data. A further report will present detailed analyses of the QL data, which have not previously been reported in a randomized trial in this disease.

If the additional data are not essential in order to interpret the main clinical results, then in the interests of brevity it may well be more appropriate to include all the data in a separate report and cross reference it in the main study report. Studies of potential new predictive factors – molecular markers for example – may be difficult to place. They will certainly be relevant to the main study results since the aim is to determine whether they can identify true interactions with treatment effect, isolating subgroups who may benefit to a substantially greater or lesser extent than patients overall. However, it will generally be the case that these are exploratory analyses, requiring independent confirmation, particularly if the trial was not specifically powered to look at treatment interactions (this will nearly always be the case, especially when tissue collection is planned in only a subset of trial patients). In this situation, it would be appropriate to publish the results separately as the overall trial result remains the most important and can be interpreted and acted upon without reference to substudy results. As the sub-study analyses would need to refer to the overall trial treatment effect, it would of course be important that analyses of sub-studies are only published after, or in parallel with, the main trial results.

It is important not to clutter reports with unnecessary data. A prime example is the common practice of including results of an analysis of clinical prognostic factors at the end of a trial report. This is only of interest if it provides new insight – for example if it includes an evaluation of new potential prognostic factors rarely if ever studied before, or if the trial is in a rare disease for which data on prognostic factors in substantial numbers of patients may be lacking. There is really no point in providing an analysis of common prognostic factors in trials in common diseases. The temptation to include an exciting p-value, however irrelevant to the trial results, somewhere in the report should be resisted.

The importance of publication guidelines for sub-studies

We discuss above some guidelines with respect to sub-studies which are an integral part of the main trial. However, within multi-centre trials, it may be that individual centres will want to publish data on their own patients within the trial – for example they may have collected additional data over and above the trial requirements, or simply wish to report historical series. It is useful to state clearly, in the protocol, guidelines on the nature and timing of such publications. The key aim is to avoid a situation where early publication of a subset of data could prejudice the publication of the full trial results. A standard paragraph from MRC protocols states 'the results from individual centres will be analysed together and published as soon as possible. No individual centre may publish data on their own patients which are relevant to the main trial results until the main study report has been published.' Another role of the independent trial monitoring/steering committee (see Section 8.10) may be to advise in situations where it may not immediately be clear that the subset results 'are relevant to the main study results.'

10.6 Disseminating results

Publications are, of course, not the only means of disseminating the results of trials, but there is little doubt they are ultimately the most important. In this section, we review other ways in which trial results are shared with the wider clinical and patient community, and suggest some good practice guidelines.

10.6.1 Conference presentations

For many trials, the first presentation of results will be at a meeting of collaborators at which there will be plenty of time to present, review and discuss the results in full. Typically, the first 'public' presentation will be at a conference, at which time is inevitably tight. Here we discuss the timing and content of conference presentations of trial results.

Timing

The general guidelines provided in Section 10.5.2 apply equally to oral presentations as to publications. It would rarely be appropriate to present results that are immature. An added difficulty with presentations is the need to submit abstracts several months in advance of the presentation date, and hence the need to predict whether the required number of events, say, will be reached by the time of the final pre-meeting analysis. Programme selection committees understandably would rather see actual results than the promise of data that 'will be presented'. However, if data are immature at the time of submission it is best to give data by randomized group only on those aspects of the trial which are complete (toxicity and compliance say), and to give overall event rates, or an estimate of the proportion of the required events seen so far. There will often be a compelling reason to present results at a particular meeting and so some flexibility is required. However, do bear in mind that the presentation of immature results runs two major risks; firstly that the results will be inconclusive, secondly that they may change with further follow-up. In both situations, any benefit gained by presenting early is lost. As a rule, aim to minimize the time between first presentation of trial results and submission for publication.

Content

The typical conference schedule allows 10–15 min for presentations with perhaps 5 min for questions. A good general rule is to allow approximately one minute per slide, however if the content is relatively simple (as in the example in Fig. 10.2) and the transition between slides is smooth (e.g. Powerpoint presentations rather than overhead transparencies) it is possible to increase this; thus for a ten-minute talk this implies having around 12–15 slides, including a title slide and acknowledgements slide. Box 10.1 gives a suggested basic format, an example (the MRC OE02 trial [11]) is given in Fig. 10.2.

Box 10.1 Suggested slides for a ten-minute presentation

1. Title, authors
2. Background bullets
3. Design – diagram and eligibility
4. Design – interventions
5. Design – outcome measures, statistics, sample size
6. Results – accrual dates, total numbers, reasons for any alteration from planned sample size
7. Results – baseline characteristics by allocated treatment
8. Results – compliance with interventions, toxicity
9. Results – primary outcome measures
10. Results – secondary outcome measures
11. Context – other relevant results
12. Conclusions
13. List of participating centres and other acknowledgements

In addition, include relevant logos and sponsor identification and, as footnotes, the date and name of the meeting at which the presentation was made.

10.6.2 Press releases

When the results of a trial have been accepted for publication, it is worth considering whether a press release to the general lay media, to coincide with their publication, would

OE02

Randomised phase III trial of surgery with or without pre-operative chemotherapy in resectable cancer of the oesophagus

PI Clark on behalf of the MRC Oesophageal Cancer Working Party

MRC Clinical Trials Unit

BACKGROUND   OE02

- A relatively common cancer of changing epidemiology
- Approximately 5000 deaths per year in the UK
- Outlook for surgery alone poor
- 20% 2-year survival
- Evidence from non-randomised studies that chemotherapy may improve results of surgery and reduce subclinical metastases
=> Does pre-op chemotherapy Prolong survival? Affect physical well-being?

MRC Clinical Trials Unit

TRIAL DESIGN   OE02

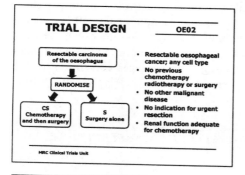

- Resectable oesophageal cancer; any cell type
- No previous chemotherapy radiotherapy or surgery
- No other malignant disease
- No indication for urgent resection
- Renal function adequate for chemotherapy

MRC Clinical Trials Unit

CHEMOTHERAPY REGIMEN   OE02

- **Two 4-day pre-operative courses, 3 weeks apart**
  - Cisplatin   80 mg/m² by 4-hr infusion on day 1
  - Fluorouracil   1g/m²/day by infusion for 4 days

MRC Clinical Trials Unit

STATISTICAL CONSIDERATIONS   OE02

- Primary outcome measure=survival
- Intended intake 800 patients in 4 years
- Enabling an increase in 2-year survival rates from 20% to 30% to be detected with a 5% significance level and 90% power

MRC Clinical Trials Unit

ACCRUAL   OE02

**March 1992 - June 1998
802 patients randomised
CS = 400   S = 402**
(from more than 40 European centres)

MRC Clinical Trials Unit

PATIENT CHARACTERISTICS   OE02

	CS	S
Age:		
Median	63 years	62 years
Range	(36 - 84)	(30 - 80)
Sex:		
Male	77%	74%
Histology:		
Adenocarcinoma	66%	67%
Site of tumour:		
Lower third	65%	63%
Level of physical activity:		
Normal	58%	55%

MRC Clinical Trials Unit

CHEMOTHERAPY RECEIVED   OE02

2 cycles with no delay/modifications	294 (76%)
2 cycles with dose delay/modification	53 (14%)
1 cycle only	22 (6%)
None given	17 (4%)
Total	386 (100%)
Details incomplete/form missing	14
Total allocated chemotherapy	400

MRC Clinical Trials Unit

Fig. 10.2 Example slides for a 10–15 min presentation.

POST-OPERATIVE COMPLICATIONS — OE02

% in patients having surgery

	CS	S
Total	40%	42%
Respiratory	16%	15%
Anastomotic	6%	8%
Infection	6%	7%
Cardiac	4%	4%
Gastro-intestinal	2%	2%
Other	8%	5%

MRC Clinical Trials Unit

SURVIVAL BY TREATMENT — OE02

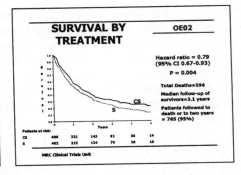

Hazard ratio = 0.79 (95% CI 0.67-0.93)

P = 0.004

Total Deaths=596

Median follow-up of survivors=3.1 years

Patients followed to death or to two years = 765 (95%)

MRC Clinical Trials Unit

SUMMARY — OE02

With 596 deaths the following benefits to chemotherapy were seen:

2-year survival:
CS: 43%
S: 34%
Difference = 9% (95% CI 3%-14%)

Median survival:
CS: 16.8 months
S: 13.3 months
Difference = 3.5 months (95% CI 1.0-6.4 months)

MRC Clinical Trials Unit

OTHER RANDOMISED TRIALS — OE02

- Literature search reveals 10 other trials
- All compare pre-operative chemotherapy plus surgery with surgery alone in cancer of the oesophagus
- 9/10 are closed to accrual
- It is possible to estimate the hazard ratio (and 95% confidence interval) for 8 of these trials

MRC Clinical Trials Unit

OTHER RANDOMISED TRIALS — OE02

Trial	Target intake	Actual intake	HR (95% CI)
Texas		39	0.79 (0.48-1.28)
Norway		121	1.12 (0.87-1.43)
Germany		46	1.09 (0.78-1.55)
Thailand		46	1.34 (0.77-2.31)
US Intergroup	450	467	1.07 (0.87-1.32)
Rotterdam	160	160	-
OESO	333	137	0.89 (0.65-1.21)
Hong Kong	147	140	0.69 (0.51-0.94)
MRC OE02	800	802	0.79 (0.67-0.93)
Italy	240	110	1.00 (0.67-1.51)
France (open)	250	150	-

MRC Clinical Trials Unit

OTHER RANDOMISED TRIALS — OE02

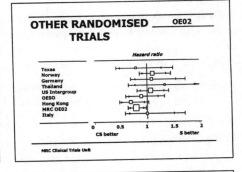

MRC Clinical Trials Unit

CONCLUSION — OE02

OE02 suggests that pre-operative chemotherapy of 2 cycles of cisplatin and fluorouracil significantly improves survival without increasing post-operative morbidity when compared with surgery alone

MRC Clinical Trials Unit

PARTICPATING CENTRES: — OE02

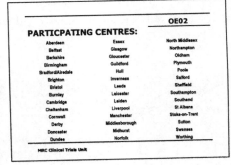

Aberdeen	Essex	North Middlesex
Belfast	Glasgow	Northampton
Berkshire	Gloucester	Oldham
Birmingham	Guildford	Plymouth
Bradford/Airedale	Hull	Poole
Brighton	Inverness	Salford
Bristol	Leeds	Sheffield
Burnley	Leicester	Southampton
Cambridge	Leiden	Southend
Cheltenham	Liverpool	St Albans
Cornwall	Manchester	Stoke-on-Trent
Derby	Middlesborough	Sutton
Doncaster	Midhurst	Swansea
Dundee	Norfolk	Worthing

MRC Clinical Trials Unit

Fig. 10.2 (Continued).

be useful or appropriate. Some trials, particularly perhaps those relating to primary care and public health, will naturally capture the public imagination and the potential for interest in the lay press will be clear. In these situations, many journals will write their own press release, making it available to the media prior to publication, although they will apply embargoes preventing discussion of the results before the publication date. For others it will be less clear if the interests of the research, or its potential to impact on the clinical community, will really be enhanced by this approach. However, for publicly funded research, press releases can be a means of showing that public money has been well spent while for research charities, it can be an excellent means of raising awareness and thus generating income.

If the results of a trial are likely to have a major impact, then it may be useful to have prepared a press release in advance of the publication which explains the results and their implications clearly, and in your own words. As a rule, these should be no more than a page long, and be written in a series of short paragraphs. The first paragraph should provide a self-contained summary of the research results and implications, with subsequent paragraphs elaborating on aspects in decreasing order of importance. The reason for this 'inverted triangle' approach is that editors will rarely have space to use an entire press release, and will inevitably precis by cutting from the bottom up. Some trials will generate a lot of interest and dealing with media inquiries can take up a great deal of time. The media particularly like attributed quotes and so a useful tip is to include a direct quote from the lead researcher in the press release which can be lifted out. Box 10.2 gives an example from a press release reporting the results of a meta-analysis of chemotherapy for malignant glioma [12].

Press releases may lead to requests for interviews, and it is helpful if one or more of the lead investigators are prepared to be interviewed. If this is likely to be a regular occurrence, then it is well worth considering a short media training course. Some general guidance for media interviews includes:

- Never reveal findings that are still provisional or confidential or that have not yet been conveyed to collaborating centres or been subjected to independent peer review.
- Do not discuss results prior to publication.
- If given the option, it is usually better to choose a live broadcast rather than a recorded one. In this way potential editorial distortion is avoided, although the experience is likely to be more nerve-racking.
- If offered only a recorded interview, then ask to see or hear the edited version before it is broadcast.

Box 10.2   Example of a direct quote in a pre-prepared press release

Lesley Stewart, Head of the MRC Clinical Trials Unit Meta-analysis Group at the Clinical Trials Unit said: 'This is a comprehensive review of trials worldwide giving the most reliable estimate of the benefit of this treatment, that patients, their families and doctors can use to help make choices about treatment options.'

- Give a fair and balanced account, emphasizing the scientific validity of the trial and the implications of its results for routine practice. Explain both the advantages and disadvantages of a new treatment policy. Avoid being enticed into using inappropriate 'major breakthrough' terminology.
- Acknowledge the importance of the patients who took part.

Finally, when any lay media interest can be anticipated, it can be very helpful to contact relevant patient support and information groups with information in advance so that they can be prepared for questions which may come their way.

10.6.3 Informing the trial patients and/or their families

The importance of the patients who volunteered to take part in a clinical trial should not be forgotten once the trial is over. It may well be appropriate to provide the patients and/or their relatives with a summary of the results of the trial, and where this is done it should be available as soon as the results are published. However, the potential impact of the results on the patients must be borne in mind, particularly in relation to the treatment the individual patient actually received. It will often be most appropriate to provide the clinicians who took part in the trial with a supply of the summaries, and for them to determine the best way to approach patients, rather than to contact patients directly. To prepare for some of the questions that a trial participant may have, it can be extremely useful to hold a meeting to discuss the trial results with relevant consumer groups before the results are published, and to involve them when producing a summary for patients. For further discussion of this issue, see Chapter 2.

10.7 Interpreting trials

When reading or reviewing a trial report, bear in mind all the aspects of relevance to good reporting. However, this alone may not be sufficient to determine whether you should agree with the conclusion. We review here some points to consider when trying to determine if a trial result or conclusion might be falsely negative, falsely positive or falsely equivalent.

10.7.1 Is the result (or conclusion) falsely negative?

A trial report may have described all the essential aspects in full detail. The result is reported as 'negative' or 'not significant.' Is that all you need to know? Almost certainly not. Firstly, the authors may simply be stating that the trial has failed to find as significant the size of difference it was designed to detect. Was the size of difference reasonable – would a smaller difference still be clinically relevant? If so, the trial may simply have been underpowered to detect the size of difference which some may consider important, and an appropriate conclusion *may* be that a larger trial is needed. However, such a conclusion, like any other, needs to consider the weight of evidence. How close was the observed difference to the desired difference? As discussed previously, this kind of judgement is much easier to make if an estimate of the treatment effect is given.

Secondly, recall that the power of a study $(1-\beta)$ is the probability of detecting a specified difference at a specified significance level, if it really exists. At the commonly used power level of 90 per cent, each trial of a truly effective treatment has a one in ten chance of being falsely negative, in other words of the play of chance alone reducing the size of difference observed. Is it possible to tell if a single, adequately powered, trial represents a false negative? Sadly no, or at least not with 100 per cent confidence, which explains why it is so important to design trials with the highest possible power. Some guidance is given by considering the trial's 'internal and external validity.' For example, are the results with respect to the main outcome measure consistent with results for other outcome measures within the same trial? For a study with survival as an outcome measure, are endpoints such as recurrence or response available? Do they show the same trends? This may give an indication of internal validity. If other relevant trials are available, a comparison with them will indicate whether the result observed in a single trial is in some sense an outlier.

One final danger with a 'negative' trial is that it may be reported as having demonstrated that two treatments are equivalent. Such a conclusion needs very careful investigation. A non-statistically significant difference alone is insufficient evidence of equivalence. One needs to consider the confidence interval for the treatment effect, and determine whether it truly excludes the possible differences which would lead one to conclude that in fact there is a clinically relevant difference between treatments. If the 95 per cent CI includes such differences, then the estimated treatment difference in the trial does not differ significantly from these relevant differences (at the 5 per cent level) and a conclusion of 'equivalence' would be inappropriate.

10.7.2   Is the result (or conclusion) falsely positive?

Authors of 'negative' trials will often spend some time discussing the possible reasons why the results were not as they had hoped, and will search for and discuss possible flaws in the design or conduct which may have contributed to the result being falsely negative. Once these have been dismissed, the discussion may move on to the quality of the evidence used to justify the study in the first place. Rather less time is generally spent by the authors of 'positive' trials discussing if their results are falsely positive. Of course this is understandable; the trial would not have been done if they had not had some reason to believe the intervention would be effective. However, the need for critical review and discussion of such trials – by both authors and 'consumers' – is just as great as for negative trials. More so in fact, since these are the trials that are most likely to change practice.

It is important therefore to consider all the important elements of trial design and conduct described in the CONSORT checklist. Specific items which tend to over-estimate a treatment benefit and therefore require particular intention include: (a) exclusion of patients who fail to complete protocol treatment (particularly in trials which compare standard treatment with or without an additional treatment component), (b) examination of multiple outcomes, with or without selective reporting of 'positive' outcomes and (c) early stopping of a trial without adherence to pre-specified stopping rules or guidelines.

Point (a) represents a failure to analyse a trial by intention to treat, and the biases this can cause are described in Section 9.4.1. Point (b) refers to the fact that the probability of a false positive increases with the number of hypothesis tests that are performed. If a trial is reported as positive on the basis of one positive result amongst an analysis of multiple outcome measures, or assessment times, then it deserves particular caution. While both these points are fairly widely understood, point (c) is perhaps less well recognized. Interim analyses represent a form of multiple testing. The size of difference in treatment effect between two treatments will fluctuate during the course of a trial, most extremely when total numbers are small, iterating to the 'correct' result as the sample size approaches the target number. The more often you examine the data the greater the chance of analysing it when there is, by chance, an extreme difference. Formal stopping rules, as described in Section 9.5, guard against this by demanding extreme p-values to justify stopping, but even so the treatment effect in a trial which stops early will generally be over-estimated. What may be less obvious, is that regular examinations of data without formal testing raise the same issues. This can be a particular problem in a single centre study, where the responsible clinicians know all the patients in the trial and are aware of their treatment allocation and their status. Effectively, such a trial is subject to almost continuous monitoring, and if a formal analysis is carried out based on concern of a difference emerging, it requires as cautious an interpretation as if regular formal analyses had been carried out.

If a trial meets all the standards of CONSORT, then is it safe to assume that it is a true positive? From trial design, we know that the probability of concluding a difference exists when in truth the treatments do not differ in efficacy is simply the significance level, α. If the trial has been designed with a two-sided hypothesis, then the probability that a trial will show a benefit to one of the treatments, when in fact it is no better than the other treatment, is $\alpha/2$. For many trials, this is 0.025, which is reassuringly small. However, another factor to bear in mind is the prevalence of truly effective treatments. Where this is high, the proportion of positive results that are true positives will be high; where it is low (more often the case in oncology), the proportion of positive results that are true positives will be low.

It is impossible to tell for sure if a given positive result is a true positive or a false positive, but considerations of internal and external validity may again give some support.

To illustrate some of these issues, we discuss a trial comparing surgery alone versus chemoradiation followed by surgery in operable oesophageal cancer patients [13], which reported significant benefits to the chemoradiation after stopping early.

The trial had a planned sample size of 190 patients, based on detecting an absolute benefit of 20 per cent (with 80 per cent power). No formal stopping rules were described, but the authors stated 'Early indications of a clinically relevant difference between treatments suggested that an interim analysis should be undertaken. The trial was closed six years after it began because a statistically significant difference between the groups was found.' At trial closure, 113 patients had been randomized. There has been much discussion of this trial, mentioning in particular the much poorer than expected results in the surgery alone group and the possibility of imbalance in the initial staging of the patients (only post-operative staging was reported). In fact, reviewing the Walsh trial against the CONSORT checklist, reveals several points that are not adequately described, including the method and timing of randomization. It is perhaps the statement about monitoring which has attracted least attention, but is a serious cause for concern. In a single centre trial such as this, it is perhaps inevitable that a form of almost subconscious continuous monitoring goes on, and understandable that in the apparent absence of formal stopping rules, concern about a possible difference should lead to a formal analysis. This could have been avoided had an independent data monitoring and ethics committee been convened to review the data regularly (see Section 8.10), or even to review the data at the point of concern and advise on a course of action. The authors, in the absence of independent advice, may have felt ethically bound to close the trial. Certainly, having done so, it was important that the results were published. What the reader can do is consider, given the circumstances, how convincing their p-value of 0.01 was in the context of what was effectively continuous monitoring. Although this trial has been cited as evidence of the benefit of pre-operative chemoradiotherapy by some, others felt the need for confirmatory trials to be performed.

Clinical versus statistical significance

A slightly different type of false positive arises when a trial result for a given outcome measure is statistically significant, but not clinically important. This can occur if the study was over-powered for that outcome measure. Clearly it is unlikely that this would ever happen for a primary outcome measure if the sample size was estimated correctly, as it would be ethically dubious to randomize more patients than are strictly necessary to detect clinically relevant differences. Such a finding may though arise with respect to a secondary outcome measure, or through a meta-analysis of the primary outcome measure in several trials. Meta-analyses in particular provide the opportunity to detect even small differences reliably, and it is important not to let extreme p-values detract from the need to consider the clinical relevance of the size of the difference observed. An example of the former can be seen in the MRC/EORTC TE20 trial of three versus four courses of BEP chemotherapy for metastatic germ cell tumours described earlier [10]. In this, the primary outcome measure was progression–free survival, and quality of life was a secondary outcome measure. Based on the primary outcome, 800 patients were required. When the quality of life data was analysed [11], the subscales were transformed to a 1–100 scale, and a change of 10 points taken as a moderate difference which would be noticeable by the patient. In fact, the study was overpowered for such differences for many of the subscales and the study generated several statistically significant results when the actual changes were much less than 10 per cent. In this case, the authors themselves point this out when discussing the interpretation of the results; had no consideration been given to the size of difference which might be clinically relevant, the authors may well have come to different conclusions.

10.8 Conclusion

This chapter describes the important issues to address when writing or reading a trial report. The widespread adoption of the CONSORT guidelines for reporting trials by medical journals is a major step forward, which should improve the quality of reporting considerably. What it cannot do is dictate how authors will interpret their results, or how 'consumers' will interpret and use them. Inevitably this will mean that positive results may be over-emphasized and negative results often explained away as a consequence of inadequate power according to the authors' pre-conceptions. It is then the responsibility of the reader to put aside pre-conceptions, to be equally critical of positive and negative results, and to know when to be cautious of either.

References

[1] Begg, C., Cho, M., Eastwood, S., Horton, R., Moher, D., Olkin, I., Pitkin, R., Rennie, D., Schulz, K.F., Simel, D., and Stroup, D.F. (1996) Improving the quality of reporting of randomized controlled trials – The CONSORT statement. *Journal of the American Medical Association*, 276(8), 637–9.

[2] Moher, D., Schulz, K.F., and Altman, D.G. (2001) The CONSORT statement: revised recommendations for improving the quality of reports of parallel-group randomised trials. *Lancet*, 357(9263), 1191–4.

[3] Altman, D.G., Schulz, K.F., Moher, D., Egger, M., Davidoff, F., Elbourne, D., Gotzsche, P.C., and Lang, T. (2001) The revised CONSORT statement for reporting randomized trials: Explanation and elaboration. *Annals of Internal Medicine*, 134(8), 663–94.

[4] Cook, R.J. and Sackett, D.L. (1995) The number needed to treat: a clinically useful measure of treatment effect. *British Medical Journal*, 310, 452–4.

[5] Altman, D.G. (1998) Confidence intervals for the number needed to treat. *British Medical Journal*, 317, 1309–12.

[6] Altman, D.G. and Anderson, P.K. (1999) Calculating the number needed to treat for trials where the outcome is time to an event. *British Medical Journal*, 319, 1492–5.

[7] Smeeth, L., Haines, A., and Ebrahim, S. (1999) Numbers needed to treat derived from meta-analyses: sometimes informative, usually misleading. *British Medical Journal*, 318, 1548–51.

[8] Hutton, J.L. (2000) Number needed to treat: properties and problems (with discussion). *Journal of the Royal Statistical Society Series A*, 163(3), 403–19.

[9] Early Breast Cancer Trialists Collaborative Group. (2000) Favourable and unfavourable effects on long-term survival of radiotherapy for early breast cancer: an overview of the randomised trials. *Lancet*, 355(9217), 1757–70.

[10] de Wit, R., Roberts, J.T., Wilkinson, P.M., de Mulder, P.H.M., Mead, G.M., Fosså, S.D., Cook, P., de Prijck, L., Stenning, S., and Collette, L. (2001) Equivalence of 3 BEP versus 4 cycles and of the 5 day schedule versus 3 days per cycle in good prognosis germ cell cancer, a randomized study of the European Organization for Research and Treatment of Cancer Genitourinary Tract Cancer Cooperative Group and the Medical Research Council. *Journal of Clinical Oncology*, 19, 1629–40.

[11] Medical Research Council Oesophageal Cancer Working Party. (2002) Surgical resection with or without preoperative chemotherapy in oesophageal cancer: a randomised controlled trial. *Lancet*, 359, 1727–33.

[12] Glioma Meta-analysis Trialists (GMT) Group. (2002) Chemotherapy in adult high-grade glioma: a systematic review and meta-analysis of individual patient data from 12 randomised trials. *Lancet*, 359(9311), 1011–18.

[13] Walsh, T.N., Noonan, N., Hollywood, D., Kelly, A., Keeling, N., and Hennessy, T.P.J. (1996) A comparison of multimodal therapy and surgery for esophageal adenocarcinoma. *New England Journal of Medicine*, 335(7), 462–7.

Chapter 11

Systematic review and meta-analysis

11.1 Introduction

It should be self-evident that healthcare decisions should be based on the best possible evidence; that effective treatments should be used whilst ineffective or harmful ones should not. Yet it is only relatively recently that the principles of evidence-based medicine have been explicitly discussed and gained widespread acceptance. There is an increasing awareness that the evidence for and against medical treatments must be evaluated properly and with appropriate scientific rigour. So far this book has set out the rationale for randomized controlled trials (RCTs) and described their role as main building blocks in clinical research. Undoubtedly, RCTs provide the most appropriate methods for the unbiased primary assessment of competing therapies. However, individual trials do not always provide the solutions that we seek and we need to look across trials at the totality of evidence. Consequently, there has been a vast increase in the number of systematic reviews and meta-analyses that have been undertaken in recent years [1] (Fig. 11.1).

Systematic reviews and meta-analyses provide an objective way of assembling, assessing and summarizing the evidence from RCTs, thereby providing a structured foundation for evidence-based medicine. The main reasons for systematic review and meta-analysis concern the need for completeness, for unbiased assessment, for synthesis and for statistical power. Probably the most important of these is the need to look at all the relevant evidence, so that evaluations and recommendations are based on the results of all trials and not just the published or well known ones. Another driving force is the need for summary and synthesis. Healthcare professionals, researchers, policy makers and indeed members of the public are relying increasingly on the process of systematic review. Faced with unmanageable amounts of information, they require reliable summaries of research on which to base clinical and policy decisions [2] and to guide future research. There

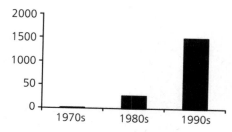

Fig. 11.1 Number of meta-analyses of randomized trials published during three decades.

simply isn't sufficient time to read all relevant primary publications. Even enthusiastic clinical teachers estimate their median reading time at only two hours per week, yet it is estimated that general physicians would need to read seventeen articles a day every day of the year in order to keep up to date in their field [3]. In the past, review articles have been the main means of synthesizing medical information, but there has been considerable criticism of this approach [4]. In contrast to reports of primary research, traditional narrative reviews rarely make their objectives and methods explicit and can represent little more than the subjective opinions of their, usually, influential authors. Reviewers are often in the difficult position of trying to evaluate conflicting or equivocal studies based on a qualitative and perhaps selective reading of the literature. Indeed, it has been suggested that:

'because reviewers have not used scientific methods, advice on some life-saving therapies has been delayed for more than a decade while other treatments have been recommended long after controlled research has shown them to be harmful [5].'

In contrast, systematic reviews use explicit methodology, aim to assess all relevant evidence objectively, and go to considerable lengths to achieve unbiased assessment [6]. Where appropriate, meta-analysis offers a quantitative means of combining this evidence and, in doing so, of increasing statistical power and precision.

11.1.1 Definitions

A number of terms are used concurrently to describe the process of systematic review and integration of research evidence. These include *systematic review, meta-analysis, research synthesis, overview* and *pooling* [7] and there is sometimes confusion in the way the terms are used. Throughout this chapter we use the term systematic review to denote the entire process of locating, assembling and appraising trials, and meta-analysis to describe the process of quantitative synthesis whereby the results of RCTs are combined.

Systematic review: Means of reviewing clearly formulated questions, using explicit methodology, to minimize bias in the location, selection, critical evaluation and synthesis of research evidence.
Meta-analysis: Means of quantitatively combining the results of research studies to provide overall summary statistics.

Thus, a systematic review may or may not include a meta-analysis element, depending on whether it is appropriate or possible, and a good quality meta-analysis should always be done in the context of a systematic review. This distinction is important as there are many examples of meta-analyses that are not products of systematic review. Throughout the chapter, discussions are restricted to reviews and meta-analyses of randomized trials, we do not cover similar explorations of epidemiological studies, although many of the issues discussed are also relevant to such projects.

11.2 Why we need systematic reviews and meta-analyses

It is generally accepted that the best primary evidence on the effectiveness of healthcare interventions comes from the results of well-designed and well-conducted RCTs. As in any scientific experiment, the observed effect in a clinical trial is composed of the true

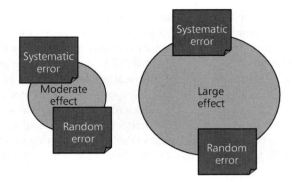

Fig. 11.2 Schematic representation of the effect of random and systematic error in a research project. Reproduced with permission from [8].

underlying effect plus the effect of both random and systematic error (Fig. 11.2) (see also Section 3.4.1).

Random error can, of course, never be eliminated, but it can be minimized by evaluating the data from large numbers of patients (see Section 3.4.1 and Chapter 5). Systematic error or bias can arise through poor design or conduct of a study, and its effects can easily be as large or larger than the size of clinically important treatment effects [9]. This is likely to be most problematic if the underlying true effect is moderate. The aim of any systematic review and meta-analysis should be to minimize both types of errors. The systematic component addresses the issue of bias and the meta-analysis element addresses the issue of numbers and random error. The observed effect should then be as close as possible to the true underlying effect, thereby providing a reliable and realistic estimate on which to base treatment policy and future research.

11.2.1 Reducing the effect of random error

In most areas of medicine, major breakthroughs are rare and we may generally anticipate that even the best new treatments will result in only modest improvements in outcome. Such benefits may, of course, be extremely important to individuals and could, in common diseases, have considerable impact on public health. Unfortunately, achieving the large numbers required is not always straightforward and many individual RCTs are too small to detect moderate but potentially worthwhile differences between treatments. A typical two-arm trial with 200–300 events is capable only of detecting absolute benefits in excess of 15 per cent, in other words improving outcome from 50 to 65 per cent or more. To detect a 5 per cent difference would require more than 2000 events (see also Section 5.4). Although there have been some notable successes in conducting large-scale trials in cancer (e.g. [10,11]), they remain very much in the minority. It seems likely that for many practical and political reasons, trials involving thousands of patients will be infeasible in many circumstances. Thus, if the underlying true effect is modest, in any group of trials addressing similar questions and with a few hundred events in each, by chance alone a few trials may have demonstrated statistically significant positive or negative results, but most will be inconclusive. However, combining the results of each of the trials in a meta-analysis might give sufficient statistical power to answer the questions reliably. The increased numbers of patients reduce the random error and narrow the confidence intervals around the result. This provides a more reliable and precise estimate of the size of any observed effect, and enables us to distinguish more easily between a real and null effect. Furthermore, narrowing the confidence intervals reduces the range of plausible treatment effects and so can aid clinical decision making considerably, especially where treatment effects are modest. For example, if we have an estimated hazard ratio of 0.85 with 95 per cent confidence interval 0.7–1.05, then we would be likely to be understandably cautious about adopting the new treatment. Although it suggests a 15 per cent relative benefit, the confidence interval is consistent with as much as a 30 per cent benefit, but also with a 5 per cent detriment. If, however, increased numbers in the trials narrow the intervals around the same estimated hazard ratio of 0.85 to 0.8–0.9, then we might adopt the new treatment more readily as the confidence intervals suggest a range between a 20 per cent benefit and a 10 per cent benefit. If the observed treatment effect is large, then we are less likely to need such tight confidence intervals before adopting treatment. If we have a hazard ratio of 0.5 in favour of the new treatment with confidence intervals 0.3–0.8, in most circumstances we would adopt the new treatment on this estimate and tightening the confidence interval would not affect clinical decision making. One use of meta-analysis is therefore to narrow confidence intervals such that similar clinical decisions would be reached based on the hazard ratio at either the lower or upper confidence limit.

11.2.2 Reducing the effect of bias

Unfortunately it is all too common for individual trials, which have produced the most striking results, to be emphasised in the medical literature. Perhaps the most important reason for performing systematic meta-analyses is to avoid this biased viewpoint. Conclusions on the relative merits of therapies should be based on the results of all relevant trials, irrespective of whether or where they have been published, or how much publicity they have received. In addition to this publication and reporting bias (Section 11.4.2), there are many aspects of the design, conduct, analysis and reporting of individual trials that may be subject to potential biases [12] and which could influence the trial results (see Chapters 4, 5 and 9). Any systematic review or meta-analysis should therefore appraise trials critically and any potential biases and problems should be noted and if possible rectified. If important problems remain, careful consideration should be given as to whether it is appropriate to include such trials in the systematic review.

11.2.3 Underlying assumptions of meta-analysis

The underlying assumption of meta-analysis is that in a group of randomized trials addressing similar questions, the true differences between treatments are likely to be in same direction. The observed size of effect may vary from trial to trial and in a small number of cases the direction may be reversed by chance alone. Although we cannot assume that the effect of a treatment given in different trials to different patient populations will be to produce exactly the same risk reduction, it is reasonable to assume that the net effect of treatment will tend to be in the same direction. Although the direction of effect may be obscured in any one trial, when all the evidence is considered, the benefit or detriment of treatment will be reflected in the overall pattern of individual trial results. The combination of these results provides an estimate of the 'average' treatment effect.

11.3   Different types of meta-analysis

All meta-analyses should be conducted in the context of a systematic review and should analyse all appropriate data in order to reduce bias. Although many papers published in the medical literature are described as meta-analyses, such projects are not all of a similar design, quality or validity. Although, there is a continuum in the effort that can be invested in ensuring that a meta-analysis is systematic and comprehensive, there are three broad types of data that can be obtained. Information can be extracted from published reports, summary data can be collected from trialists, or individual patient data (IPD) can be obtained from trialists. These IPD projects involve the central collection, validation and re-analysis of, usually updated, 'raw' data, from all clinical trials, worldwide, that have addressed a common research question; obtained from those responsible for the original trials [13]. Although they are less common than other types of review, they are becoming increasingly used in a wide range of healthcare areas. IPD meta-analyses have an established history in cardiovascular disease and cancer, where the methodology has been developing steadily since the late 1980s. In cancer, for example, more than fifty IPD meta-analyses of screening and treatment across a wide range of solid tumour sites and haematological malignancies have been completed [14]. IPD has also been used in systematic reviews in a number of other fields including Alzheimers disease [15], dyspepsia, epilepsy [16], malaria, HIV infection [17] and hernia [18,19].

However, meta-analyses which use aggregate data either supplied directly by trialists, or more frequently extracted from published reports, are less resource-intensive and more common.

11.3.1   Comparing IPD and other approaches

Given the extra resource and commitment required, it is reasonable to question the need for the IPD approach. There is evidence that meta-analyses based only on data extracted from published papers may give estimates of treatment effects, and of their significance, that are not confirmed when all the randomized evidence is re-analysed in an IPD meta-analysis [20–22]. For example, a comparison of an IPD meta-analysis in advanced ovarian cancer (of platinum-based combination chemotherapy versus single-agent non-platinum drugs) [23] with a similar analysis using only data that could be extracted from the published papers (Table 11.1), found that the IPD analysis gave less encouraging results [20].

In this study the aim was to compare the overall differences in outcome between the approaches; comparing the policy of extracting data from published reports with the policy of collecting IPD. The analysis of published summary data, which included eight trials and 788 patients, favoured combination chemotherapy with an estimated improvement in survival at thirty months of 7.5 per cent. This was marginally significant at conventional levels ($p = 0.027$). The IPD meta-analysis which was based on eleven trials and 1329 patients suggested only a 2.5 per cent improvement and this did not reach conventional levels of significance ($p = 0.30$). Further investigation revealed that the

Table 11.1 Comparison of meta-analysis approaches using an example in advanced ovarian cancer

	Individual patient data from trialists	Data extracted from publications
Trials	11	8
Patients	1329	788
Odds ratio	–	0.71
Hazard ratio	0.93	–
95 per cent confidence interval	0.83–1.05	0.52–0.96
p-value	0.30	0.027
Absolute benefit at thirty months	2.5%	7.5%
Comments	Median follow up 6.5 years	Point estimate at 30 months

differences between the two approaches were attributable to a number of factors. These included:

- missing trials (unpublished plus those which did not publish the required information),
- excluded patients,
- the point in time at which analyses using data from publications were based,
- method of analysis,
- additional long-term follow-up which was available with the IPD approach.

None of these factors were found to be very much more important than the others. Rather they each contributed cumulatively to the difference. The analysis based on the summary data available from published reports not only provided a conventionally statistically significant result but gave an estimated benefit three times larger than that suggested by the IPD. Given the poor prognosis for advanced ovarian cancer, when balanced against other factors such as toxicity, ease of administration and cost, the clinical interpretation of the results from the two approaches could well be different.

A similar investigation, comparing the results of an IPD review with analyses using data from published papers of trials comparing ovarian ablation with control in the treatment of breast cancer also found differences in the results obtained by the two approaches [24]. However, in this case, it was the IPD that gave the strongest evidence in favour of the intervention. The meta-analysis of published data available in 1990 was inconclusive about the effect of ovarian ablation. However, the meta-analysis using IPD, largely because of prolonged follow up, showed a significant reduction in the annual odds of death with an absolute improvement in overall survival of 10.2 per cent at fifteen years for women randomized to ovarian ablation.

In contrast, an investigation comparing the results of different types of meta-analysis of trials investigating selective decontamination of the digestive tract (a form of antibiotic

Table 11.2 Comparison of meta-analysis approaches using an example in selective decontamination of the digestive tract [25]

Type of meta-analysis	Deaths/Patients	Odds ratio	95% CI
Data extracted from publications	762/3142	0.87	0.74–1.03
Summary data obtained from trialists	975/3564	0.92	0.80–1.08
IPD obtained from trialists	829/3357	0.89	0.76–1.05

prophylaxis for patients in intensive care units) found that there was little difference between three types of approach (Table 11.2) [25]. This comparison used data from seventeen trials for which all three methods of systematic review (data extracted from publications, tabular summary data provided by trialists or IPD provided by trialists) could be used, out of a total of twenty-five trials including 4310 patients identified as relevant to the therapeutic question.

In this case the authors concluded that despite the advantages of IPD, the approach is costly and that analysis of summary data provided by study investigators is a valid alternative to IPD, when categorical data are used and censoring is not relevant. Here the authors aimed to compare the differences attributable only to the data type used and exactly the same trials were used in each analysis. It is not clear how the additional eight trials (where data were not available in all three formats) would have affected the outcome in terms of the estimates achieved with the most comprehensive and inclusive analysis possible with each of the three approaches.

These examples illustrate the difficulties of trying to generalize and extrapolate from literature-based analyses. In most cases, it will not be possible to estimate whether the results of such analyses will differ from analyses based on the full IPD, and if so in which direction and to what extent they will be changed, until the IPD has been collected and analysed.

11.3.2 Potential benefits of the IPD approach

As implied in the conclusions of the above study, a major benefit of IPD is that it allows time-to-event analysis (see Section 11.5.7). Although there are methods that allow us to estimate and combine time-to-event summary statistics from published reports [26], in practice this can prove extremely difficult as the required information is seldom presented in a usable format. Thus, the ability to conduct time-to-event analyses across all trials might be reason in itself for collecting IPD in illnesses, including many cancers, where prolongation of survival, or time to recurrence of disease or onset of symptoms is important. The IPD approach is the only practical way to carry out analyses to investigate whether any observed treatment effect is consistent across well-defined groups of patients, indeed this might be the only context in which it is reasonable to explore subgroups (see Section 11.5.7).

Where trials have used different classifications or scales of measurement e.g. different tumour staging systems, or different units for recording haemoglobin, IPD may provide the opportunity to translate between scales and combine data, a process that might not otherwise be feasible. It also allows detailed data checking to ensure consistency and quality of randomization and follow-up. Importantly, it also means that up-to-date follow-up information can be collected and thereby provides a valuable opportunity to look at longer-term outcomes. Some additional advantages of direct collaboration with trialists, when collecting either IPD or summary data from source, is that this contact can result in more complete identification of relevant trials and better compliance in providing missing data. Discussions with the trialists during the project can also aid interpretation and wider endorsement and dissemination of the results and to better clarification of, and collaboration in, further research. For these reasons IPD meta-analyses are considered by many to be the 'yardstick' against which other forms of systematic review should be measured [27].

11.3.3 Potential costs of the IPD approach

It is often said that IPD reviews are much more time-consuming and expensive than other forms of systematic review [28]. However, this assumption is often based on comparison with meta-analyses of the published data that have been done with minimum effort, rather than with high quality systematic reviews, such as those carried out by the Cochrane Collaboration [6]. Furthermore, since resource comparisons were first discussed, technological progress has enabled some of the labour-intensive aspects of IPD meta-analysis to be done more easily, quickly and cheaply.

Most organizations now store their trial data on computer and most researchers have access to e-mail. This makes data collation and provision less time-consuming both for trialists providing data and for the team receiving it. Both the time taken to transfer data and the effort involved in assembling the meta-analysis database are reduced. Queries about data can easily be done by e-mail. Maintaining contact is also much easier using e-mailing lists and website bulletins. Software advances have also meant that data are now much more easily transferred between different types of database package, and that the format in which data are supplied is seldom a problem. Packages themselves have become more adaptable with many useful features. Little specialist programming expertise is now required to set up and run new IPD projects.

A key but time-consuming aspect of IPD meta-analysis is contacting trialists and persuading them to participate and provide data. However, the time taken to negotiate the provision of summary data is likely to be similar and time spent on this activity can be partially offset against time taken to contact authors for clarification of information presented in published reports. One aspect of IPD meta-analyses that adds to the cost and which is not encountered in other forms of review is funding collaborators' meetings where the collaborative group of trialists providing data and the researchers organizing the project meet to discuss the results. Although not normal practice, such meetings could also be useful where trialists supply summary data.

11.3.4 Choosing which approach is appropriate

Although, on balance, IPD reviews are likely to be more costly and time-consuming, the difference in resource requirements for different types of well-conducted systematic reviews may not be as great as is often thought. It is, of course, not always necessary to

Table 11.3 Factors that may influence the systematic review approach. Modified and reproduced with permission from [29]

When IPD may be beneficial	When IPD may not be beneficial
Poor reporting of trials. Information inadequate, selective or ambiguous	Detailed and clear and unbiased reporting of trials (CONSORT quality)
Long-term outcomes	Short-term outcomes
Time-to-event outcome measures	Binary outcome measures
Multivariate or other complex analyses	Univariate or simple analyses
Differently defined outcome measures	Outcome measures defined uniformly across trials
Subgroup analyses of patient-level characteristics important	Patient subgroups not important
IPD available for high proportion of trials/individuals	IPD available for only a limited number of trials
High proportion of individuals excluded from analyses	Reported analyses include almost all individuals

go to the lengths of collecting IPD. For example, if we are interested in binary outcomes that are likely to occur relatively quickly, where all relevant trials are published and data presented in a comprehensive and compatible way, then the most straightforward of meta-analyses based on data presented in trial publications, is probably all that is required. However, such an extreme is likely to be rare and usually unpublished trials will need to be assessed and trialists contacted to provide at least some additional summary data.

At the outset of any systematic review, the methodological factors likely to influence the results in that particular situation should be considered together with resource and time constraints so that an active decision can be taken about which approach to adopt. Table 11.3 gives some of the factors likely to influence this decision. The proportion of data available, in each of the formats, may also be a major factor in deciding which approach to take. For example, there would be little point collecting IPD if it were only available for very few trials, nor would it be useful to extract data from publications if only a very small proportion presented usable data.

11.4   Methodological principles of systematic review

There are a few underlying principles of methodology that should be adhered to when conducting a systematic review of RCTs, relating to the need to obtain complete data on all the randomized evidence.

11.4.1 Include *only* randomized trials

Randomized trials provide the best means of obtaining an unbiased and fair comparison between medical treatments and the problems associated with non-randomized studies are well-documented [30]. As discussed in Chapter 4, prospective allocation by a method that ensures that treatment assignment cannot be known in advance, ensures that individuals cannot be selected to receive a particular intervention, and the process of randomization minimizes the likelihood of systematic differences between patient groups. Therefore, any observed differences should be due to differences in treatment and not to differences in the characteristics of the patients in the two groups. Therefore, most systematic reviews and meta-analyses of treatment interventions in cancer are restricted to 'properly' randomized trials, and any trials allocating treatment by quasi-random methods such as date of birth are excluded. Unfortunately, few published reports give adequate descriptions of randomization. For example, an examination of the first twenty RCTs reported in four leading general medical journals during 1987 found that only 40 per cent described the randomization process adequately [31]. Consequently, not all studies described in published reports as randomized can be assumed to be free of bias in the allocation of treatment. On further inquiry, it can turn out that 'randomization' has been done by birth-date, date of clinic visit, by alternate allocation, or by using pre-prepared lists with treatments correctly assigned randomly, but to which clinicians entering patients had free access. All of these could lead to bias. Furthermore, there is evidence that the method of concealment (how difficult it is to know or guess the next treatment to be allocated) is correlated with trial outcome, such that those trials with the most secure methods of allocation tend to give the least positive results [32]. It is therefore important that all systematic reviews of RCTs should ensure that included trials are indeed randomized.

11.4.2 Include *all* randomized trials

It is widely acknowledged that RCTs with statistically significant results are more likely to be published than those with non-significant results (publication bias). This arises from both editorial policy and because investigators themselves often do not submit negative or inconclusive results for publication [33]. As a consequence of selective publication, the medical literature can give a skewed or biased picture of the evidence on a particular question. Thus, to obtain a balanced view, it is important that all the randomized evidence is considered, irrespective of whether or not it is published.

Some would argue that unpublished trials should not be included in a systematic review as they have not been subject to peer review and are therefore unreliable. However, for IPD reviews, this criticism can be countered by obtaining the trial protocol, and by careful checking of the IPD supplied by the trialist. In fact, checking IPD should be considerably more rigorous than is possible during peer review of a manuscript. Checking unpublished summary data provided by trialists may be more difficult and will depend on the level of detail of the information supplied. Care must therefore be taken with this type of data, which has neither the benefit of peer review nor the extensive data checking that is possible with IPD. It should be noted that publication of a well-written paper in a high profile journal does not necessarily guarantee the quality of the trial data.

Any meta-analysis that relies on the published literature alone will always be at risk of bias towards the positive which will be reflected in the review and, potentially, could lead to unjustified conclusions and to inappropriate decisions about patient care, health policy and future clinical research. To deal with this, even when a researcher is unable to obtain and/or review information from unpublished sources, they should identify and list as many of such trials as possible. This then gives some indication as to the possible effect that these might have on an analysis of published trials alone. For example, we would have more confidence in the results of a meta-analysis of published trials including 5000 patients and lacking 500 patients from unpublished sources than in one of 2000 patients but where a further 1500 patients from unpublished trials were missing.

Conversely, an ongoing issue is what to do about trials for which IPD are not available, for whatever reason (e.g. loss or destruction of data, or unwillingness to collaborate). If unavailability is related to the trial results; for example, if trialists are keen to supply data from trials with promising results but reluctant to provide data from those that were less encouraging, then ignoring the trial could bias the results of the IPD analysis. If a large proportion of the data have been obtained, we can be relatively confident of the results, but with less information we need be suitably circumspect in drawing conclusions. Sensitivity analysis combining the results of any unavailable trials (as extracted from publications) and comparing these with the main IPD results can be a useful aid to interpreting the data (Section 11.5.7). As for other types of systematic review, IPD meta-analyses should clearly state what trials were not included and the reasons why.

11.4.3   Include trials once only

Individual trials are often reported several times, and it is important to ensure that each eligible trial is included only once in the systematic review and meta-analysis [34]. In practice, it can be quite difficult to determine when multiple publications refer to the same trial because authors may change, different numbers or subgroups of patients may be analysed and reported and the trial may be described differently. As it is likely to be the results of trials favouring new treatments that are reported and presented most often, this could exaggerate the influence of publication bias. It is therefore important to scrutinize publications extremely carefully to spot papers that are updates or duplicate reports of trials already represented in the systematic review.

In full papers, clues may be obtained by matching the trial accrual dates, lists of participating centres and details of treatment scheduling as well as the authors, patient numbers and general descriptions. However, it is almost impossible to do this with abstracts. Since trials are very likely to be presented at several meetings this can make things difficult and it is advisable to seek clarification from authors if trials appear similar. In an IPD meta-analysis, direct contact and collaboration with trialists should identify duplicate publications especially as they will ultimately need to supply the underlying dataset.

In future, if the unique identifying schemes currently in development (Box 11.1), become adopted widely then the problem of duplicate publication bias should be solved. As all publications should include the unique trial identifying number it will make it easy to spot at a glance where reports refer to the same trial.

Box 11.1 The International Standard Randomized Controlled Trial Number (ISRCTN)

For researchers conducting systematic reviews, difficulties can arise in determining publications that refer to the same trial, as, for example, authors differ, or numbers included in analyses vary between publications. Similar difficulties may occur where a trial is included in more than one register. Such problems could lead to double counting; including trials more than once in a systematic review, and consequently such trials receiving undue weight in any quantitative analyses. An internationally accepted, uniform system of unique trial identifiers would therefore be extremely useful to reviewers, making it immediately apparent where multiple reports or register entries refer to the same trial.

Although the concepts underpinning the ISRCTN scheme are not new, it represents the first time unique identifiers have been assigned to RCTs on an international basis. The ISRCTN scheme was launched in 2001 concentrating initially on UK cancer trials and on other UK MRC funded trials. However, funding organizations and individual trialists worldwide will be invited to participate in the scheme. The scheme, overseen by an independent advisory group, is managed by Current Controlled Trials, who are also responsible for the metaRegister of Controlled Trials (*m*RCT).

- The ISRCTN is an 8-digit number that is assigned to an RCT. It is used to uniquely identify a trial and remains with it through its duration, from funding, through the entirety of the trial process to eventual publication.

- The ISRCTN should be included in trial protocols, documentation and publications and presentations. It should also be recorded within online bibliographic databases and trial registers.

- The ISRCTN is issued to trials by the trial sponsor. Where sponsors do not administer ISRCTNs for the trials that they support, an ISRCTN can be obtained by the principal investigator on registering the trial with the *meta*Register.

The ISRCTN should, in future, promote widespread prospective registration and provide a more complete public record of RCTs, through the *m*RCT and contributing registers. The numbering system should facilitate identification of trials that appear on more than one register, and so help to prevent 'double-counting' of trials. As the scheme progresses, it is envisaged that journal editors will require ISRCTNs for all trials submitted for publication. This should further facilitate trial searching and allow reviewers to more easily identify duplicate publications of individual trials.

11.4.4 Include *all* and *only* randomized patients

All individuals who were randomized in a trial should be included in the analysis, and any patients who were not randomized should be excluded. Failure to do this could result in unpredictable bias. Unfortunately, not all trials follow this policy when reporting their results, and patients can be excluded (sometimes covertly) from published analysis for a number of reasons. Such patient exclusions, if related to treatment, could

Table 11.4 Sensitivity analysis – excluding certain pre-specified types of individual – from an IPD meta-analysis in soft tissue sarcoma. Modified and reproduced with permission from [36]

Patients included	Deaths / Patients	Hazard ratio	p-value
All patients	709 / 1568	0.90	0.157
All except patients: Less than 15 years With metastatic disease That received induction chemotherapy	691 / 1544	0.89	0.121
All except patients: With locally recurrent disease Less than fifteen years With metastatic disease That received induction chemotherapy	597 / 1366	0.91	0.278

seriously bias the results, for example, if patients are excluded because they are unable to tolerate the allocated therapy or follow the treatment schedule. An empirical study evaluating the impact of patient exclusion using information from several cancer IPD meta-analyses, comprising data from over 100 RCTs and thousands of patients found that meta-analyses that maintained the investigators' exclusions were more likely to favour the investigational treatment than those that analysed all randomized patients [35].

As IPD meta-analyses, or those collecting summary data from source, do not rely on the trialists' original analyses, trialists should be asked to provide data on all patients. Any randomized patient excluded from the original trial analyses can then be reinstated in the meta-analysis and any non-randomized patients can be removed from the dataset (in some cases non-randomized patients may be included in published analyses, for example, by including patients from a non-randomized pilot phase of the trial). Although not all trials may keep records of excluded patients, experience in the cancer field has been good and it has been possible to recover information from the majority of excluded patients. For example, in an IPD meta-analysis in soft tissue sarcoma [36], data were recovered on 99 per cent of the 344 patients that had been excluded from the investigators' own analyses. In a more recent meta-analysis in high-grade glioma data from 83 per cent of the 253 patients that had been excluded from the original analyses were recovered [37].

There can be good clinical reasons for excluding certain types of individuals from analyses. However, to be unbiased, any exclusions should be pre-specified and applied objectively and uniformly across trials. Ideally, their impact should be assessed by sensitivity analyses (including and excluding patients to determine whether it influences the estimated treatment effect) (see Section 11.5.7). In the soft tissue sarcoma IPD meta-analysis [36], in such pre-specified sensitivity analyses, exclusions made no appreciable impact on the estimated effect of chemotherapy (Table 11.4). A further advantage of having done these analyses is that it re-assures us as to the robustness of the results.

11.5 Practical methods for systematic review and meta-analysis

Whatever approach is taken, using data from publications, obtaining summary data directly from trialists or collecting IPD, it is vital that every effort is made to obtain all

Data from Publications

Data from Trialists
(IPD and Summary Tables)

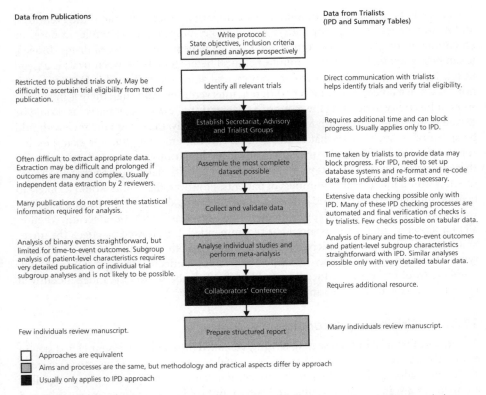

Restricted to published trials only. May be difficult to ascertain trial eligibility from text of publication.

Direct communication with trialists helps identify trials and verify trial eligibility.

Requires additional time and can block progress. Usually applies only to IPD.

Often difficult to extract appropriate data. Extraction may be difficult and prolonged if outcomes are many and complex. Usually independent data extraction by 2 reviewers.

Time taken by trialists to provide data may block progress. For IPD, need to set up database systems and re-format and re-code data from individual trials as necessary.

Many publications do not present the statistical information required for analysis.

Extensive data checking possible only with IPD. Many of these IPD checking processes are automated and final verification of checks is by trialists. Few checks possible on tabular data.

Analysis of binary events straightforward, but limited for time-to-event outcomes. Subgroup analysis of patient-level characteristics requires very detailed publication of individual trial subgroup analyses and is not likely to be possible.

Analysis of binary and time-to-event outcomes and patient-level subgroup characteristics straightforward with IPD. Similar analyses possible only with very detailed tabular data.

Requires additional resource.

Few individuals review manuscript.

Many individuals review manuscript.

Write protocol: State objectives, inclusion criteria and planned analyses prospectively

Identify all relevant trials

Establish Secretariat, Advisory and Trialist Groups

Assemble the most complete dataset possible

Collect and validate data

Analyse individual studies and perform meta-analysis

Collaborators' Conference

Prepare structured report

☐ Approaches are equivalent

▨ Aims and processes are the same, but methodology and practical aspects differ by approach

■ Usually only applies to IPD approach

Fig. 11.3 Stages of a systematic meta-analysis – modified and reproduced with permission from [29].

the relevant data and that appropriate methodology is used at all stages of the project (Fig. 11.3). The underlying principles are the same and, irrespective of the approach adopted, the same methods should be used by each up to the point of data collection.

As with a clinical trial, a good deal of planning and organization is required before a systematic review can be started. A good deal of resource is involved in this pre-data collection planning stage, which may take several months. During this time the research question will be refined, a prospective protocol will be developed and the required collaborative and organizational structures put in place. This will be followed by a period of data collection or abstraction, data verification and finally any quantitative analyses that are appropriate. Like a trial, the final phases of a systematic review involve the dissemination of results through presentation and publication.

11.5.1 Defining the question

Any systematic review should pose sensible questions that are clinically meaningful and methodologically appropriate. Although meta-analyses often emphasize the large numbers of individuals that are included, it is important that these numbers are not achieved at the expense of combining trials inappropriately. There is always likely to be a degree of trade-off between achieving statistical power and addressing tightly defined questions.

It will rarely be possible to combine trials comparing exactly the same interventions, and it is inevitable and appropriate to accept some variation, for example, in doses or scheduling of drugs or in the composition of regimens within a class of drugs. Indeed, it can be argued that a certain amount of clinical heterogeneity between trials is a good thing, because it is likely to be more representative of the real world. However, it is not usually sensible to combine very different interventions. Although there is inevitably some subjectivity in defining the scope of a systematic review, the comparisons should be driven by the clinical question to be addressed. Put simply, the systematic review should be specified in such a way that results will be clinically meaningful. For example, if a review of the role of palliative therapy in advanced lung cancer compared any palliative therapy including chemotherapy, radiotherapy, or nutritional support versus no treatment, it would include large numbers of patients. However, the results would be likely to be difficult to interpret. If good evidence of an effect was shown by the meta-analysis, it would not be clear which therapy or therapies were responsible for the effect and whether all or a subset of interventions should be recommended. If it showed no effect, the meta-analysis could be rightly criticized on the grounds that the results of trials of effective types of therapy may have been swamped by trials of ineffective therapies. So although numbers would be much reduced it would probably be better to look independently at each individual palliative therapy.

11.5.2   Writing a protocol

As with any formal clinical research, writing a detailed protocol is an essential first step in any systematic review. Developing a protocol makes a systematic review more rigorous as the methodology is specified at the outset. For example, rules concerning eligibility are made in advance of any results, and subset and subgroup analyses are pre-planned rather than *ad hoc*. Any deviations from the protocol should be explained in the completed review. Protocols are also valuable in helping to identify problems and clarify issues early in the project. A good protocol can also be invaluable in explaining and promoting the proposed review to potential collaborating trialists, serving to demonstrate the importance of the question, the appropriateness of methodology and competence of those undertaking the review, all of which can be important in persuading them to participate. Specifying inclusion criteria means that trials can be evaluated for suitability at an early stage. Although there may be a temptation to obtain data from all trials at the outset of the meta-analysis, a more measured approach makes it less likely that trials will have to be withdrawn or excluded after data have been prepared and provided. Time spent at this stage more than makes up for itself later, although it does mean that initiating collaborations may be delayed. Box 11.2 shows some of the items that should be considered for inclusion in a systematic review protocol.

11.5.3   Organizational structures

Although systematic reviews can be undertaken by individuals as one-off projects, they are more usually done by of a research group or organization. Those carried out as part of the Cochrane Collaboration (see Section 11.8) may be done by individual reviewers or by a group of co-reviewers. In either case the infrastructure provided by the collaboration, from the (disease/problem oriented) Collaborative Review Group, provides training, support and advice to the reviewer(s) as well as ensuring quality standards are met.

Box 11.2   Suggested items to be included in a systematic review protocol

- Rationale for systematic review
    Underlying biology and epidemiology
    Review of trials
- Objectives
- Main aims of review
    Main comparisons to be made
- Search strategies
- Inclusion/exclusion criteria
- Data to be collected
- Brief description of data checking procedures
- Analyses
    Main analyses to be performed
    Primary outcome measures
    Additional outcome measures
    Subset analyses and planned categories (Section 11.5.7.5)
    Subgroup analyses and planned categories (Section 11.5.7.6)
- Organization
    Organizational structures, e.g. Steering/Advisory Committee Personnel
- Sources of support
- Conflict of interest
- Publication policy
- Provisional timetable
- Provisional list of trials to be included
- Example data collection forms
- Data coding information

IPD meta-analyses are usually carried out as collaborative projects whereby all trialists contributing information from their studies, together with those managing the project, become part of an active collaboration. They are usually managed by a small local organizing group or secretariat, which may be aided in important and strategic decision making by a larger advisory group. Such an advisory group will usually comprise medical and possibly statistical or methodological experts relevant to the question addressed in the meta-analysis, and will often have international representation. The political and communication aspects of running these large collaborative projects are where they differ most from, and where they may be more time consuming than other types of systematic review. For example, during the initiation phase of an IPD project, a secretariat, advisory group and trialists group all need to be established. Moreover, throughout the project communication is essential to ensure that good relationships are developed and maintained with all collaborators, which can sometimes run to over a hundred individuals. The secretariat will usually also organize a face-to-face meeting of all collaborators, to bring individuals together to discuss the preliminary results. All publications and presentations are made in the name of the collaborative group, with members of the group and participating organizations usually listed in an appendix to the text. Prior to this, manuscripts are reviewed by the full collaborative group, which, if large, can be time-consuming.

11.5.4 Identifying trials

Systematic reviews should attempt to locate information on all pertinent trials and will almost always need to go beyond a simple search of bibliographic databases for relevant publications. Not only are positive trials more likely to be published than negative or inconclusive ones, but particularly striking results are perhaps more likely to be published in those English language [38] high-impact journals indexed by bibliographic databases. Furthermore, such databases do not cover all medical journals – MEDLINE, for example, indexes less than 4000 out of around 16,000 biomedical journals and EMBASE indexes 4000.

Systematic reviews that restrict trial identification to searches of bibliographic databases and exclude unpublished trials, trials published in non-English language journals, or those reported in the 'grey' literature (meeting abstracts, theses, etc.) can lead to exaggerated estimates of intervention effectiveness [39–41]. It is therefore important to employ a well thought out strategy for identifying trials. Failure to do so is likely to result in only a proportion of all eligible trials being identified (Fig. 11.4) and could bias the results of any systematic review. Box 11.3 lists various ways to search for trials depending on the question posed and the type of systematic review planned.

The Cochrane Collaboration has been responsible for a number of initiatives to make it easier for reviewers to identify RCTs. Since 1994 it has contributed to the retrospective re-tagging and indexing of 100,000 trials that were not previously indexed appropriately as RCTs in MEDLINE and has also been involved in a project to identify and re-tag trials within EMBASE. It is also responsible for compiling the Cochrane Controlled Trials Register (CENTRAL) that contains details of and citations to all reports of controlled trials that have been identified through its extensive systematic searches of the world medical literature, including searches of MEDLINE, EMBASE and an extensive programme of handsearching. CENTRAL is already the largest single source of RCT

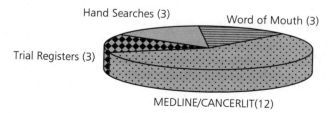

Fig. 11.4 Methods of identifying trials at initiation of a meta-analysis of neo-adjuvant chemotherapy for cancer of the uterine cervix [42].

Box 11.3   Methods to identify and locate RCTs

◆ Search Cochrane Controlled Trials Register (CENTRAL)

◆ Search MEDLINE, CANCERLIT, EMBASE

◆ If appropriate, search other bibliographic databases [43]
  e.g. Allied and Alternative Medicine, Biological Abstracts (BIOSIS) CAB Health, Cumulative Index to Nursing and Allied Health Literature (CINAHL), Derwent Drug File, Phychological Abstracts, Science Citation Index/Current Contents

◆ Hand search relevant un-indexed journals

◆ Hand search meeting proceedings

◆ Cross check bibliographies of identified trials

◆ Consult general registers

◆ Consult relevant specialist registers

◆ Consult pharmaceutical industry if appropriate

◆ Consult authors of identified trials

citations. At the end of 2001 it contained records of over 250,000 reports of controlled trials and it is the first place that many reviewers seek trials. At present, others prefer to use MEDLINE (or other commercial databases) as it has more sophisticated searching facilities and does not contain duplicate citations.

Even if CENTRAL is consulted as the primary source of trials, it is recommended that MEDLINE should also be searched for recent publications [43]. This is because RCTs are downloaded to CENTRAL from MEDLINE and other bibliographic databases by searching for those with the indexing term RCT. Recent trials will not have benefited from the additional safety net of the re-tagging exercise. Consequently, some RCTs may not be tagged appropriately and will therefore not be downloaded to CENTRAL. For the same reason reviewers should employ the Cochrane Collaboration search strategies [43] rather than rely on selection by the RCT index term. A free version of MEDLINE is available at www.ncbi.nlm.nih.gov/pubmed.

To gain a fuller coverage of journals, EMBASE should also be searched, the overlap with MEDLINE in indexed journals is only 34 per cent [44] and whereas MEDLINE indexes mostly journals published in the US, EMBASE has more of a European focus and includes a large number of non-English language journals. It also has a good coverage of pharmaceutical journals. Although searching bibliographic databases is often seen as a straightforward task, it requires both skill and experience to obtain the best results and inexperienced searchers should seek expert help. As an example, a modified (simplified) version of the Cochrane Collaboration search strategy for locating RCTs, combined with specific terms to locate trials of chemotherapy, radiotherapy or surgery in lung cancer is shown in Box 11.4.

Appropriate journals and meeting abstracts that are not indexed by the bibliographic databases selected and have not already been searched by a Cochrane group (in which

Box 11.4   Search strategy for MEDLINE to locate RCTs of chemotherapy, radiotherapy or surgery in lung cancer

1	randomized controlled trial.pt.	18	(lung adj cancer$).ab,ti.
2	exp Randomized Controlled Trials/	19	(lung adj neoplasm$).ab,ti.
3	exp Random Allocation/	20	cancer with lung.ab,ti.
4	exp Double Blind Method/	21	carcinoma with lung.ab,ti.
5	exp Single Blind Method/	22	16 or 17
6	1 or 2 or 3 or 4 or 5	23	18 or 19 or 20 or 21 or 22
7	clinical trial.pt.	24	exp Drug Therapy/
8	exp Clinical Trials/	25	drug therapy.ab,ti.
9	clin$ with trial.ab,ti.	26	chemotherapy.ab,ti.
10	(sing$ or doubl$ or trebl$ or tripl$ with blind$ or mask$).ab,ti.	27	25 or 26 or 27
		28	exp Radiotherapy/
11	exp Placebos	29	radiotherapy.ab,ti.
12	placebo$.ab,ti.	30	29 or 30
13	random$.ab,ti.	31	exp Surgery/
14	exp Research Design/	32	surgery.ab,ti.
15	7 or 8 or 9 or 10 or 11 or 12 or 13 or 14	33	32 or 33
16	exp Carcinoma/	34	28 or 31 or 34
17	exp Lung Neoplasms/ (lung adj carcinoma$).ab,ti.	35	6 or 15
		36	36 and 24 and 35

case they would already be included in CCTR) should be searched by hand for relevant trials. A master-list of journals searched by Cochrane groups can be found on their web-site at www.cochrane.org/srch.htm.

The bibliographies of identified trials should be cross-checked for references to further trials and the bibliographies of appropriate review articles and books should also be searched (in the awareness that the most cited references are also likely to be the ones that favour investigational interventions). General trial registers and relevant specialist registers should also be searched (Table 11.5). Details of registers can be found as an appendix to the Cochrane handbook at www.cochrane.org/cochrane/hbook.htm. Where appropriate, providers of trial data and other experts in the field, and the pharmaceutical industry may be consulted and asked to supplement a provisional list of trials. This is likely to be useful in identifying unpublished trials.

Trial registration   Trial registers provide an extremely useful source of information for those undertaking systematic reviews. Some registers are simply retrospective lists of completed trials which provide a useful record of trial publications that other researchers have found by searching bibliographic databases, handsearching and other methods of identification. Others register trials at inception and therefore contain information about trials that are underway and actively recruiting patients, trials that have closed to accrual but are not yet published as well as completed and published trials.

Table 11.5 Web addresses for some bibliographic databases and trials registers

UKCCCR cancer trials register	http://www.ctu.mrc.ac.uk/ ukcccr/	Managed by the MRC Clinical Trials Unit, the UKCCCR Register is a comprehensive, fully searchable database of UK randomized controlled trials in all types of cancer.
PDQ (physicians data query)	http://www.cancer.gov/ search/clinical_trials/	Produced by the National Cancer Institute (USA), the main site is comprehensive covering latest information about cancer treatment, screening, prevention, genetics and supportive care. It includes PDQ, a searchable database of ongoing and closed international clinical trials (Phase I–III), both government and industry sponsored.
NHMRC clinical trials registry	http://www.ctc.usyd.edu.au./ 6registry/reg1.shtml	Australian national registry, ultimately intended to include all disease areas, but currently restricted to cancer. Includes unpublished and ongoing trials.
Current controlled trials	http://www.controlled-trials.com	A 'metaRegister' encompassing a number of registers of controlled trials managed and produced by the Current Science Group.
National research register (UK)	http://www.doh.gov.uk/ research/nrr.htm	Details a large number of NHS-supported randomized trials in all disease areas. Incorporates the MRC Clinical Trials Directory amongst other databases. Searches of the NRR will retrieve trials from these sources.
Centerwatch: clinical trials listing service	http://www.centerwatch.com/	A listing of clinical trials in all disease areas. Mostly USA-based industry and government-sponsored trials.

These prospective registers have the additional advantage of providing an unbiased sample because trials are submitted to the register when they are started and are therefore recorded even if they are not ultimately published. They therefore do not suffer from publication bias, which makes them particularly valuable for research purposes. Such registers usually provide simple-to-access and comprehensive information on the design, objectives, eligibility, interventions and accrual of clinical trials, together with details of any associated publications. They fulfil a variety of roles including helping to overcome unnecessary duplication of trials, promoting trials generally and increasing public awareness of trials that are currently being conducted (Box 11.5), as well as being an invaluable source of trials to the reviewer.

There is an ethical imperative for all trials to be registered, thereby providing a public record of research in which people are being enrolled, and enabling information about all trials to contribute to the evidence base for healthcare decisions concerning both clinical practice and further research. There is now a groundswell of opinion recognizing the value of trial registration [45] and increasing calls for it to become a legal and ethical requirement worldwide.

Box 11.5 Prospective registers of clinical trials

Prospective registration of a clinical trial means putting on public record some basic data at the time a trial starts. The aim is to provide the public, health providers, researchers and funding bodies with reliable information about research in progress. Once completed, trial information remains in the register database.

◆ Registers are an invaluable source of information for those conducting systematic reviews or meta-analyses as they provide a valuable method of identifying unpublished and ongoing trials. Because trials are registered at the outset, this avoids the problems of publication bias.

◆ Registers provide a straightforward way for clinicians and researchers to learn about trials in their area of interest, to find out what new treatments are being investigated and potentially to decide whether they want to collaborate in such trials as participants.

◆ Anyone planning a new trial can find out whether anything similar has already been done or is currently ongoing. Such planning can help avoid unnecessary duplication of effort, or alternatively help aid trial design where confirmatory trials are required, as researchers can learn valuable lessons from previous studies.

◆ Funding bodies can make use of information from registers when assessing applications for future trials. They can check whether similar trials exist and can then take an informed decision about whether the planned new trial will contribute useful information.

◆ Registering trials may actually save effort for those running trials; if the information contained in the register provides sufficient information to answer routine queries, for example whether the trial is open or closed and how it is recruiting.

◆ Registering trials has the potential to improve recruitment as it can increase the level of awareness about the trial, both within the medical profession and in the patient population.

◆ Registration provides a means of assigning unique identifying numbers to trials (see Box 11.1).

The US government led the way with the FDA modernization act (1997) which required the establishment of a prospective database of all trials of new treatments for serious or life-threatening diseases (www.clinicaltrials.gov). In the UK, the Medical Research Council requires investigators to register their trials within their own directory of trials before it releases funds. Information from this directory is available through the meta-register of trials and its cancer trials via the UKCCCR register (Table 11.5). A further advantage of trial registration is that it provides a mechanism for assigning unique identifying numbers to RCTs. The international initiative to assign ISRCTNs – International Standard Randomized Controlled Trial Number – (see Box 11.1) to all new trials as they are registered, and to include this number in all publications, reports and presentation about the trial, will make it easy for reviewers to tell at a glance where multiple publications refer to the same trial (see Section 11.4.3). Openness about trials in progress reduces the impact of publication bias, prevents duplication of effort, promotes collaboration and can ultimately save lives [45]. Trial registration is therefore of value to all those involved in trials and research and to the general public. A list of web addresses for both cancer-specific and more general trial registers is given in Table 11.5.

11.5.5 Data collection

Data collection, collation and verification are time-consuming aspects of any systematic review or meta-analysis. For those that use data extracted from published reports, several weeks may be required to allow time to read each paper carefully and extract the appropriate data. This stage may take many months for those that use IPD. The trialists need to be contacted and invited to provide the desired information. The data then need to be transferred checked and verified before any analyses can be done. The value of writing a clearly specified protocol (see Section 11.5.2) cannot be over-emphasized, as collecting the wrong data or finding out that additional information is required during the data collection phase can be both costly and time-consuming. Thus, a clear idea of what questions may be reasonably addressed, which endpoints will be used and usually a clear idea of how any final analyses will be organized is an essential precursor to data collection.

Data solely extracted from publications

Where analyses are to be based on information taken from published papers or reports, articles must be read in meticulous detail to ensure that the appropriate information is used. Data should be abstracted in a structured way, either onto standard paper forms (Box 11.6) or directly into an electronic database. There is usually no contact with the authors and consequently no opportunity for those responsible for the trials to verify that the data used are accurate and appropriate. It is therefore considered good practice for data extraction to be performed independently by two reviewers. Any discrepancies are resolved by discussion or by adjudication by a third party. Identifying multiple publications originating from the same trial can be particularly problematic. Often, it is not straightforward to determine whether multiple papers have reported the same trial, because authors and patient numbers may change between reports. Additional individuals may have been accrued to trials that are reported whilst ongoing, or different subsets of patients described. Ultimately the use of unique identifying numbers will distinguish multiple publications of the same report (see Box 11.2). In the meantime, it would be beneficial if reviewers tried to contact authors in cases where there is doubt about duplication to ensure that data from any one trial are represented only once in the meta-analysis.

Aggregate data supplied by investigators

With this approach trialists are asked to supply summary data from their trial, usually by completing data tables for each endpoint of interest. It has the advantage that data may be obtained from unpublished trials and that additional data that were not included in the published report may also be collected. If a number of outcomes or subgroups are to be investigated then it will usually be necessary to complete many different tables.

Individual patient data supplied by investigators

With this approach, trialists are asked to provide individual details on all patients included in their trial. The minimum data that can be collected are the patient identifier,

Box 11.6   Example pages from data extraction form [46]

Concomitant Chemotherapy and Radiotherapy for Cancer of the Cervix
Cochrane ID:

Study ID _____   Data collection form no. _____
Study source(s) _____
Study notes _____
_____
_____
_____
Reviewer _____

Verification of study eligibility

1. Is the study a randomised controlled trial? 0=no, 1=yes, 2=unclear

2. Has the trial compared concomitant cytotoxic chemotherapy plus radiotherapy (± surgery) with radiotherapy (± surgery) alone? 0=no, 1=yes, 2=unclear

3. Has the trial took place between 1 January 1980 and 1 January 2000 now closed to patient accrual? 0=no, 1=yes, 2=unclear

Is the trial eligible for inclusion, i.e. the answer to each of questions 1-3 is yes (=1)?

Trial Methods

Was the concealment of treatment allocation? 0=inadequate, 1=adequate, 2=unclear, 3=not used

Date trial opened (ddmmyy) _____   Minimum follow-up (months)
Date trial closed (ddmmyy) _____   Maximum follow-up (months)
Number of centres _____   Median follow-up (months)

	Treatment	Control
No. of patients randomised		
No. of patients analysed		
No. of patients excluded		

Reason(s) for exclusions _____
_____
_____
_____
_____

Interventions: Surgery

Was a hysterectomy performed?   0=no, 1=yes
If yes, what was the type of hysterectomy?
0=simple, 1=radical, 2=radical with lymphadenectomy, 3=exenteration

1

Concomitant Chemotherapy and Radiotherapy for Cancer of the Cervix
Cochrane ID:

Interventions: Radiotherapy

Is the local radiotherapy given the same in both arms?   0=no, 1=yes

Patients to which the following radiotherapy refers (e.g. all, stage II etc.)
External beam RT
RT total dose (Gy) ____   No. of fractions ____   Dose per fraction (Gy) ____
Intracavitary RT
How was the dose rate described?   0=not clear or not stated, 1=low-dose rate, 2=high-dose rate
Dose Point A (Gy) ____   No. of insertions ____

	Treatment	Control
No. of patients completing radiotherapy as planned		
No. of patients who did not start radiotherapy		
No. of patients who did not finish radiotherapy		
No. of patients experiencing delay		

Patients to which the following radiotherapy refers (e.g. all, stage II etc.)
External beam RT
RT total dose (Gy) ____   No. of fractions ____   Dose per fraction (Gy) ____
Intracavitary RT
How was the dose rate described?   0=not clear or not stated, 1=low-dose rate, 2=high-dose rate
Dose Point A (Gy) ____   No. of insertions ____

	Treatment	Control
No. of patients completing radiotherapy as planned		
No. of patients who did not start radiotherapy		
No. of patients who did not finish radiotherapy		
No. of patients experiencing delay		

Interventions: Chemotherapy

Mode of delivery   1=intravenous, 2=intraarterial
Sequence of delivery   1=concurrent only, 2=concurrent & sequential
Treatment

	Dose per cycle (mg/m²)	Cycle length (days)	No. of cycles
Drug			
Drug			
Drug			

Control

	Dose per cycle (mg/m²)	Cycle length (days)	No. of cycles
Drug			

2

Concomitant Chemotherapy and Radiotherapy for Cancer of the Cervix
Cochrane ID:

Participants
Please supply the number of patients in each category:

Age (supply groups, if required)

	Treatment	Control
Median		
Range		

Stage

	Treatment	Control
IB		
IIA		
IIB		
IIIA		
IIIB		
IVA		

Histology

	Treatment	Control
Squamous		
Adeno		
Mixed		
Other		

Grade

	Treatment	Control
Well differentiated / I		
Moderately differentiated / II		
Poorly differentiated / III		
Unknown		

Performance status (supply codes)

	Treatment	Control
PS scale used		

Outcomes: Patterns of failure

	Treatment	Control
No of patients with local recurrence		
No of patients with distant recurrence		
No of patients with both local and distant recurrence		

Outcomes: Progression-free Survival

	Treatment	Control
% at 1 years		
% at 2 years		
% at 3 years		
% at 4 years		
% at 5 years		
% overall		

Outcomes: Survival

	Treatment	Control
% at 1 years		
% at 2 years		
% at 3 years		
% at 4 years		
% at 5 years		
% overall		

3

Concomitant Chemotherapy and Radiotherapy for Cancer of the Cervix
Cochrane ID:

Outcomes: Late Toxicity

Toxicity scale used ____
Treatment
Please supply the number of patients in each category (worst side effects):

	Grade 1	Grade 2	Grade 3	Grade 4
Genitourinary				
Gastrointestinal				
Neurological				
Fistula				
Other				
Overall				

Control
Please supply the number of patients in each category (worst side effects):

	Grade 1	Grade 2	Grade 3	Grade 4
Genitourinary				
Gastrointestinal				
Neurological				
Fistula				
Other				
Overall				

Outcomes: Quality of Life

Quality of life assessed   0=no, 1=yes
Main conclusions of QoL assessment _____
_____
_____

Conclusions of Trial Publication
Main conclusions/recommendations of the trial publication _____
_____
_____
_____
_____
_____

5

treatment allocated and outcome, together with the date of randomization and date of outcome, if time-to-event is to be calculated. However, it is often important to collect additional baseline or prognostic variables. As well as providing the opportunity for sub-group analyses and a richer understanding of the trials, these covariates are also extremely useful in checking the integrity of the randomization process. In practical terms there is likely to be a trade-off between requesting a minimal dataset with least inconvenience for trialists and obtaining a wide range of variables for further analysis at the risk of discouraging participation in the meta-analysis. However, most trialists (or their data centres) are usually able to supply information on the most common prognostic variables with little additional effort.

Those conducting an IPD meta-analysis should be prepared to accept data in a variety of high-tech and low-tech formats, ranging from electronic transfer of databases to photocopies of anonymized patient notes. For most trial organizations, recent trials will be supplied on floppy disk or sent by e-mail. However, for old or archived trials it may be easiest for trialists to complete paper data collection forms (Fig. 11.5).

Patient identifier	Date of birth dd/mm/yyyy or age	Sex	Tumour stage	Histology	Perf status	Treatment arm	Randomised dd/mm/yyyy	Survival status	Death/ Last follow-up dd/mm/yyyy	Cause of death
001	67	M	ll	3	1	1	15/05/1992	D	13/02/1993	1
002	76	M	lll	2	1	1	22/05/1992	D	07/03/1993	1
003	78	M	lll	3	2	2	06/06/1992	D	11/11/1992	3
004	62	M	ll	2	1	1	28/06/1992	A	30/11/2001	
005	69	F	lll	3	1	2	17/07/1992	D	14/10/1996	1
006	71	M	lll	9	1	2	21/07/1992	D	31/05/1994	9
007	68	F	lll	2	2	1	14/08/1992	D	19/04/1994	1

Fig. 11.5 Example data form for collecting IPD.

In our experience, an increasing amount of data is being sent by e-mail (Fig. 11.6), which reduces considerably the amount of resource required for data entry and checking, and makes communicating and querying data considerably easier. Every effort should be made to reduce the burden on the trialist or data centre providing the information.

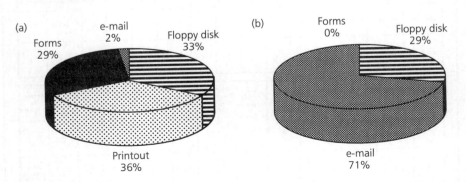

Fig. 11.6 Method of supplying data for (a) a meta-analysis initiated 1989 [23,47] and (b) a meta-analysis initiated 1994 [36].

Box 11.7 Example coding instructions for an IPD meta-analysis

Meta-Analysis of Chemotherapy in Locally Advanced Bladder Cancer

Suggested Coding

Sex
1 male
2 female
9 unknown

CLINICAL STAGE
T Category
1 T1
2 T2
3 T3
4 T4a
5 T4b
7 other
9 unknown

N Category
0 N0
1 N1
2 N2
9 unknown

M Category
0 M0
1 M1
9 unknown

PATHOLOGICAL STAGE
pT Category
Please code as suggested for Clinial Stage
PN Category
Please code as suggested for Clinial Stage
pM Category
Please code as suggested for Clinial Stage

Allocated Treatment
1 chemotherapy
2 control

Local Treatment — Surgery
0 no surgery
1 radical cystectomy
2 partial cystectomy
7 other surgery
9 unknown

Local Treatment – Radiotherapy
0 no radiotherapy
1 radical radiotherapy
2 pre-operative radiotherapy
3 post-operative radiotherapy
4 pre- and post-operative radiotherapy
7 other radiotherapy
9 unknown

Grade
Code as convenient, but please give details of the system used (e.g. UICC etc)

Performance Status
Code as convenient, but please give details of the system used (e.g. WHO etc)

Tumour Diameter
Please supply as the largest single dimension of the tumour in mm
unknown = 999

Renal Function
Code as convenient, but please give details of the measurement used (e.g. creatinine clearance, glomerular filtration rate etc.)

Pre-treatment Haemoglobin
Please supply giving details of the measurement used (e.g. g/dl, mmol/l etc.)

Local Recurrence/Progression
0 no evidence of recurrence / progression
1 local recurrence
2 local progression

Distant Metastases
0 no distant metastases
1 distant metastases
9 unknown

Treatment on Recurrence/Progression
1st digit – Surgery
0 no surgery
1 surgery
8 not applicable
9 unknown

2nd digit – radiotherapy
0 no radiotherapy
1 radiotherapy
8 not applicable
9 unknown

3rd digit – chemotherapy
0 no chemotherapy
1 chemotherapy
8 not applicable
9 unknown

Survival status
0 alive
1 dead

Bladder cancer present at death
0 no
1 yes
8 not applicable
9 unknown

Cause of death
1 bladder cancer
2 chemotherapy-related toxicity
3 radiotherapy-related toxicity
4 surgical complications
5 secondary tumour
6 other chronic disease
7 other
8 not applicable
9 unknown

Excluded from most recent Analysis
0 no
1 yes

Example of Data Form

Patient ID	Centre ID	Date of Birth (dd/mm/yyyy or dd/mm/yy)	Age	Sex	T category	N category	M category	pT category	pN category	pM category	Grade	Performance Status	Tumour Diameter (mm)	Renal Function	Pretreatment Haemoglobin	Allocated Treatment
1234	1	01/05/1943	49	1	3	9	0	3	9	0	2	2	50	55	10.5	1
1235	2	12/09/32	64	2	2	1	1	2	1	1	1	1	34	67	96.0	2

Local Treatment (surgery)	Local Treatment (radiotherapy)	Local Recurrence Status	Date of local Recurrence / Progression (dd/mm/yyyy or dd/mm/yy)	Distant Metastases	Date of Distant Metastases	Treatment on Recurrence / Progression (3 digits)	Survival Status	Date of Death / Last follow up (dd/mm/yyyy or dd/mm/yy)	Bladder Cancer Present at Death	Cause of Death	Excluded from most recent Analysis	Reason for Exclusion
1	0	1	30/06/1995	0	//	001	1	24/03/1997	1	1	0	
2	2	0	//	1	31/10/98	011	0	12/04/2000	8	8	1	didn't complete treatment

The meta-analysis coordinators should provide details of the desired coding of variables (Box 11.7) but will generally accept data in whichever form it is most convenient for trialists to supply it. Provision of data may entail considerable work for the trialist and so good communication is essential, both to convince them of the value of the project, and to explain what is required of them.

11.5.6 Data checking

Data extracted from publications

Checking summary data taken from publications is limited to ensuring that data have been extracted and entered to the meta-analysis database appropriately. It may be useful for each of the reviewers who extract data from the publications to enter information separately into the database or analysis package. This 'double' data entry may provide a useful check against inputting error.

Summary tabular data provided by trialists

For summary data supplied by trialists, data tables should be scrutinized for any obvious errors or inconsistencies and where possible cross-checked with any publications. However, where data have been brought up-to-date or subdivided by patient types that were not reported in the publication, this may not be possible. These types of data are undoubtedly the most difficult to scrutinize as they have neither the benefit of peer review nor the detailed checking possibilities of IPD. Where such data supplement published data, common elements should be cross-checked with publications for consistency. Where summary data are from unpublished trials, the information supplied has largely to be taken at face value although some checks for internal consistency can be carried out. For example, the total numbers of individuals and total numbers of events should be the same for different subgroups supplied. It has been noted that there have been instances of meta-analyses of unpublished summary (and therefore unchallengeable) data, that show more favourable results than similar analyses of published data, and that have been produced in situations where there are vested financial interests [48].

Individual patient data

The main aims of data checking procedures are to ensure the accuracy of data, integrity of randomization and completeness of follow up. For any one trial the results of all the data checks should be considered together to build up an overall picture of that trial and any associated problems. Where there are concerns about the data supplied, these should be brought to the attention of the trialist and sympathetic efforts made to resolve them.

Range and consistency checks should be carried out for all data irrespective of whether they were supplied electronically or were entered manually into the meta-analysis database (in which case it is important to audit the data entry process). Any missing data, obvious errors, inconsistencies between variables or extreme values should be queried and rectified as necessary. If details of the trial have been published, these also should be checked against the raw data and any inconsistencies similarly queried. All of the changes made to the data originally supplied by the trialists, and the reasons for these changes, should be recorded.

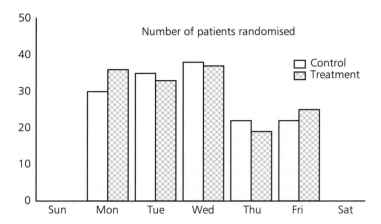

Fig. 11.7 Example of pattern of randomization anticipated for non-acute conditions. The day of week can be calculated from a date by most standard database packages.

As part of a series of investigations to check the validity of the treatment assignment process (i.e. that the trial is in fact randomized), the distribution of patient-related variables can be checked for balance across treatment arms and across major baseline characteristics. This can be done using a chi-square test. It is, however, important to remember that imbalances may occur by chance alone especially for non-stratified variables and when trials are small. Other checks that can be done include looking at the weekday of randomization (Fig. 11.7). For example, for UK cancer trials we would expect very few randomizations at the weekend. In studies from other countries it is important to appreciate cultural differences in working patterns. Similarly, randomizations in trials of acute disease would be expected on all days of the week.

The pattern of randomization can also be checked by producing simple plots of cumulative accrual. Figure 11.8 illustrates this for a trial with a 1:1 assignment carried out by minimization, showing the numbers allocated to the two treatments to be close throughout and crossing frequently. Figure 11.9 (which has been made public with the trialists' permission [13]) illustrates how illuminating such plots can be. The curve is from an unpublished trial of radiotherapy versus chemotherapy in multiple myeloma.

Here we see that from the start of the trial until early 1985 the pattern is similar to that of Fig. 11.8. However, in the middle of 1985 the curves diverge and remain apart – the cumulative accrual to the chemotherapy arm continues to rise, whereas the radiotherapy arm remains flat for a period. On further enquiry, it transpired that in this trial the radiotherapy equipment was unavailable for six months during the trial, but during this time patients continued to enter the chemotherapy arm. It was only when the individual patient data were provided for a meta-analysis that this problem was brought to the attention of the trialist who agreed that the appropriate solution was to exclude this small number of non-randomized chemotherapy patients from the analysis.

Where survival (or another time-dependent variable) is the primary outcome it may be important that trial follow-up is as up-to-date as possible since an increased follow-up

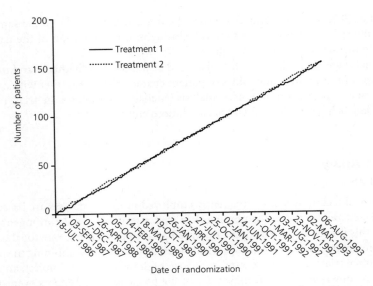

Fig. 11.8 Example plot of cumulative numbers of patients randomized to two treatment arms.

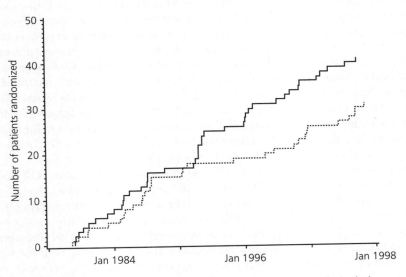

Fig. 11.9 Cumulative randomization plot for a trial with a non-random phase during recruitment. Reproduced with permission from [13].

may see a reduction in treatment effect if the survival curves are converging, or an increased treatment effect if the curves are diverging. Thus, where appropriate, data should be checked to ensure that follow-up is up-to-date and that it is balanced across treatment arms. Balance in follow-up can be checked by selecting all patients outcome-free and using the date of censoring as the event to carry out a 'reverse survival' analysis (see Section 9.3.4). This produces censoring curves, which should be the same for all arms of the trial. Any imbalance should be brought to the attention of the trialist and updated information should be sought.

As a final stage of checking, each trial should be analysed individually and the trialist sent a copy of the analyses and tables of patient characteristics, together with a printout of their data as included in the meta-analysis database. This allows the trialist to verify that the data being used from their trial are indeed correct.

11.5.7 Analyses

Binary data

The statistical techniques most frequently employed in meta-analyses are based on the Mantel–Haenszel method of combining data over a series of 2×2 contingency tables. Basically this involves comparing the observed and expected event rate for the 'experimental' treatment and control groups within each trial and then combining the results of the individual trials. There are a number of ways of doing this. The simplest, an example of which is shown in Box 11.8, makes use of the proportion of patients event-free at a given time point. For each individual trial the overall number of events within the study is used to calculate the expected number of events that would occur if there were no difference between the two arms of the trial. The difference between the actual observed (O) and the expected (E) number of events is then calculated for the 'experimental' arm, giving the $O-E$ value. A negative $O-E$ value indicates that the 'experimental' treatment group has fared better than the control group, whilst a positive $O-E$ value indicates the opposite. If the 'experimental' treatment has no effect, then each individual $O-E$ could be either positive or negative and will differ only randomly from zero. Likewise, the summed $O-E$ from all the studies will differ only randomly from zero if there is no difference between the 'experimental' and control groups. If, however, the treatment does have a beneficial effect, then there will be a trend for individual $O-E$ values to be negative, and the overall summed value to be clearly so.

The $O-E$ and its variance can then be used to calculate odds ratios (OR) for each trial. This OR gives the ratio of the odds of an event among the 'experimental' group to the corresponding odds of an event among the control group patients. An OR value of 1.0 represents equal odds or no difference between treatments, while a value of 0.5 indicates a halving of the odds of an event measured for patients in the 'experimental' arm. An OR across trials can be calculated by summing the individual $O-E$ and variance values in such a way that the pooled OR represents a weighted average of the individual ORs, with the individual trials that contain most information (usually the largest trials) having the greatest influence. This approach is known as the fixed effect model. An alternative approach where the pooled estimate of effect takes account of both the within trial variance and the between trial variance is known as the random effect model. The pros and cons of each are discussed in Section 11.6.1.

Time-to-event data

A major advantage of collecting IPD is that it allows a more appropriate analysis of time-to-event data. Usually this involves carrying out standard log rank analyses (see

Box 11.8 Calculating an odds ratio – hypothetical example

Suppose there are four trials comparing 'experimental' treatment versus control, and that the numbers of deaths on each arm of these trials are as below:

	'Experimental'	Control	p-value
Trial A	29/67	39/72	0.20
Trial B	3/23	10/30	0.09
Trial C	7/39	11/28	0.05
Trial D	45/145	64/172	0.30

Individually, none of these trials show a statistically significant difference between the number of deaths on the 'experimental' and control arm. For trial A, there are sixty-seven patients on the treatment arm, of whom twenty-nine have died. The expected number of deaths on the 'experimental' arm (E), O–E value (O–E), variance (V) and odds ratio (OR) can be calculated:

	'Experimental'	Control	Total
Dead	29	39	68 (D)
Alive	38	33	71
Total	67 (nt)	72	139 (N)

$$E = (D/N)nt \qquad O\!-\!E = 29 - 32.78$$
$$= (68/139)67 \qquad = -3.78$$
$$= 32.78$$

$$OR = \exp[(O\!-\!E)/V] \qquad V = [E(1 - nt/N)(N - D)]/(N - 1)$$
$$= \exp(-3.78/8.74) \qquad = [32.78(1 - 67/139)(139 - 68)]/138$$
$$= 0.65 \qquad = 8.74$$

Similar values can be calculated for trials B, C and D:

	O–E	Variance	Odds ratio
Trial A	−3.78	8.74	0.65
Trial B	−2.64	2.46	0.34
Trial C	−3.48	3.25	0.34
Trial D	−4.86	17.81	0.76

Combined or pooled OR can now be calculated as follows:

$$OR = \exp\left[\Sigma(O\!-\!E)/\Sigma V\right] \quad 95\%\,CI = \exp\left[(\Sigma(O\!-\!E)/\Sigma V) \pm \left(1.96/\left(\sqrt{\Sigma V}\right)\right)\right]$$
$$= \exp(-14.76/31.56)$$
$$= 0.63 \ (95\% \ CI \ 0.45 - 0.89)$$

The combined OR is conventionally significant in favour of treatment with a 36 per cent reduction in the odds of death for the treatment group patients. Adapted and reproduced with permission from [50].

Section 9.3.4) on individual trials and then using the stratified log rank $O-E$s and their variances to calculate a hazard ratio (HR). Rather than summarizing the overall number of events as in an odds ratio, the HR makes use of the time (from randomization) until each individual event takes place, and also uses information from patients who have not yet experienced the event (censored patients).

In this way, the HR summarizes the entire 'survival' experience. The calculations follow through in exactly the same way as for calculation of an OR, simply by substituting the log rank $O-E$ and variance for those calculated from the crude number of events. These hazard ratios represent the instantaneous risk of failure on treatment as opposed to control. An HR of less than 1.0 favours treatment whereas an HR of more than 1.0 favours control. For example, when measuring survival, an HR of 0.8 indicates a 20 per cent reduction in the overall risk of death when receiving treatment as compared to control. Such time-to-event analyses can be extremely important in chronic illness where a prolongation of survival, time without evidence of disease, or time without symptoms is important.

While not all systematic reviews of survival-type endpoints have time and resource available to collect and analyse IPD, they should make the most efficient use of the summary statistical data available. Where meta-analyses are based on published information, provided that trials are sufficiently well reported, it may be possible to estimate HRs from a variety of statistical summary measures rather than calculating odds ratios [25] at fixed timepoints, as is usually done for this type of meta-analysis. Where log HRs, HRs or log rank $O-E$s plus variances are presented, these can be used directly in the calculation of an overall HR. Even when these are not presented, manipulation of the chi-square value, p-value or variance can be used to calculate an HR indirectly. Some of the methods of doing these calculations are shown in Box 11.9 opposite. The particular method used will depend on what information is presented for particular trials, and different methods can be used for different trials as appropriate. If there is not sufficient information to obtain an estimated HR from summary statistics then the HR can be estimated by splitting the published survival curves into discrete time intervals, calculating an OR for each of these periods and then combining the ORs over time. This is often the only practical way to proceed as few papers present sufficient information to permit manipulation of summary statistics by either the direct or indirect method. For example, a study using information from fourteen IPD meta-analysis comparisons, involving a number of cancers and a total of 138 RCTs found that only 60 per cent of published trial reports had estimatable HRs [49].

Graphical representation of meta-analyses

Results of meta-analyses are usually presented as plots, often called forest plots, illustrating the HR (or OR) for each individual trial and for the overall combined results (Fig. 11.10). The vertical line of equivalence drawn through unity indicates the point at which there is no difference between 'experimental' treatment and control groups. Trials favouring the 'experimental' treatment will have an HR of less than 1.0 and lie to the left-hand side of this line and those favouring control will fall on the right-hand side. Each individual trial is illustrated by a box drawn with a horizontal line and tick marks

Box 11.9　Estimating HRs from summary statistics

To calculate a HR we require estimates of the observed minus expected ($O–E$) number of events and its variance (V).

$$HR = \exp[(O–E)/V]$$

If the variance is presented, then O–E may be calculated by simple manipulation of the χ^2 or p-value.

$$O–E = \sqrt{\chi^2} \times \sqrt{V}$$

$$O–E = \sqrt{V} + (1 – P/2)$$

If the variance is not given, but confidence intervals (CI) for the HR are, then V may be estimated:

$$V = \left[\frac{\text{Upper CI–Lower CI}}{2\Phi^{-1}(1 – \alpha/2)} \right]^2$$

In practice, the denominator inside the square brackets will be 2×1.96 for the 95% CI and 2×2.58 for the 99% CI, e.g. for 95% CI.

$$V = \left[\frac{\text{Upper CI–Lower CI}}{3.92} \right]^2$$

If CIs are not given but the total number of events E is known then V may be estimated as $E/4$ (provided that the treatment effect is not too large and the randomization ratio is $1:1$).

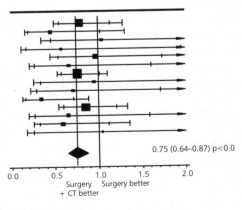

	(no. events/no. entered) Surgery + CT	Surgery	O–E	Variance
GOG	52/113	62/112	−6.75	28.42
MDAH	12/18	15/17	−4.65	5.88
Mayo	12/22	11/23	0.21	5.71
NCI4	9/17	5/8	−1.42	2.64
NCI5	22/38	24/41	−0.33	11.47
NCI6	9/21	11/20	−2.00	4.90
EORTC	92/193	105/188	−13.31	48.84
DFCI	7/21	8/25	−0.20	3.74
ECOG	9/24	11/23	−1.70	4.96
Bergonie	11/28	19/26	−7.60	6.96
SSG	65/121	69/119	−5.35	32.72
Rizzoli	7/16	13/22	−2.10	4.85
IGSC	14/40	25/46	−5.09	9.73
SAKK	4/12	4/12	0.08	2.00
Total	325/684	382/682	−50.21	172.83

0.75 (0.64–0.87) p<0.0

0.0　0.5　1.0　1.5　2.0
Surgery　Surgery better
+ CT better

Fig. 11.10 Example HR plot from a meta-analysis of chemotherapy in soft tissue sarcoma. Reproduced with permission from [36].

indicating the 95 per cent and 99 per cent confidence intervals. The size of the box is proportional to the statistical variance in the trial such that, the bigger the box, the greater the number of events and, usually, the bigger the trial. A trial reaches conventional levels of significance if the 95 per cent confidence intervals do not cross the equivalence line.

The diamond at the bottom of the plot illustrates the combined results for all trials, with the edges denoting the 95 per cent confidence interval. An overall result reaches significance at the 5 per cent level if the edge of the diamond does not cross the equivalence line. Trials are often ordered chronologically with the oldest trial at the top.

Sensitivity analyses

Sensitivity analyses can be done to test the robustness of the main results of the meta-analysis. These are often done by running analyses with and without the inclusion of certain trials, and then comparing the results. They can be used to test assumptions made in the meta-analysis, for example decisions made about the eligibility of certain trials or types of trials. If results are changed substantially, depending on whether or not a particular trial, or group of trials, with questionable eligibility are included in the meta-analysis, the decision regarding eligibility will need thoughtful justification. The final results will also need to be treated with suitable circumspection. When using data extracted from publications, sensitivity analyses can be used to explore the influence of trial quality by carrying out analyses with and without trials of dubious quality. Where results comprise one or two large trials and a number of smaller trials, they can also be used to see to what extent the result is driven by the largest trial. Likewise, sensitivity analyses can be done to assess the potential impact of publication bias by removing the smallest trials. Although sensitivity analyses are usually done as described above, in many cases it may be preferable and more informative to look at differences between trials in the form of subset analysis, particularly when looking at issues of eligibility. It may also be informative to use the order of trials on the forest plot to explore possible patterns of trends. For example, ordering trials by intended dose may give an insight to issues relating to inadequate/adequate dosing.

Subset analyses

There is inevitably some subjectivity in setting the question to be posed in a systematic review (see Section 11.5.1) and there is likely to be a trade-off between pooling only very similar trials, and achieving high statistical power. One way of dealing with this dilemma is to group trials by important characteristics in subset analyses. By grouping similar trials together we are attempting to minimize the clinical and statistical variability within the subsets of trials. This approach allows us to look for consistency and inconsistency between subsets of trials. We are hoping to partition any overall heterogeneity in such a way that it is explained mostly by differences between subsets of trials rather than by variation within subsets (see also Section 11.6.2). Individual meta-analyses are done and pooled results calculated, for each subset of trials, and if appropriate, an overall pooled result calculated for all trials. For example, in an IPD meta-analysis of chemotherapy in non-small cell lung cancer [51], it was decided *a priori* to split the trials according to the type of chemotherapy that was used. This was because it was thought that older chemotherapies might be less effective than newer regimens. In fact the results indicated

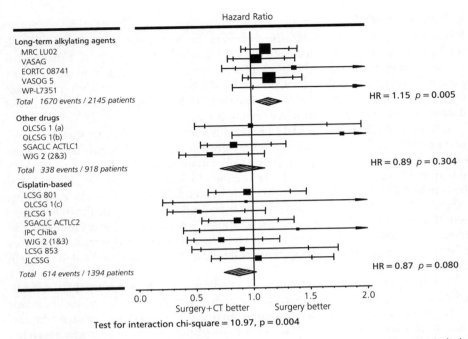

Fig. 11.11 Surgery+chemotherapy versus surgery alone in non-small cell lung cancer–survival analysis. Modified and reproduced with permission from [50].

that rather than just the quantitative differences that were anticipated, there was evidence of a qualitative difference (difference in direction of effect) between the types of chemotherapy. Long-term administration of oral alkylating agents appeared to be detrimental, whereas other more modern types of cisplatin-based chemotherapy were suggestive of a benefit. (Fig. 11.11).

The top subset of trials using long-term alkylating agents lie to the right-hand side of the line and the pooled result for this subset of trials indicated by the hatched diamond immediately below indicates a significant detriment of the intervention. In contrast, the bottom subset of trials using cisplatin-based chemotherapy lie mostly to the left hand side of the line and the pooled estimate denoted by the hatched diamond immediately below this group indicates a result in favour of chemotherapy, although this is not conventionally statistically significant. The results for these subsets of trials are clearly different, shown formally by the chi-square test for interaction (see Section 9.4.8), which is conventionally significant. In this case it is not sensible to combine the results of all trials, statistically it would be improper and clinically it would be meaningless, so there is no solid black diamond at the foot of the plot. In other circumstances, where there is no difference between subsets of trials it may be appropriate to show an overall pooled result.

With this type of analysis, because trials are simply grouped by trial level characteristics, it is possible to subset trials irrespective of whether summary or individual patient data are used. Planned subset analyses should, of course, be pre-specified in the systematic review protocol.

Subgroup analyses

When assessing the role of any new treatment, an important additional question is whether the treatment is equally effective in well-defined subgroups of patients. For example, is the treatment more or less effective in males or females, or in old or young patients? As discussed in Chapter 9, the results of subgroup analyses can be very misleading because of the multiplicity of testing and there is a high probability that any observed difference is due solely to chance (see Section 9.4.8.9).

In individual trials it is unusual to have sufficient numbers and statistical power to permit reliable subgroup analyses. However, provided that such data have been collected uniformly across studies, a meta-analysis of all trials may achieve sufficient power in each subgroup to permit a more reliable exploration of whether the effect is, in fact, larger (or smaller) for any particular type of patient. Although still potentially misleading, subgroup analysis within the context of a large meta-analysis may be the only reliable way of performing such exploratory investigations. Not only do the greater numbers give increased statistical power, but we can also look for consistency across trials. In all types of systematic review any subgroup analyses should be pre-specified and stated clearly in the review protocol.

In contrast to what we have termed subset analysis, which groups whole trials, subgroup analysis groups individuals according to characteristics such as age, sex or tumour stage. In a meta-analysis setting, subgroup analyses are carried out for each trial and then the trial level summary statistics for each subgroup are combined to give an overall pooled effect. For example, the effect of treatment compared to control is calculated for men, and the effect of treatment compared to control is calculated for women, within each trial. The individual trial results for men can then be combined to give a pooled estimate of treatment effect for men and the same done for women.

In conventional meta-analyses using aggregate data from publications, it is usually extremely difficult to extract sufficient compatible data to undertake meaningful subgroup analyses. It is unlikely that separate results would be presented for each of the characteristics of interest (e.g. presenting separate results for men and for women, for stage II stage III and stage IV tumours, etc.) for every trial. Meta-regression has been proposed as a method of identifying significant relationships between the treatment effect and covariates of interest, based on the type of information that may be available in a trial publication. However (in the absence of IPD) the unit of regression is restricted to the trial and there are many problems with the approach (see Section 11.6.3). Consequently, it is unlikely that practically useful analysis of subgroup data will be possible in the context of a systematic review based on just summary data extracted from publications.

Subgroup analyses can be done using tabulated data supplied by trialists, for example, if separate data tables for men, for women and for each specific age group are provided for each trial. It is worth noting that this could be extremely time consuming for trialists, especially if the necessary cross-tabulations were not done for their own analyses. It is conceivable for a small trial that a trialist may have to generate as many data tables as there are patients. To look at categories of patients defined by more than one baseline characteristic, for example, post-menopausal women with oestrogen-receptor-positive and node-negative status, is likely to prove impractical for both trialist and reviewer.

In contrast, IPD permits straightforward categorization of individuals for subgroup analysis defined by single or multiple factors. For example, because age is collected for each individual patient, it is straightforward to categorize patients into the same age bands in all trials (say younger than sixty-five and sixty-five years and older) and then to look at whether the effect of treatment differs between the older and younger age group. It is important to note that these subgroup analyses, based on IPD, remain stratified by trial.

When interpreting the results of subgroup analysis plots, we should look at the overall pattern of results and note firstly to what extent the confidence intervals for each of the subgroups overlap. Where there are large overlaps there is generally no indication of a difference in the effect of treatment in the subgroups. This is tested formally by the test for trend or interaction (see Section 9.4.8). It is important not to use subgroup analysis to focus on individual subgroups of patients where the result for that group reaches significance. For example, in the hypothetical example below (Fig. 11.12) it would be incorrect and unwise to conclude that the investigational treatment worked in those with brown eyes, but not in those with blue or green eyes. There are simply larger number of individuals with brown eyes and there is no indication that the treatment is any more or any less effective according to eye colour.

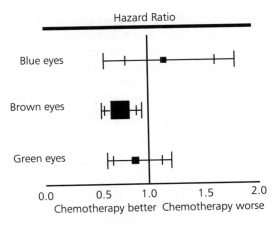

Fig. 11.12 Hypothetical example of a forest plot for subgroup analysis.

Example of subgroup analysis in meta-analysis

An IPD meta-analysis of thoracic radiotherapy for small-cell lung cancer [52] showed an overall benefit of combined radiotherapy and chemotherapy over chemotherapy alone ($p = 0.001$), equivalent to a 14 per cent reduction in the mortality rate. In addition, there was a significant trend ($p = 0.01$) towards a larger relative effect of radiotherapy on the mortality of younger patients than older ones. The relative risk of death in the treated group ranged from 0.72 for patients younger than fifty-five years to 1.07 for patients older than seventy years, with a very clear pattern of a decreasing benefit of radiotherapy across the five increasing age categories that were investigated. Although the authors suggested that the smaller effect of treatment in older patients could be explained by toxicity, they were sensibly cautious in interpreting the result of this subgroup analysis.

Relative and absolute differences

The HR or OR provides a measure of the chance of dying on the 'experimental' treatment compared to control. This is a relative benefit, giving an overall idea of how the experimental treatment compares to the standard treatment. It does not, however, provide information on what this means in absolute terms (see Section 10.4). Although there may be a large relative effect of an intervention, if the absolute risk is small, it may not be worth adopting the intervention because the change in absolute terms is minimal (a big percentage of a small amount is still a small amount). Therefore it is generally useful to convert this relative difference to absolute differences at given points in time. This depends on both the baseline (control group) survival and the HR, and the way that the two inter-relate is not intuitively obvious.

The formulae required to convert HRs and ORs to absolute differences are shown below:

$$A = [\exp(\log_e Pb \times HR)] - Pb,$$

$$A = Pb[(1 - Pb)(1 - OR)/(Pb + OR(1 - Pb))],$$

where A is the absolute difference, Pb the baseline event rate on control group.

Table 11.6 provides examples of how HRs translate to absolute differences at various event rates. For example an HR of 0.7 will give a 6 per cent benefit on a baseline of 80 per cent, improving survival from 80 to 86 per cent. With a baseline of 50 per cent the same HR gives an absolute benefit of 12 per cent taking survival from 50 to 62 per cent and on a baseline of 5 per cent, survival will be improved by 7 per cent from 5 to 12 per cent.

Table 11.6 Absolute benefits (%) calculated for various HRs and baseline event rates

HR	Baseline survival (%)				
	80	50	20	10	5
0.7	6	12	12	10	7
0.8	4	7	8	6	4
0.95	1	2	2	1	1

Evaluating results

When evaluating the results of any meta-analysis, it is usually informative to consider the results in a number of formats. The relative difference given by the HR and (where IPD are available) illustrated by the survival curve, gives a good overall impression of the results. Absolute differences and baseline event rates give a good indication of the results specific to clinically important points in time. This is also very important when considering the results of subgroup analyses. Even where there is no evidence that there is a differential relative effect of treatment (as measured by an HR or OR) in patient subgroups, if the underlying event rates for different categories of patients differ, then the effect of treatment in absolute terms will be different. For example, if young patients have a baseline survival of 80 per cent at two years then an HR of 0.7 in favour of treatment is equivalent to a 6 per cent benefit in survival improving the survival rate from 80 to 86

Table 11.7 Baseline survival and equivalent absolute increases in survival from an IPD meta-analysis of chemotherapy in high-grade glioma. Reproduced with permission frm [36].

HR = 0.84		One year survival rate		Two year survival rate	
		Baseline (%)	Absolute increase (%)	Baseline (%)	Absolute increase (%)
Age	≤ 40	78	3	50	5
	41–59	45	6	14	5
	≥ 60	22	6	4	2
Sex	Male	45	6	18	5
	Female	40	6	16	5
Histology	AA	58	5	31	6
	GM	35	6	9	4
	Other	72	4	52	5
Performance status	Good	54	5	22	6
	Poor	31	6	9	4
Extent of Resection	Complete	50	5	19	5
	Incomplete	40	6	16	5
	Biopsy	36	6	19	5

per cent. For old patients with a 20 per cent, two-year survival rate, the same HR of 0.7 translates to a 12 per cent benefit improving survival from 20 to 32 per cent. All of these, together with the nature of the treatment and other clinical factors should play a part in interpreting the results. It is often useful to present a table of absolute effects according to the baseline event rate for important prognostic variables. For example, Table 11.7 illustrates how the overall HR of 0.84 translates to different absolute effects ranging from 2 to 6 per cent at two years depending on the characteristics of patients with high-grade glioma.

11.5.8 Reporting and disseminating results

Publishing results of systematic reviews and meta-analyses

Dissemination of the results of a systematic review should be similar to that of a clinical trial and much of the guidance presented in Chapter 10 concerning publication and presentation of RCTs also applies to systematic reviews.

As discussed in Section 11.1, one of the advantages of systematic review is that objective and pre-specified methodology is used. Transparency of process should ensure that other researchers can easily reproduce the results. It is therefore essential that reports and publications should be consistent with this aim, and so should report analyses and results in sufficient detail to permit reproduction and present results and discussion in an unbiased format. It is important that any potential weaknesses of the review are brought to the attention of the reader. For example, if the review did not consider unpublished data, it should be stated that publication bias might be a problem.

The methods section is particularly important. In the same way that the report of a trial should provide details of the types of patients who were considered for the trial, so the report of a systematic review should report what the inclusion and exclusion criteria for the review were. It is important to give details of all trials that were considered for inclusion (as distinct from trials that were clearly irrelevant) and to provide details of why any particular trials were excluded. It should also be clear which of the eligible trials were able to be included in any analyses, as well as details of and reasons why any could not be included; for example, if publications did not report sufficient data to be included in quantitative analysis, or if trialists would not supply individual patient data. The search strategies used to locate trials should be reported, and it should be stated whether attempts were made to locate unpublished trials and the method for doing so. Methods used to screen trials and extract or obtain data should also be given. Similarly, the quantitative methods should be described fully. The fact that analyses were pre-specified should be stated, as should an outline of planned analyses.

The main characteristics of eligible trials should be reported (it is often easiest to do this in tabular format) and an overall description of patient characteristics given. The results of all analyses should be reported, though some may be dealt with briefly. Ideally, any planned analyses that were not ultimately possible should also be mentioned. As discussed previously, it is often useful to present results in a variety of formats, reporting for example both relative and absolute effect sizes. The robustness of the meta-analyses in terms of sensitivity analyses should also be reported, and any heterogeneity and its implications noted.

The discussion section of a systematic review often may be relatively brief. The position that many researchers involved in the field take is that their role is to conduct the review to the highest possible standards and to simply present the results. Many argue that unless the results are overwhelming, interpretation should be left to the reader.

Authorship

As systematic reviews are often done as collaborative projects, joint or group authorship is usual. Certainly, for IPD systematic reviews and meta-analyses, most groups have adopted the convention that primary publications should be in the name of the collaborative group responsible for the meta-analysis rather than individual authors. This emphasizes the collaborative nature of the project and engenders continued collaboration.

QUORUM

Following the initiative to improve the quality of reporting of RCTs and the CONSORT statement (see Section 10.3.1), similar guidance has been produced to improve the quality of reporting of systematic reviews and meta-analyses. The QUORUM statement consists of a checklist and flow diagram that encourages authors to provide readers with information about literature searches, inclusion/exclusion, validity assessment, data abstraction, study characteristics and data synthesis [53], although it does not require assessment of how well things have been done. Authors, editors and peer reviewers are encouraged to use the checklist to ensure that the important aspects of study design and analysis are covered in reports. It remains to be seen whether QUORUM, or any of the other similar checklists, become adopted as the international standard. The QUORUM statement and checklist can be found at http://www.consort-statement.org/QUORUM.pdf.

11.6 Some statistical issues in meta-analysis

11.6.1 Fixed versus random effect model

The examples discussed in Section 11.5.7 use the fixed effect model, which is the most straightforward and easiest to understand method of analysis. However, some would argue that a random effect model is a more appropriate way to analyse the data. In the simplest fixed effect model the contribution of each trial to the combined estimate is proportional to the amount of information in it. Weighting each trial by its variance is intuitively appealing. However, in this approach only *within-trial* variability is considered and no allowance is made for any *between-trial* variability. Random effect models explicitly allow for between-trial variability by weighting trials using a combination of their own variance and the between-trial variance.

Where there is little between-trial variability, the within-trial variance will dominate and the random effect weighting will tend towards the fixed effect weighting. If, however, there is significant between-trial variability, this will dominate the weighting factor and within-trial variability will contribute little towards the weighting factor. In this way all trials will tend towards contributing equally towards the overall estimate and small trials may unduly influence the results. There are strong proponents of both approaches. Those in favour of the random effect model argue that it formally allows for between-trial variability, and that the fixed effect approach unrealistically assumes a single effect across all trials and thus can give over-precise estimates. Those in favour of the fixed effect approach argue that the random effect model is using a statistical model to address a clinical problem. In particular, it gives no insight into the source of between-trial variability. In practice, it is common to find that the estimates from the two approaches are similar, but in the presence of statistical heterogeneity the confidence interval for the random effects estimate will be much wider than the confidence interval for the fixed effect estimate. Whichever model or approach is adopted, the aim should always be to minimize obvious sources of heterogeneity by carefully specifying questions and not combining obviously heterogeneous trials within a comparison, so that it becomes almost irrelevant which model is used.

11.6.2 Heterogeneity

There is inevitably a certain amount of clinical heterogeneity between trials, because of differing protocols, treatments, and patient characteristics and this will be true irrespective of whether any statistical test for heterogeneity is significant. If statistical heterogeneity is observed, then the possible reasons for this should be explored [54]. Perhaps the treatments are sufficiently different and can be split into less heterogeneous subsets of trials. If such a source of heterogeneity is found and trials can be subdivided according to the appropriate characteristic, separate analyses can be performed. In fact, this may enable us to address questions such as which particular treatments perform best or which types of patient will benefit most. Indeed, it could be argued that modeling such heterogeneity using the random effect approach (see Section 11.6.1) is effectively throwing away valuable information. The example of chemotherapy in non-small cell lung cancer described in Section 11.7 provides an example of this. There is statistical heterogeneity if all the trials are grouped together irrespective of chemotherapy type, but because the trials were split into subsets by type of chemotherapy, the heterogeneity was explained mostly by the differences between subsets. Splitting the trials in this way, according to a good clinical rationale minimized the heterogeneity within the subsets and maximized the interaction term between subsets. It suggested a different effect according to the type of chemotherapy used and in this particular example it would not be informative to combine all trials in a random effect model. As in this example, it is useful to consider possible sources of heterogeneity at the outset rather than trying to explain it after the fact. Otherwise, in the search for the clinical source of statistical heterogeneity, there is likely to be some *post hoc* reasoning in the explanation, so that only cautious conclusions should be drawn.

Heterogeneity can be investigated fully only when IPD are available, particularly when the endpoint is the time to an event. Although reported trial characteristics may give some insight, for example by employing meta-regression techniques, it is unlikely that all reasonable possible sources of heterogeneity can be investigated in a meta-analysis based on data extracted from publications.

11.6.3 Meta-regression

For meta-analyses that use summary data, meta-regression has been proposed as a means of exploring observed heterogeneity [55]. As in any regression analysis, meta-regression tries to identify significant relationships between the outcome and covariates of interest. Clearly when IPD are not available, the unit of regression is restricted to the trial. The covariates may be constant for the entire trial, e.g. the protocol dose of drug, or a summary measure of attributes describing the patient population, e.g. mean age or percentage of males. Several variables may be modelled together and provided that reasonable data are available, the technique may be a useful exploratory tool. However, there are limitations. Not all publications will report on all the covariates of interest (and there could be potential bias associated with selective presentation of data that have shown a positive association within the trial). If a trial is missing a covariate it drops out of the regression, limiting the power and usefulness of the analysis, which is already likely to be based on relatively few data points. Furthermore, summary data may misrepresent individual patients [1]. This is known as the ecologic fallacy or regression to the mean. What is true of a trial with a median age of sixty may not necessarily be true for a 60-year-old patient. Potentially all the benefit could have been shown in the seventy year olds and none in the fifty year olds. It should always be borne in mind that a significant association does not prove causality and should rather be regarded as hypothesis generating.

11.6.4 Investigating publication bias

Funnel plots have been suggested as a means of investigating whether publication bias is likely to be a particular problem within individual meta-analyses. These plots are based on the fact that precision in estimating treatment effect increases with sample size. Thus if we plot estimated treatment effect against size or number of events in a group of similar trials, we would expect to see a wide scatter in the results for small trials with the spread narrowing as the trial size increases. If there is no bias then we would expect the shape of the plot to resemble a funnel (see Figs 11.13 and 11.14).

If there is publication bias, then we would expect the plot to be skewed, effectively with a gap where the small negative studies ought to be. Although formal tests for evaluating asymmetry have been proposed, observed asymmetry in a funnel plot could

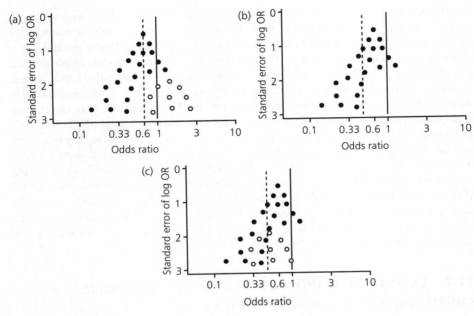

Fig. 11.13 Hypothetical funnel plots (a) symmetrical in the absence of bias (b) asymmetrical plot in the presence of publication bias smaller studies showing no statistically significant effects are missing (c) asymmetrical plot in the presence of bias due to low methodological quality of small studies (open circles show small studies of poor quality whose results are biased towards larger effects). Reproduced with permission from [56].

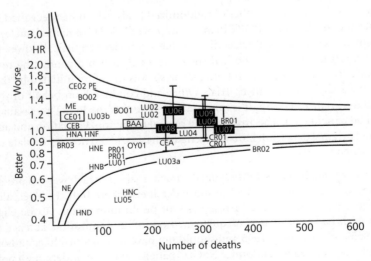

Fig. 11.14 Example funnel plot illustrating British MRC trials of interventions in solid tumours. Trials are included irrespective of publication status and so illustrate the type of pattern expected where there is unlikely to be publication bias. Reproduced with permission from [57].

be attributable to a number of factors other than publication bias [1]. For example, odds ratios overestimate risk reduction if event rates are high. If smaller trials were conducted in higher risk populations that might benefit differentially from treatment and larger trials in more general populations (as can happen if new cancer treatments are first explored in small trials of patients with advanced disease), then the estimated effect will be greater in smaller trials thereby leading to asymmetry. Similarly, hazard ratios tend to migrate towards unity over time (if the event rate remains constant). Thus larger trials that tend to follow up patients for longer will produce lower estimates of efficacy, again potentially leading to funnel plot asymmetry. Furthermore, it is likely to be particularly difficult to observe and measure asymmetry if, as is commonly the case, meta-analyses are based on only a moderate number of trials. In practice, interpretation is very difficult, and although funnel plots may serve as a useful exploratory tool, asymmetry in a funnel plot does not necessarily indicate publication bias. Conversely, symmetry cannot be taken as proof that publication bias (or indeed other forms of heterogeneity) do not exist. Ultimately there is no substitute for attempting to identify unpublished trials, and funnel plots should not be used as an excuse for avoiding doing so.

11.7 Example of an IPD meta-analysis: Postoperative radiotherapy in non-small-cell lung cancer

Introduction Worldwide, over half a million new cases of lung cancer are diagnosed each year [58] and it is the leading cause of cancer deaths. Surgery is the treatment of choice for non-small-cell lung cancer (NSCLC), and around one fifth of tumours are suitable for potentially curative resection [59]. However, even for patients with apparently completely resected disease, survival rates are disappointing – around 40 per cent at two years. In an effort to improve both local control and survival, the use of adjuvant post-operative radiotherapy (PORT) has been explored.

Despite the conduct of a number of randomized trials, which had recruited a total of over 2000 patients, the role of PORT in the treatment of NSCLC remained unclear. Owing to their small size, individual trials did not have sufficient statistical power to detect moderate survival differences and had shown inconclusive and conflicting results. An international systematic review and meta-analysis was therefore initiated by the British Medical Research Council Cancer Trials Office and conducted on behalf of the PORT Meta-analysis Trialists' Group. It is important to note that the PORT meta-analysis was of individual patient data. This involved the central collection, validation and analysis of the updated original data from individual eligible trials and did not rely on data extracted from published papers.

Methods The main methods underlying the meta-analysis, which were all pre-specified in a formal protocol, are presented in more detail elsewhere [60]. In brief, all eligible randomized trials were included irrespective of publication status. To be eligible for inclusion, trials had to have used adequate methods of randomization, accrued between January 1965 and December 1995 and should not have used orthovoltage radiotherapy. They should have aimed to randomize NSCLC patients who had undergone a potentially curative resection. Analyses were done on an intention-to-treat basis using the log rank test stratified by trial. Expected numbers of events and variance for individual trials were combined according to a fixed effect model. In this way individual patient survival times were used to calculate hazard ratios giving the overall chance of dying on PORT at any time compared to surgery alone. This is a relative difference and so absolute effects at various points were also calculated by applying the HR to the survival rate on the surgery arm (see Section 11.5.7).

Data   Data were available from all nine eligible trials and 2128 patients representing 99 per cent of patients from all known eligible randomized trials. Table 11.8 shows the main trial characteristics. Further details of the radiotherapy techniques used can be found elsewhere [60]. Total radiotherapy doses ranged from 30 to 60 Gy, given in between 10 and 30 fractions and there was considerable diversity in other aspects of radiotherapy planning. Patients were mostly male and had stage II or III tumours with squamous cell histology and good performance status. Updated follow up was obtained for most trials such that the overall median was around four years, with a range of 2–10 years in individual trials.

Survival   Survival data were available for all trials and included information from 2128 patients and 1368 deaths. Results are shown in Fig. 11.15 where trials are ordered from earliest to most recent and Fig. 11.6 shows the corresponding survival curves for all patients. Although the confidence intervals (CI) for individual trial results are wide, there is a clear pattern of results in favour of surgery alone and there is no clear evidence of statistical heterogeneity ($p = 0.11$) between trials. The combined results show a significant adverse effect of PORT on survival ($p = 0.001$). The hazard ratio of 1.21 indicates a 21 per cent greater chance of death on PORT than on surgery alone (95 per cent CI 1.08–1.34). This is equivalent to an absolute detriment of 7 per cent at two years (95 per cent CI 3–10 per cent) reducing overall survival from 55 per cent to 48 per cent.

Table 11.8 Characteristics of trials included in the PORT meta-analysis.

Trial	Recruitment	Patients	Disease stage	Radiotherapy dose		
				Total (Gy)	Fractions	Weeks
Belgium	1966–77	202	I,II,III	60	30	6
LCSG 773	1978–85	230	II,III	50	25–27.5	5–5.5
CAMS	1981–95	317	II,III	60	30	6
Lille	1985–91	163	I	45–60	22.5–30	6
EORTC 08861	1986–90	106	II,III	56	28	5.5
MRC LU11	1986–93	308	II,III	40	15	3
GETCB 04CB86	1986–94	189	I,II,III	60	24–30	6
Slovenia	1988–92	74	III	30	10–12	2
GETCB 05CB88	1988–94	539	I,II,III	60	24–30	6

LCSG = Lung Cancer Study Group, CAMS = Chinese Academy of Medical Sciences, EORTC = European Organization for Research and Treatment of Cancer, MRC = Medical Research Council, GETCB = Groupe d'Etude et de Traitement des Cancers Bronchiques Twenty small-cell patients excluded.

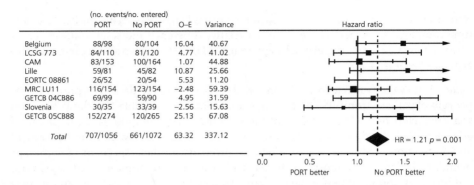

Fig. 11.15 Hazard ratio plot for survival in the PORT meta-analysis. Reproduced with permission from [42].

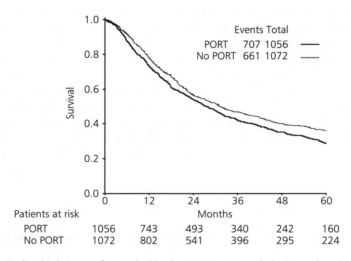

Fig. 11.16 Kaplan-Meier curve for survival in the PORT meta-analysis. Reproduced with permission from [42].

The cause of this detriment was not apparent from these analyses, although the limited cause-of-death information available suggested that the excess mortality on PORT might be the result of causes of death other than cancer. The addition of radiation treatment post-operatively may exert a deleterious effect by virtue of acute or delayed radiation effects, such as radiation pneumonitis or cardiotoxicity, on lungs likely to be already damaged by surgery and perhaps smoking.

Additional outcomes   For recurrence-free survival, that is the time from randomization to the first event – local recurrence, distant recurrence or death – a total of 1447 events were observed. Of these, 402 first events were deaths, 252 were local recurrences and 793 were distant recurrences. The overall pattern of results is similar to survival and there is no evidence of gross statistical heterogeneity between trials ($p = 0.21$). The HR of 1.13 indicates a 13 per cent relative detriment of PORT equivalent to an absolute detriment of 4 per cent at two years, reducing the recurrence-free survival rate from

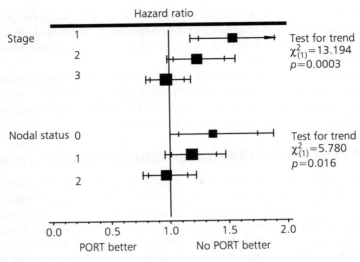

Fig. 11.17 Survival by stage and nodal status. Reproduced with permission from [42].

50 to 46 per cent. Analyses of local and distant recurrence-free survival also indicated an adverse effect of PORT with HRs of 1.16 (95 per cent CI 1.05–1.29) and 1.16 (95 per cent CI 1.04–1.29), respectively. As the observed detriment was somewhat less for these outcomes, this perhaps suggests that there may be anti-tumour activity attributable to radiotherapy and that the increased risk of death from PORT may be attributable to other mechanisms. Taken as a whole, the results suggest that although PORT may be beneficial in terms of preventing local recurrence, the effect is likely to be small and outweighed by the deleterious effect on survival.

Subgroups Analyses were also performed to determine whether there was evidence of a differential effect of PORT in pre-defined subgroups of patients. For survival there was no evidence to suggest that PORT was differentially effective in any group of patients defined by age, sex or histology.

However, as shown in Fig. 11.17, there was some evidence that the effects of PORT were more detrimental in patients with stage I than in those with stage II disease. Considering the results for stage III patients alone, there was no clear evidence of a detriment. Similarly, there was a trend that PORT was increasingly detrimental with lower nodal status. However, the confidence intervals are wide indicating that there is no clear evidence of a difference between treatments for stage III or N2 patients.

PORT conclusions This meta-analysis has demonstrated an adverse effect of PORT on survival for NSCLC patients with completely resected tumours. The 21 per cent relative increase in the risk of death associated with PORT represents a considerable hazard. Although exploratory analyses by stage and by nodal status suggested that this effect was most pronounced for earlier stage patients and those with lower nodal status, it is important to note that no patient group showed evidence of a clear benefit from PORT.

Although based on data from trials that used different radiotherapy doses and schedules, there was no indication from the meta-analysis that any of these individual schedules were less detrimental than others. There could still be scope for investigating more modern techniques, such as conformal or hyper-fractionated radiotherapy. However, there would need to be a clear expectation that these newer techniques would not produce similar adverse effects.

As for any such study, this meta-analysis can only provide average estimates of the effect of PORT. Nevertheless, it is probably the best available evidence on which to base future treatment policy. The results indicate that PORT should not be used routinely to treat patients with early stage, completely resected NSCLC.

11.8 The Cochrane Collaboration http://www.cochrane.org

The Cochrane collaboration is a worldwide organization committed to evidence-based medicine and the rigorous evaluation of healthcare interventions [61]. Although a relatively young organization, it has already produced a great many high quality systematic reviews and put in place mechanisms for their widespread dissemination and updating, both to healthcare professionals and to the public. It has also done much to promote lay involvement in the organization and in the development and appraisal of systematic review and meta-analysis methodology.

The collaboration is named after Archie Cochrane who, in 1972 published a now classic monograph [61] suggesting that because healthcare resource would always be limited, it should be used to provide, equitably, treatments which had been shown to be effective by properly designed evaluation. In particular he stressed the importance of using evidence from RCTs as these were likely to provide much more reliable information than other sources of evaluation. He noted that even though the results of trials may have been published, valid evidence about the effects of healthcare was not always readily available to those who needed it. He wrote:

> It is surely a great criticism of our profession that we have not organised a critical summary, by specialty and subspecialty, adapted periodically, of all relevant randomized controlled trials [62].

These ideas that treatment should be based on interventions that have been shown to be effective by properly controlled research and that systematic, up-to-date summaries of this information should be widely and easily available, comprise the central philosophy and ultimate goal of the Cochrane Collaboration. Founded upon an ambitious vision to put Cochrane's ideas into practice, and building on the experience of the international collaborative development of the Oxford Perinatal Trials Database, the first Cochrane Centre opened in Oxford in 1992. The Cochrane Collaboration, which was founded in 1993, is a worldwide endeavour, the importance of which has been likened to the Human Genome Project [63]. Internationally, thousands of health professionals, consumers and researchers are working together using the principles of systematic review and evidence-based medicine to address unresolved health problems. The collaboration, which has ten key principles (Box 11.10), aims to prepare, maintain, and promote the accessibility of high quality systematic reviews of all aspects of healthcare, based largely, though not exclusively, on the results of RCTs. However, like the Human Genome Project, this will take time. It has been estimated that up to a million RCTs have been published and it is estimated that it will take about twenty years to reach a stable state, where all existing information has been assessed and summarized, so that new primary research can be

Box 11.10   The Cochrane Collaboration's ten key principles

- *Collaboration,* by internally and externally fostering good communications, open decision-making and teamwork.
- *Building on the enthusiasm of individuals,* by involving and supporting people of different skills and backgrounds.
- *Avoiding duplication,* by good management and co-ordination to maximise economy of effort.
- *Minimising bias,* through a variety of approaches such as scientific rigour, ensuring broad participation, and avoiding conflicts of interest.
- *Keeping up to date,* by a commitment to ensure that Cochrane Reviews are maintained through identification and incorporation of new evidence.
- *Striving for relevance,* by promoting the assessment of healthcare interventions using outcomes that matter to people making choices in health care.
- *Promoting access,* by wide dissemination of the outputs of the Collaboration, taking advantage of strategic alliances, and by promoting appropriate prices, content and media to meet the needs of users worldwide.
- *Ensuring quality,* by being open and responsive to criticism, applying advances in methodology, and developing systems for quality improvement.
- *Continuity,* by ensuring that responsibility for reviews, editorial processes and key functions is maintained and renewed.
- *Enabling wide participation in the work of the Collaboration* by reducing barriers to contributing and by encouraging diversity.

easily assimilated into existing systematic reviews [64]. New systematic reviews are being completed rapidly. These are published quarterly as part of the 'Cochrane Library' and are disseminated in CD/disk format [65] and over the Internet (http://www.update-software.com, http://www.updateusa.com).

11.9   Conclusions

Systematic reviews and meta-analyses formally appraise and, where appropriate, combine the results of trials that have considered similar questions. The methods aim to reduce the potential influence of both random error and bias, and to establish more reliably whether there is a real difference between treatments. This can be done in a relatively short period of time compared to initiating new prospective studies. Given that in many cases there may already be sufficient evidence to resolve therapeutic issues, it could be considered both scientifically inappropriate and unethical not to carry out a formal systematic review of existing information, before embarking upon a new prospective study. However, a systematic review is not a quick fix and if done properly, is likely to take many months to complete.

The overall results of a well conducted systematic review should provide the most comprehensive and least biased appraisal of a therapeutic question, the meta-analysis element providing an estimate of the average effect of a treatment. This is probably the most reliable and best available evidence to guide treatment policy for future patients. Further information from subgroup analyses and knowledge of underlying risks for different types of patient may also guide decision making. However, when interpreting the results of any systematic review, it is important to remember that neither individual trials nor meta-analyses can provide prescriptions on how individual patients should be treated. The estimated average treatment effect is, however, an essential piece of information to be considered by both patients and doctors alongside other factors, such as toxicity, cost, patient preference and quality of life, when making individual treatment choices.

In summary, there are very many advantages of systematic review and meta-analysis. The process enables us to take a more global perspective as the value of any individual study depends on how well it fits with or expands other work as well as its own merits [66]. Not only are the power and precision of estimated benefit and risk improved and the influence of bias limited by adopting appropriate methodology, but we can also assess whether findings are consistent and can be generalized across different populations, settings and treatment variations [2]. The process can be thought of as being like assembling a well-worn jigsaw puzzle, whereby all the individual pieces have to be found, checked that they are for the correct puzzle and where necessary repaired before all the individual pieces can be put together. The resulting big picture should provide us with far greater insight than any single piece (no matter how new and shiny) in its own right. Despite the many advantages, it is important that systematic reviews and meta-analyses are neither used nor interpreted blindly. We must not be fooled by the apparent authority of large numbers but critically appraise the quality and value of the evidence on which any systematic review or meta-analysis is based and ensure that the methodology used is appropriate. In this way we can use the process both to obtain valuable answers to unresolved questions that can be put into clinical practice and to establish baselines and the basis on which future research can be built.

References

[1] Lau, J., and Ioannidis, J. (1998) Summing up evidence: one answer is not always enough. *Lancet*, 351, 123–7.

[2] Mulrow, C. (1994) Rationale for systematic reviews. *British Medical Journal*, 309, 597–9.

[3] Davidoff, F., Haynes, B., Sackett, D., and Smith, R. (1995) Evidence-based medicine. A new journal to help doctors identify the information they need. *British Medical Journal*, 310, 1085–6.

[4] Mulrow, C. (1987) The medical review article: state of the science. *Annals of Internal Medicine*, 106, 485–8.

[5] Antman, E.M., Lau, J., Kupelnick, B., Mosteller, F., and Chalmers, T.G.A. (1992) Comparison of results of meta-analyses and randomized controlled trials and recommendations of clinical experts. *Journal of the American Medical Association*, 268, 240–8.

[6] Chalmers, I., Enkin, M., and Keirse, J.N.C. (1993) Preparing and updating systematic reviews of randomized controlled trials of healthcare. *Milbank Q*, 71, 411–33.

[7] Egger, E., and Davey-Smith O'Rourke, K. (2001) Rationale, potentials and promise of systematic reviews. In *Systematic Reviews in Health Care. Meta-analysis in Context*, pp. 3–19. BMJ Books, London.

[8] Tierney, J. (1999) Meta-analysis in the research and treatment of cancer. *Principles and Practice of Oncology*, 13, 1–12.

[9] Collins, R., Gray, R., Godwin, J., and Peto, R. (1987). Avoidance of large biases and large random error in the assessment of moderate treatment effects: The need for systematic overviews. *Statistics in Medicine*, 6, 245–50.

[10] The ICON Collaborators. (1998) ICON2: randomized trial of single-agent carboplatin against three-drug combination of CAP (cyclophosphamide, doxorubicin and cisplatin) in women with ovarian cancer. *Lancet*, 352, 1571–6.

[11] Gray, R., James, R., Mossman, J., and Stenning, S. (1991) AXIS – a suitable case for treatment. *British Journal of Cancer*, 63, 841–5.

[12] Stewart, L.A., and Parmar, M.K.B. (1996) Bias in the analysis and reporting of randomized controlled trials. *International Journal of Technology Assessment in Healthcare*, 12, 264–75.

[13] Stewart, L.A., and Clarke, M.J. (1995) Practical methodology of meta-analyses (overviews) using updated individual patient data. *Statistics in Medicine*, 14, 2057–79.

[14] Clarke, M., Stewart, L., Pignon, J.P., and Bijnens, L. (1998) Individual patient data meta-analyses in cancer. *British Journal of Cancer*, 77, 2036–44.

[15] Qizilbash, N., Whitehead, A., Higgins, J., Wilcock, G., Schneider, L., and Farlow, M. (1998) Cholinesterase inhibition of Alzheimer disease: a meta-analysis of the tacrine trials. *Journal of the American Medical Association*, 280(20), 1777–82.

[16] Marson, A.G., Williamson, P.R., Clough, H., and Hutton, J.L. (2002) Carbamazepine versus valproate monotherapy for epilepsy. *Epilepsia*, 43, 505–13.

[17] HIV Trialists Collaborative Group. (1999) Zidovudine, didanosine, and zalcitabine in the treatment of HIV infection: meta-analyses of the randomised evidence. *Lancet*, 353, 2014–25.

[18] EU Hernia Trialists Collaboration. (2000) Laparoscopic compared with open methods of groin hernia repair – systematic review of randomised controlled trials. *British Journal of Surgery*, 87, 860–7.

[19] EU Hernia Trialists Collaboration. (2000) Mesh compared with non-mesh methods of open groin hernia repair – systematic review of randomised controlled trials. *British Journal of Surgery*, 87, 854–9.

[20] Stewart, L.A., and Parmar, M.K.B. (1993) Meta-analysis of the literature or of individual patient data: is there a difference? *Lancet*, 341, 418–22.

[21] Pignon, J.P. and Arriagada, R. (1993) Meta-analysis. *Lancet*, 341, 964–5.

[22] Jeng, G.T., Scott, J.R., and Burmeister L.F. (1995) A comparison of meta-analytic results using literature vs individual patient data: paternal cell immunization for recurrent miscarriage. *Journal of the American Medical Association*, 274, 830–6.

[23] Advanced Ovarian Cancer Trialists' Group (1991) Chemotherapy in advanced ovarian cancer: an overview of randomized clinical trials. *British Medical Journal*, 303, 884–93.

[24] Clarke, M. and Godwin, J. (1998) Systematic reviews using individual patient data: a map for the minefields? *Annals of Oncology*, 9, 827–33.

[25] D'Amico, R., Pifferi, S., Leonetti, C., Torri, V., Tinazzi, A., and Liberati, A. (1998) Effectiveness of antibiotic prophylaxis in critically ill adult patients: systematic review of randomized controlled trials. *British Medical Journal*, 316, 1275–85.

[26] Parmar, M.K.B., Torri, V., and Stewart, L.A. (1998) Meta-analyses of the published literature for survival endpoints. Some methods, problems and solutions. *Statistics in Medicine*, 17, 2815–34.

[27] Chalmers, I. (1993) 'The Cochrane Collaboration: preparing, maintaining and disseminating systematic reviews of the effects of healthcare'. *Annals of the New York Academy of Science*, 703, 156–65.

[28] Stern, J.M., and Simes, R.J. (1997) Publication bias: evidence of delayed publication in a cohort study of clinical research projects. *British Medical Journal*, 315, 640–5.

[29] Stewart, L.A., and Tierney, J.F. (2002) To IPD or not IPD? Advantages and disadvantages of systematic reviews using individual patient data. *Evaluation of the Health Professions*, **25**, 79–100.

[30] Pocock, S.J. (1993) *Clinical Trials: A Practical Approach*. John Wiley, New York.

[31] Altman, D.G., and Doré, C. (1990) Randomization and baseline comparisons in clinical trials. *Lancet*, **335**, 149–53.

[32] Schultz, K.F., Chalmers, I., Haynes, R.G., and Altman, D.G. (1994) Empirical evidence of bias: Dimensions of methodological quality associated with estimates of treatment effects in controlled trials. *Journal of the American Medical Association*, **273**, 1408–12.

[33] Dickersin, K., Min, Y.I., and Meinert, C.K. (1992) Factors influencing publication of research results. *Journal of the American Medical Association*, **267**, 374–8.

[34] Tramèr, M.R., Reynolds, D.J.M., Moore, R.A., and McQuay, H.J. (1997) Impact of covert duplicate publication on meta-analysis: A case study. *British Medical Journal*, **315**, 635–40.

[35] Tierney, J.F., and Stewart, L.A. (2000) Investigating Patient Exclusion Bias in Meta-analysis. *The 8th Cochrane Colloquium*, Cape Town.

[36] Sarcoma Meta-analysis Collaboration (1997) Adjuvant chemotherapy for localized resectable soft-tissue sarcoma of adults: meta-analysis of individual data. *Lancet*, **350**, 1647–53.

[37] Glioma Meta-analysis Trialists (GMT) Group. (2002) Chemotherapy in high-grade glioma: A systematic review and meta-analysis of individual patient data from 12 randomised trials. *Lancet*, **359**, 1011–18.

[38] Egger, M., Zellweger-Zahner, T., Schneier, M., Junker, C., Lengeler, C., and Antes, G. (1997) Language bias in randomized controlled trials published in English and German. *Lancet*, **350**, 326–9.

[39] Burdett, S., Stewart, L.A., and Tierney, J.F. (2002) Publication bias and meta-analyses: a practical example. *International Journal of Technology Assessment in Health Care*, In press.

[40] Juni, P., Holenstein, F., Sterne, J., Bartlett, C., and Eggar, M. (2002) Direction and impact of language bias in meta-analysis of controlled trials: empirical study. *International Journal of Epidemiology*, **31**, 115–23.

[41] McAuley, L., Pham, B., Tugwell, P., and Moher, D. (2000) Does the inclusion of grey literature influence estimates of intervention effectiveness reported in meta-analyses? *Lancet*, **356**, 1228–31.

[42] Neoadjuvant chemotherapy for locally advanced cancer of the uterine cervix. A meta-analysis using individual patient data. An MRC protocol.

[43] Lefebvre, C., and Clarke, M.J. (2001) Identifying randomised trials In *Systematic Reviews in Health Care. Meta-analysis in Context*, pp. 69–86, BMJ Books, London.

[44] Smith, B.j., Darzins, P.J., Quinn, M., and Heller, R.F. (1992) Modern methods of searching the medical literature. *Medical Journal of Australia*, **157**, 603–11.

[45] Tonks, A. (1999) Registering clinical trials. *British Medical Journal*, **319**, 1565–8.

[46] Green, J.A., Kirwan, J.M., Tierney, J.F., Symonds, P., Fresco, L., Collingwood, M., Williams, C.J. (2001) Survival and recurrence after concomitant chemotherapy and radiotherapy for cancer of the uterine cervix: a systematic review and meta-analysis. *Lancet*, **358**, 781–6.

[47] Advanced Ovarian Cancer Trialists' Group. (1998) Chemotherapy in advanced ovarian cancer: four systematic meta-analyses of individual patient data from 37 randomized trials. *British Journal of Cancer*, **78**, 1479–87.

[48] Eggar, M., Dickersin, K., and Davey Smith. (2001) Problems and limitations in conducting systematic reviews. In *Systematic Reviews in Health Care. Meta-analysis in Context*, pp. 43–68, BMJ Books, London.

[49] Tierney, J., Rydzewska, L., Burdett, S., and Stewart, L. (2001) Feasibility and reliability of using hazard ratios in meta-analyses of published time-to-event data. *The 9th Cochrane Colloquium*, Lyon, [abstract].

[50] Stewart, L.A. (1992) The role of overviews. In *Introducing New Treatments for Cancer: Practical, Ethical and Legal Problems*. John Wiley, New York.

[51] Non-small Cell Lung Cancer Collaborative Group (1995) Chemotherapy in non-small cell lung cancer: a meta-analysis using updated data on individual patient data from 52 randomized clinical trials. *British Medical Journal*, 311, 899–909.

[52] Pignon, J.P., Arriagada, R., Ihde, D., Johnson, D., Perry, M., and Souhami, R. (1992) A meta-analysis of thoracic radiotherapy for small-cell lung cancer. *New England Journal of Medicine*, 327, 1618–24.

[53] Moher, D., Cook, D., Eastwood, S., Olkin, I., Rennie, D., and Stroup D for the QUORUM Group. (1999) Improving the quality of reports of meta-analyses of randomised controlled trials: The QUORUM statement. *Lancet*, 354, 1896–90.

[54] Thompson, S. (1994) Why sources of heterogeneity in meta-analysis should be investigated. *British Medical Journal*, 309, 1351–5.

[55] Berlin, J.A., and Antman, E.M. (1994) Advantages and limitations of meta-analytic regressions of clinical data. *Online Journal of Current Clinical Trials*, doc. no. 134.

[56] Eggar, M., Davey Smith, G., Schneider, M., and Minder, C. (1997) Bias in meta-analysis detected by a simple graphical test. *British Medical Journal*, 315, 629–34.

[57] Machin, D., Stenning, S., Parmar, M., Fayers, P., Girling, D., Stephens, R., Stewart, L., and Whaley, J. (1997) Thirty years of Medical Research Council randomized trials in solid tumours. *Clinical Oncology*, 9, 100–114.

[58] Parkin, D.M., and Saxo, A.J. (1993) Lung cancer: worldwide variation in occurrence and proportion attributable to tobacco use. *Lung Cancer* (suppl), 9, 1–16.

[59] Silverberg, E., Boring, C.C., and Squires, T.S. (1990) Cancer Statistics. *CA: A Cancer Journal for Clinicians*, 40, 9–26.

[60] PORT Meta-analysis Trialists Group. (1998) Postoperative radiotherapy in non-small cell lung cancer: A systematic review and meta-analysis of individual patient data from nine randomized controlled trials. *Lancet*, 352, 257–63.

[61] Clarke, M., and Langhorne, P. (2001) Revisiting the Cochrane Collaboration. Meeting the challenge of Archie Cochrane – and facing up to some new ones. *British Medical Journal*, 13, 323, 829–32.

[62] Cochrane, A.L. (1972) Effectiveness and Efficiency: Random reflections on health services. The Nuffield Provincial Hospitals Trust, London.

[63] Naylor, C. (1995) Grey zones of clinical practice: some limits to evidence-based medicine. *Lancet*, 345, 840–2.

[64] Chalmers, I., and Haynes, B. (1994) Reporting, updating and correcting systematic reviews of the effects of heath care. *British Medical Journal*, 309, 862–5.

[65] The Cochrane Library (database on disk and CD-ROM) (1996) The Cochrane Collaboration. Oxford: Update Software – updated quarterly.

[66] Cooper, H.M. (1994) *The Integrative Research Review: A Systematic Approach*. Beverly Hills, CA: Sage Publications.

Chapter 12

Benefits of an established trials centre and research group

12.1 Introduction

In this book, we have described the conduct of cancer clinical trials, systematic reviews and meta-analyses. Some trials will be conducted by a single centre or small group of collaborating hospitals with a separate grant for each study, others as part of a long-term programme of research by an established trials centre and research group with some core funding. In this final chapter, we describe the advantages of such an established group. These include the strategic planning of coherent programmes of clinical studies and meta-analyses; undertaking large multi-centre and multi-group trials nationally and internationally; having a team of well-trained and experienced core staff thoroughly familiar with locally developed and well tested procedures, who have built up a group of centres conversant with the practicalities of collaborating in trials over many years; developing long-term collaboration with patient-advocacy groups; training and teaching; fulfilling advisory and consultative roles, and conducting a programme of trials-associated and methodological research.

12.2 The characteristics of an established trials centre

The functions of trials coordinating staff in running individual trials and as members of site-specific groups, planning groups and trial management groups have been described in earlier chapters. However, an established trials centre has additional benefits that apply across its entire programme of trials and related research (see Box 12.1). These particularly relate to having an internationally recognized centre of excellence with accumulated experience and expertise in all aspects of conducting cancer trials.

12.3 International collaboration between trials centres

We discuss the practicalities of collaboration between trials groups in Section 7.10. Established trials centres can readily collaborate internationally to undertake trials that might otherwise not be feasible, as they provide a focus for many clinical centres within a country, and have defined procedures and infrastructures for such collaborative efforts. From time to time, therefore, established trials centres can organize international meetings to discuss areas of research in which international planning is likely to be needed. These areas can include broad clinical research strategy aimed at encouraging complementarity

Box 12.1 The additional benefits accruing to an established trials centre

- An internationally recognized centre of excellence which can collaborate with other international trials groups
- Coherent programmes of clinical trials planned strategically and run cost-effectively
- Cross-fertilization of ideas and experience across trials in different cancer sites
- An established network of collaborating centres, expert advisers and independent assessors
- A team of experienced core staff with statistical, medical, computing, trial coordinating, management, administrative and secretarial expertise
- Continuity of staff, permitting the development of disease-specific expertise
- A programme of systematic reviews and meta-analyses linked to the trials
- Long-standing links with patient advocacy groups
- Established procedures for relating to sponsors and for collaboration between industrial and non-industrial partners
- Availability of data from trials for many years after publication for meta-analyses and other research
- A clear focus for the 'ownership,' follow-up and long-term retention of trial data
- A programme of methodological and trials-associated research to improve trials and make productive use of large amounts of accumulated data

Box 12.2 Circumstances in which international planning is needed

- To achieve adequately large and sufficiently rapid intakes into trials in rare cancers
- To study uncommon treatment situations in common cancers
- To achieve rapid intakes into large trials

in centres' programmes of trials, avoiding undesirable duplication, and collaboration in a single trial or a joint analysis of trials to be run in parallel (see Box 12.2).

International collaboration is essential for achieving rapid, adequately sized intakes into randomized trials in uncommon cancers, and has been highly productive in trials in advanced bladder cancer, testicular cancer, gliomas, ovarian cancer, osteosarcoma and lymphoma. International collaboration is also helpful in studying uncommon therapeutic situations related to common cancers and in achieving rapid intakes into large trials. For example, colorectal cancer is common, but only occasionally is it thought that resection of an isolated liver or lung metastasis should be undertaken. When such resection is considered desirable, it is not known whether giving post-operative chemotherapy might benefit the patient. The European Organization for Research and Treatment of Cancer, the National Cancer Institute of Canada, and the Gruppo Interdisciplinare Valutazione Interventi in Oncologia therefore collaborated in a comparison of chemotherapy versus no chemotherapy following potentially curative resection of liver or lung metastases from colorectal cancer (EORTC protocol 40923); 478 patients were randomized during forty-four months.

An example of a large pragmatic trial involving international collaboration is the ICON3 trial. This compared paclitaxel plus carboplatin versus non-paclitaxel control chemotherapy as first-line treatment for advanced ovarian cancer; 2074 patients were randomized from 132 hospitals in eight countries during forty-three months [1].

12.4   Coherent programmes of trials

Over the years, an established trials centre builds up a large network of collaborating clinicians and other people who collaborate in many trials. This enables the group to plan coherent programmes of trials strategically, to run them cost-effectively, and to prioritize within and across cancer sites.

12.4.1   Framing clinically relevant hypotheses

Trials centres create channels for receiving and developing ideas for new trials and, if appropriate, putting them to the test within a relevant programme.

Ideas for new trials can arise from anyone within the medical research community, from the results of ongoing or recently completed trials, from other clinical research such as phase I and phase II studies, from meta-analyses, and from meetings of experts and patient-advocacy groups organized by the centre for the purpose of identifying the questions that most urgently need to be answered.

12.4.2   Example of a strategically planned programme of clinical research

A coherent programme of research can certainly be achieved on an *ad hoc* basis by independent groups and individuals who are aware of other trials, and plan their own to be complementary. There can be additional advantages, however, from having a single trials group with the capacity to run trials in all the relevant stages of a particular cancer, where good trial ideas exist. In this way, it is possible to ensure that there is no unintentional overlap in eligibility for trials. For example, in developing their trials in germ-cell cancer in the late 1980s, the MRC Testis Cancer Group were able to ensure that all patients with metastatic germ-cell cancer were eligible for one, and only one, trial. At that time, trials were ongoing in virtually every stage of disease, which had the added advantage that collaborating clinicians could consider every patient they saw for a suitable trial. This may well have contributed to the very high proportion of newly diagnosed patients (over 50 per cent of the national annual incidence) going into these trials.

12.5 Maintaining a network of collaborating centres

Trials centres are able to establish, maintain and continue to develop a network of collaborating clinical investigators and their teams, expert advisers, independent assessors, and local data managers throughout the programme. For example, in testicular cancer, a series of three successive MRC trials in stage I seminoma showed how the base of collaborating clinicians expanded over time, the first trial recruiting approximately 500 patients from twenty centres over four years, the second 600 patients from forty-five centres over three years, and the third 1500 patients from seventy-two centres over five years.

An efficient trials centre is able to keep collaborators informed of progress in all aspects of the programme, and to respond promptly and positively to any ideas, comments, criticisms or queries that collaborators may raise.

It is understandably difficult, however, for collaborators in a large programme of multi-centre trials to feel that they share in the ownership of the programme. They need to be shown that they are not just recruiting patients and providing data for the benefit and prestige of the trials centre, but that their views and their advice, often based on many years of experience, are not only valued but are actively sought and acted upon. This can be achieved in a number of ways by centre staff.

♦ Maintain personal links with collaborators, by telephone, at visits to centres, at meetings and conferences. Send them copies of annual reports, newsletters and reprints, and encourage them to visit the centre and comment on any aspects of the programme and the ways it is conducted.

♦ Contact the organizers of appropriate scientific conferences and, if acceptable, arrange to have a stand providing newsletters and displaying posters and information on all trials relevant to the conference. Arrange for someone always to be available at the stand to answer queries, to provide details of trials and outline protocols, and to record the names and addresses of potential collaborators.

♦ Offer to speak about one or more open trials, recently completed trials, and future plans at meetings organized locally by centres or by regions.

♦ Keep patient advocacy groups informed of the progress of all trials relevant to them, reminding them of the purposes and possible benefits.

In addition, there are a number of societies, some quite informal, concerned with particular cancers or areas of cancer research. These, too, can keep members informed about new developments and can generate productive discussion and new ideas. In conjunction with established trials centres, representatives of research groups for each of the main cancer sites or types can meet regularly to (1) review where matters stand in therapeutic research internationally, (2) discuss ideas for new trials, and (3) suggest how new trials can best be developed and activated. Small meetings of relevant researchers can then discuss particular issues in depth. In the United States, the National Cancer Institute, and in the United Kingdom, the National Cancer Research Institute provide forums for airing, discussing and developing new ideas, reviewing proposed trials, and setting priorities.

Meetings needed for developing and conducting multi-centre research programmes are likely to be of two main types: large collaborators' meetings and smaller planning group meetings. Regular newsletters and annual reports also help to maintain interest.

12.5.1 Collaborators' meetings

Collaborators' meetings are large meetings, involving all types of specialists treating cancers grouped according to the programmes of trials in particular cancer sites. A collaborators' meeting thus involves a whole programme of trials and might take place once every one to two years. Participants might include clinicians collaborating in the current programme or with an interest in doing so, expert advisers, and representatives from other groups conducting trials in the same area.

The main purpose of these meetings is for soliciting, documenting and considering collaborators' comments on the progress of open trials and their ideas for the future (see Box 12.3). They therefore fulfill an invaluable role in helping to frame clinically relevant hypotheses for new trials and in assessing the level of interest new ideas are likely to attract. They also help to give collaborators a sense of corporate identity.

Each meeting has a number of typical agenda items. It is useful to include the agenda and a summary of background information and data to be discussed in a brochure which those attending can take away with them and which can be sent to those unable to attend. A brochure is helpful in keeping collaborators fully informed and enabling them subsequently to discuss the research programme and the meeting with their colleagues. Not all the agenda items will need to be discussed in detail at the meeting: some of them can more appropriately be dealt with mainly through the brochure and briefly discussed at the meeting. For example, presentations made to scientific meetings and full publications since the previous meeting can be listed in the brochure and their abstracts reproduced, collaborators being invited to raise questions or make comments if they wish. This approach enables maximum time to be spent on items that require full discussion.

The progress of the current research programme is summarized and recent results presented, attention being drawn to any matters of particular interest or importance. In presenting the progress of trials still open to patient intake (see also Section 8.6.2), recruitment should be shown, centre by centre, in the brochure to enable discussion. It is important to say what is going well but also to air any problems. The experiences of different centres will vary and centres can often usefully share experiences with each other. If the intake to a trial is going well and any problems are being dealt with efficiently, then clinicians not yet participating are more likely to decide to do so.

Box 12.3 The aims of collaborators' meetings

- ◆ To summarize the progress of the clinical research programme
- ◆ To bring collaborators up-to-date on the progress of the currently open trials
- ◆ To discuss any problems and how they can best be tackled
- ◆ To encourage those not entering patients into current trials to do so
- ◆ To discuss ideas for new trials and to explore likely levels of interest
- ◆ To coordinate with other trials groups over clinical research strategy
- ◆ To provide an update on developments in new treatment policies or associated research from invited experts

The results of recently completed trials will often suggest ideas for new trials. Ideas for new trials also emerge from the results of trials conducted by other groups discussed at meetings. Indeed, it is important to involve representatives from other groups for this purpose and also to consider collaborative or parallel trials, if appropriate, and to avoid unnecessary duplication.

It adds greatly to the interest in a collaborators' meeting if one or more experts on either clinical or basic scientific issues is invited to give a talk to bring the meeting up to date on the latest developments in the field. Topics might include, for example, national priorities, improved methods of staging, basic scientific studies and translational research on potential new treatment modalities, new developments in established treatments, and the assessment of quality of life.

The most important function of a collaborators' meeting is to provide an opportunity for discussion about ongoing trials and those being planned and ideas for future trials, and to get some feel for the level of support that new trials are likely to attract.

12.5.2   Planning group meetings

Planning groups are characteristically highly focused. Their purpose is to discuss ideas in depth and to develop the details of a new outline proposal. They meet as and when necessary.

12.5.3   Newsletters and annual reports

An excellent way for a trials centre to keep a large number of collaborators, interested individuals, sponsors and other trials centres and groups generally informed about its whole programme of trials and related research is to produce regular newsletters and annual reports and to circulate these widely.

Newsletters typically relate to specific areas of the programme, such as individual cancer sites. They keep collaborating clinicians and others informed about the progress of the relevant trials and encourage collaboration.

Annual reports provide an overall picture of the work of the centre, helping readers to decide which trials they might like to join. The most helpful reports are set out attractively and logically, for easy reference, and show, at a glance, whom to contact for further information on any particular topic or trial.

12.6   Trials centre staff

The staff of a trials centre comprise a team who have acquired considerable experience and specialized expertise, often over many years. This is an invaluable resource that greatly facilitates the conduct of substantial long-term research programmes.

12.6.1   Staff and expertise

The staff include statistical, medical and computing scientists, clinical trials managers, data managers and assistants, and administrative and secretarial staff. Clinical expertise is essential and can be provided by medically qualified full-time or part-time members of the centre, by clinicians working in close collaboration with the centre, or both. Expert advice on, for example, histopathology, quality of life assessment, and health economics, may more appropriately be provided from outside the centre, depending on the size of the centre and the nature of its programme.

All staff members are fully trained in their own area of expertise and keep up-to-date on all aspects of their work, including progress in the treatment of the cancers with which they deal and developments in computing software and trials methodology. In addition to undergoing in-house training, staff can be encouraged to attend appropriate training courses, including relevant higher degrees and diplomas, and to participate in specialist conferences and clinical and scientific meetings.

The variety of expertise that a single trial requires illustrates another benefit of an established trials centre. An individual trial of modest size may well require a full-time trials manager, but only fractions of other staff: perhaps 10 per cent of a statistician, for example. We have emphasized the benefits of continuity of staff from design through to analysis, but this is hard to achieve when only fractions of staff are required. A trials centre conducting a substantial programme of trials is much more likely to be able to justify half-time or full-time members of staff working across several trials, and such posts are much easier to fill. When at least some of these staff are core-funded they are also able to work on developing new trials; a great deal of work can be required in putting together a trial grant application before any trial-specific funding can be obtained.

12.6.2 Standard operating procedures

Trials centres should develop standard operating procedures (SOPs) that state the general principles adhered to by the centre in conducting its research programmes and provide general instructions on the conduct of trials. They thus establish a scientific and administrative policy applied across all trials, ensuring a high level of efficiency in working practices, greatly assisting the training of new staff, and enabling staff members to take over others' trials with minimum disruption. SOPs will obviously differ between centres in detail and in the way they are organized and set out, but the general topics and the principles should be very similar from centre to centre.

Typical SOPs cover many of the topics dealt with in this book, including trial conduct, grant applications, costings, protocol design, informed consent, contracts between industrial and non-industrial partners, ethics committees, collaborators' responsibilities, data management, and publication. They should be kept under constant review and updated as often as is necessary.

12.7 Links with patient advocacy groups

Patient advocacy groups include general groups which have the aims of involving consumers in the prioritization and commissioning of research and development in all areas of medicine, and of ensuring that the results of research are appropriately disseminated. The major cancer charities play an invaluable role in providing information on all aspects of cancers and their management through booklets, telephone conversations, personal contact and web sites. There is also a wide variety of organizations concerned with particular types of cancer. Box 12.4 indicates the roles of patient advocacy groups that are relevant to cancer trials.

Box 12.4   Roles of patient advocacy groups relevant to cancer trials

Providing potential patients with information on

- The treatment modalities used to treat cancer and their adverse effects and how they can be avoided or ameliorated
- Clinical trials and what is involved in agreeing to enter a trial
- Why randomized trials are needed
- Ethical issues, including patients' rights to withdraw from a trial without having to give reasons

Providing cancer trials centres and research groups with advice on

- Patients' concerns and perceived priorities
- The wording of patient information leaflets and consent forms

Cancer trials centres and clinical research groups are able to establish long-term links with such organizations. They can assist greatly in providing cancer patients and their families with information on the types of treatment and their adverse effects, on the sorts of investigations that are likely to be needed, and on current randomized trials, and can explain why treatments being compared often need to be assigned at random. They can provide many other forms of support as well. They are a source of independent advice on patients' concerns and on what agreeing to take part in a trial is likely to involve for patients. They relay, to cancer researchers, patients' concerns and views on research priorities. They can also be of great help in advising on the wording of patient information sheets and consent forms for randomized trial protocols.

When good collaborative relationships have been established with patient advocacy groups, these groups can make informed and practical suggestions about proposed new trials and how they are likely to be perceived by patients.

12.8   Long-term follow-up, ownership and retention of data

A further benefit of an established trials centre with core-funded staff is that it provides a natural 'home' for trial data, both electronic and paper-based, to be retained in the long term. Issues to be aware of in this respect include the need to:

- continue long-term follow-up of trial patients,
- retain data securely for a specified period after completion of a trial as required by GCP,
- provide access to trial data for relevant research projects including systematic reviews and meta-analyses, which may happen as many as twenty years or more after the trial was completed.

Where funding for an individual trial is attached to a person – perhaps the principal investigator – rather than an institution or group with a long-term commitment, all these issues can be problematic. It is difficult to secure funding for long-term follow-up of trials when individual trials are grant-funded, whereas it is likely to be easier to justify as part of a rolling programme of trials. It may also be unclear who is responsible for trial data should the principal investigator move or change jobs. It is therefore important to ensure that guidelines with respect to these issues are produced at an early stage.

12.9 Methodological and trials-associated research

Perhaps the greatest benefit of established trials centre staff conducting a series of trials is the potential this gives for developing practical and theoretical methodology that can enhance past trials and underpin future ones. A programme of clinical trials generates large amounts of data and can therefore be backed up by relevant trials-associated and methodological research to the benefit of the trials programme. Such research also provides further opportunities to involve, in a different capacity, some of the clinical collaborators who provided patients for the trials. The randomized controlled trial itself is not the only research tool the clinical researcher has to hand [2], and the appropriate tool has to be chosen according to the nature of the question being asked. Much valuable trials-associated research involves tools other than the randomized trial. Such research can include, for example, developing quality of life questionnaires [3]; undertaking surveys of clinicians' practice and attitudes; studying factors of prognostic influence; improving staging definitions; and methodological and statistical research.

Each trials centre is likely to have a programme of methodological and trials-associated research, the results of which can help to improve the design, conduct, analysis and interpretation of trials. Such a programme is likely to involve prospective methodological studies and retrospective analyses of accumulated data from large numbers of patients in many trials. Research in our own unit includes, for example, refining tumour staging and thereby greatly assisting the design of testis cancer trials [4], surveys of practice and opinions which provided invaluable information for planning future trials, particularly in lung cancer [5–8], investigating prognostic factors [9–12], long-term survival [13], and adverse effects [14], Bayesian data monitoring [15,16], and many aspects of quality of life assessment (see Chapters 6 and 9).

Part of the success of the programme of MRC testis cancer trials is attributable to the parallel programme of associated, retrospective research. While being valuable in its own right, this has, for example, provided a means by which many people, with disparate ideas about how testicular cancer should be treated, could be brought together in a large collaborative project, and become involved in planning future trials. In addition, the fact that the majority of patients are seen in a relatively small number of cancer centres makes it feasible to involve the majority of people treating the disease in the decision-making process. Two examples of how retrospective studies led on to programmes of trials are illustrated below.

Example 1: Stage I non-seminomatous germ-cell tumours (NSGCT). Until the 1980s, treatment for stage I NSGCT was typically orchidectomy with post-operative radiotherapy or extensive lymph-node dissection at the time of surgery. A policy of surveillance following orchidectomy alone with further treatment only at relapse was, however, used in some centres, with long-term survival rates apparently comparable with those in patients receiving adjuvant therapy.

In 1984, the MRC initiated both a retrospective (TE01) [17] and prospective (TE04) [18] study of patients on surveillance. The aim was, in TE01, to assess the overall relapse rate and survival rate, and to investigate possible prognostic factors to indicate if any patients were at sufficiently high risk of relapse to justify adjuvant therapy, and, in TE04, to validate any hypotheses generated by the retrospective study. In addition, in TE04, data were collected on the timing of radiological investigations. These studies together enabled a prognostic index to be defined that identified a group of patients (20–25 per cent of all stage I patients on surveillance) with a 50–60 per cent risk of relapse within two years.

As a result of these studies, the MRC conducted one of the first studies of post-operative short-course chemotherapy in these patients (TE05), which showed that two courses of bleomycin, etoposide and cisplatin (BEP) virtually eliminated the risk of relapse in high-risk patients [19]; and launched a randomized trial (TE08) investigating the impact of different CT scan schedules on stage of disease at relapse and timing of relapse, based on hypotheses formed in the TE04 study.

Example 2: Metastatic germ-cell tumours. There is a long-established practice of dividing patients with metastatic germ-cell tumours according to prognosis, and tailoring treatment accordingly. However, all the major groups worldwide had established their own prognostic criteria in different ways and considered use of their own criteria to be a prerequisite for clinical trials. This naturally inhibited collaboration. The MRC had resolved one long-running dispute by showing in a retrospective study of patients treated mainly prior to the platinum era (TE02), that volume of disease and tumour markers were complementary prognostic factors [20]. Once platinum-based chemotherapy had become established, a further retrospective study (TE07) was carried out with the specific intention of devising a prognostic classification for future trials in the platinum era [21]. The European Organization for Research and Treatment of Cancer (EORTC) were looking at data with a similar aim, and, through collaboration, the eligibility criteria for two subsequent randomized trials were developed, and the trials (TE09, TE13) run as a successful collaborative effort [22,23].

Though the MRC and EORTC were now collaborating, wider collaboration was still hindered by lack of a universally agreed prognostic classification. The MRC therefore initiated an international study to develop just such a classification. All the major germ-cell cancer treatment centres worldwide were invited, and agreed to collaborate under the name of the International Germ Cell Cancer Collaborative Group. The classification of metastatic germ-cell tumours that resulted (known as the International Germ Cell Consensus Classification) [4] was adopted by the International Union Against Cancer to form the basis of the latest TNM classification of germ-cell tumours, leading them to introduce non-anatomical factors (tumour markers) for the first time.

The basis for collaboration that this work produced has enabled large, reliable trials to be carried out rapidly, despite the rarity of the disease. Subsequently, many trials groups internationally now use the IGCCC to determine eligibility for trials. TE20, comparing three versus four courses of BEP in good-risk patients, recruited over 800 patients from twelve countries in less than three years [24]. Trials in intermediate-risk and poor-risk patients involve many of the countries collaborating in the IGCCCG project.

A further example of how involvement in a trials-related research project led on to successful new trials is the individual-patient-data meta-analysis in advanced ovarian cancer [25], the first such project to be undertaken by the MRC Clinical Trials Unit. The collaborators' meeting for the meta-analysis, held to present and discuss the results and where they should lead, brought together an international group of clinicians with a specific interest in clinical trials in ovarian cancer. Directly from discussion of the results came proposals for trials in early and advanced disease (ICON1, ICON2) which had a captive group of potential, and in due course actual, collaborators. The ICON (International Collaborative Ovarian Neoplasm) collaborative group thus formed has continued to expand and has conducted some of the largest trials in ovarian cancer ever undertaken.

In a trials centre with a programme of research in a number of types of cancer, scientific staff will be aware of many aspects of the centre's programme, not just those in which they are directly involved. This can be very beneficial, as much research can be conducted across cancer sites or is relevant to sites other than the one in which it was undertaken. Examples from the programme in our own unit include studies of hypoxic cell sensitizers, continuous hyperfractionated accelerated radiotherapy, chemotherapy dose-intensification, pre-operative chemotherapy, immediate versus delayed treatment, cytokines, the accuracy of histological reporting, comparisons of quality of life instruments, evaluation of haematological toxicity as a prognostic factor and defining quality of life endpoints.

12.10 Conclusion

The established cancer trials centre occupies a crucial scientific and organizational position, facilitating not only the planning, conduct and reporting of individual trials but also the strategic planning of long-term programmes of research nationally and internationally. There are many such groups throughout the world. There is, however, much scope for closer collaboration between them to achieve rapid intakes into large trials with a higher level of international strategic planning. Such enhanced collaboration will lead to more rapid improvements in treatment to the benefit of patients with cancer worldwide.

References

[1] The International Collaborative Ovarian Neoplasm (ICON) Group. (2002) Paclitaxel plus carboplatin versus standard chemotherapy with either single-agent carboplatin or cyclophosphamide, doxorubicin, and cisplatin in women with ovarian cancer: the ICON3 randomised trial. *Lancet*, **360**, 505–15.

[2] Sackett, D.L., and Wennberg, J.E. (1997) Choosing the best research design for each question. *British Medical Journal*, **315**, 1636.

[3] Sprangers, M.A.G., Cull, A., Bjordal, K., Groenvold, M., and Aaronson, N.K., for the EORTC Study Group on Quality of Life (1993) The European Organization for Research and Treatment of Cancer approach to quality of life assessment: guidelines for developing questionnaire modules. *Quality of Life Research*, **2**, 287–95.

[4] International Germ Cell Cancer Collaborative Group. (1997) International germ cell consensus classification: a prognostic factor-based staging system for metastatic germ cell cancers. *Journal of Clinical Oncology*, **15**, 594–603.

[5] Stephens, R., and Gibson, D. (1993) The impact of clinical trials on the treatment of lung cancer. *Clinical Oncology*, 5, 211–19.

[6] Crook, A., Duffy, A., Girling, D.J., Souhami, R.L., and Parmar, M.K.B. (1997) Survey on the treatment of non-small cell lung cancer (NSCLC) in England and Wales. *European Respiratory Journal*, 10, 1552–8.

[7] Hopwood, P., Harvey, A., Davies, J., Stephens, R.J., Girling, D.J., Gibson, D., and Parmar, M.K.B., on behalf of the Medical Research Council Lung Cancer Working Party and the CHART Steering Committee (1998) Survey of the administration of quality of life (QL) questionnaires in three multicentre randomised trials in cancer. *European Journal of Cancer*, 34, 49–57.

[8] Sambrook, R.J., and Girling, D.J. (2001) A national survey of the chemotherapy regimens used to treat small cell lung cancer (SCLC) in the United Kingdom. *British Journal of Cancer*, 84, 1447–52.

[9] Mead, G.M., and Stenning, S.P., for the Medical Research Council Testicular Tumour Working Party (1993) Prognostic factors in metastatic non-seminomatous germ cell tumours: the Medical Research Council studies. *European Urology*, 23, 196–201.

[10] Reading, J., Hall, R.R., and Parmar, M.K.B. (1995) The application of a prognostic factor analysis for Ta.T1 bladder cancer in routine urological practice. *British Journal of Urology*, 75, 604–7.

[11] Feld, R., Abratt, R., Graziano, S., Jassem, J., Lacquet, L., Ninane, V., Paesmans, M., Rocmans, P., Schiepers, C., Stahel, R., and Stephens, R. (1997) Pretreatment minimal staging and prognostic factors for non-small cell lung cancer. *Lung Cancer*, 17(Supplement 1), S3–S10.

[12] Fossa, S.D., Oliver, R.T.D., Stenning, S.P., Horwich, A., Wilkinson, P., Read, G., Mead, G.M., Roberts, J.T., Rustin, G., Cullen, M.H., Kaye, S.B., Harland, S.J., and Cook, P. (1997) Prognostic factors for patients with advanced seminoma treated with platinum-based chemotherapy. *European Journal of Cancer*, 33, 1380–7.

[13] Stephens, R.J., Bailey, A.J., and Machin, D. (1996) Long-term survival in small cell lung cancer: the case for a standard definition. *Lung Cancer*, 15, 297–309.

[14] Macbeth, F.R., Wheldon, T.E., Girling, D.J., Stephens, R.J., Machin, D., Bleehen, N.M., Lamont, A., Radstone, D.J., and Reed, N.S., for the Medical Research Council Lung Cancer Working Party (1996) Radiation myelopathy: estimates of risk in 1048 patients in three randomized trials of palliative radiotherapy for non-small cell lung cancer. *Clinical Oncology*, 8, 176–81.

[15] Parmar, M.K.B., Spiegelhalter, D.J., Freedman, L.S., and the CHART Steering Committee. (1994) The CHART trials: Bayesian design and monitoring in practice. *Statistics in Medicine*, 13, 1297–312.

[16] Fayers, P.M., Ashby, D., and Parmar, M.K.B. (1997) Tutorial in biostatistics: Bayesian data monitoring in clinical trials. *Statistics in Medicine*, 16, 1413–30.

[17] Freedman, L.S., Parkinson, M.C., Jones, W.G., Oliver, R.T.D., Peckham, M.J., Read, G., Newlands, E.S., and Williams, C.J., on behalf of the Medical Research Council Testicular Tumour Subgroup (Urological Working Party) (1987) Histopathology in the prediction of relapse of patients with stage I testicular teratoma treated by orchidectomy alone. *Lancet*, ii, 294–8.

[18] Read, G., Stenning, S.P., Cullen, M.H., Parkinson, M.C., Horwich, A., Kaye, S.B., and Cook, P.A. (1992) MRC prospective study of surveillance for stage I testicular teratoma. *Journal of Clinical Oncology*, 10, 1762–8.

[19] Cullen, M.H., Stenning, S.P., Parkinson, M.C., Fossa, S.D., Kaye, S.B., Horwich, A., Harland, S.J., Williams, M.V., and Jakes, R., for the MRC Testicular Tumour Working Party (1996) Short course adjuvant chemotherapy in high risk stage I NSGCT: an MRC study report. *Journal of Clinical Oncology*, 14, 1106–13.

[20] MRC Working Party on Testicular Tumours. (1985) Prognostic factors in advanced non-seminomatous germ cell tumours: results of a multicentre study. *Lancet*, i, 8–11.

[21] Mead, G.M., Stenning, S.P., Parkinson, M.C., Horwich, A., Fossa, S.D., Wilkinson, P.M., Kaye, S.B., Newlands, E.S., and Cook, P.A. (1992) The second MRC study of prognostic factors in NSGCT. *Journal of Clinical Oncology*, 10, 85–94.

[22] Horwich, A., Sleijfer, D., Fossa, S.D., Kaye, S.B., Oliver, R.T.D., Cullen, M.H., Mead, G.M., de Wit, R., de Mulder, P.H.M., Dearnaley, D.P., Cook, P.A., Sylvester, R.J., and Stenning, S.P. (1997) A randomised trial of bleomycin, etoposide and cisplatin compared to bleomycin, etoposide and carboplatin in good prognosis metastatic non-seminomatous germ cell cancer: a multi-institutional MRC/EORTC trial. *Journal of Clinical Oncology*, 15, 1844–52.

[23] Kaye, S.B., Mead, G.M., Fossa, S., Cullen, M., de Wit, R., Bodrogi, I., van Groeningen, C., Sylvester, R., Collette, L., Stenning, S., de Prijck, L., Lallemand, E., and de Mulder, P. (1998) BEP vs BOP/VIP for poor prognosis non-seminomatous germ cell tumours: results of an MRC/EORTC randomised trial. *Journal of Clinical Oncology*, 16, 692–701.

[24] de Wit, R., Roberts, J.T., Wilkinson, P.M., de Mulder, P., H.M., Mead, G.M., Fosså, S.D., Cook, P., de Prijck, L., Stenning, S., and Collette, L. (2001) Equivalence of 3 BEP versus 4 cycles and of the 5 day schedule versus 3 days per cycle in good prognosis germ cell cancer, a randomized study of the European Organization for Research and Treatment of Cancer Genitourinary Tract Cancer Cooperative Group and the Medical Research Council. *Journal of Clinical Oncology*, 19, 1629–40.

[25] Ovarian Cancer Trialists Group. (1991) Chemotherapy in advanced ovarian cancer – an overview of randomized clinical trials. *British Medical Journal*, 303, 884–93.

Index

either they would have to be substantial or a randomized study may involve different ... Secondary outcome measures could be important ... collecting such data may be appropriate.

- *The trial population was highly selective.* Perhaps a treatment is particular type of patient, or perhaps in a particular setting, and the question arises as to whether the results can be extrapolated to other patients or settings. Sometimes treatments pass through the broad stages of efficacy ...

... have been found resistant to all treatment ... the effect on more resistant types of ... re-discussed further ...

... this ... the systematic review indicates ... proven benefit, or the ... for it against a clinically ... result, then a further trial is unlikely to be needed. But ... data that may be obtained will augment the number ... is insufficient to be conclusive, then a new trial ... the systematic review may be of benefit in designing ... situations in which a meta-analysis was used ... about future trials.